# Albumin-Based Drug Delivery Systems

# Albumin-Based Drug Delivery Systems

Editor

**Gábor Katona**

MDPI • Basel • Beijing • Wuhan • Barcelona • Belgrade • Manchester • Tokyo • Cluj • Tianjin

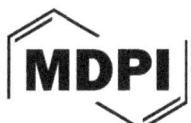

*Editor*
Gábor Katona
Institute of Pharmaceutical
Technology and Regulatory
Affairs
University of Szeged
Szeged
Hungary

*Editorial Office*
MDPI
St. Alban-Anlage 66
4052 Basel, Switzerland

This is a reprint of articles from the Special Issue published online in the open access journal *Pharmaceutics* (ISSN 1999-4923) (available at: www.mdpi.com/journal/pharmaceutics/special_issues/albumin_DDS).

For citation purposes, cite each article independently as indicated on the article page online and as indicated below:

LastName, A.A.; LastName, B.B.; LastName, C.C. Article Title. *Journal Name* **Year**, *Volume Number*, Page Range.

**ISBN 978-3-0365-4108-2 (Hbk)**
**ISBN 978-3-0365-4107-5 (PDF)**

© 2022 by the authors. Articles in this book are Open Access and distributed under the Creative Commons Attribution (CC BY) license, which allows users to download, copy and build upon published articles, as long as the author and publisher are properly credited, which ensures maximum dissemination and a wider impact of our publications.

The book as a whole is distributed by MDPI under the terms and conditions of the Creative Commons license CC BY-NC-ND.

# Contents

About the Editor . . . . . . . . . . . . . . . . . . . . . . . . . . . . . . . . . . . . . . . . . . . vii

Preface to "Albumin-Based Drug Delivery Systems" . . . . . . . . . . . . . . . . . . . . . . ix

**Junyong Park, Mijeong Bak, Kiyoon Min, Hyun-Woo Kim, Jeong-Haeng Cho and Giyoong Tae et al.**
Effect of C-terminus Conjugation via Different Conjugation Chemistries on In Vivo Activity of Albumin-Conjugated Recombinant GLP-1
Reprinted from: *Pharmaceutics* **2021**, *13*, 263, doi:10.3390/pharmaceutics13020263 . . . . . . . . . 1

**Gábor Katona, Bence Sipos, Mária Budai-Szűcs, György Tibor Balogh, Szilvia Veszelka and Ilona Gróf et al.**
Development of In Situ Gelling Meloxicam-Human Serum Albumin Nanoparticle Formulation for Nose-to-Brain Application
Reprinted from: *Pharmaceutics* **2021**, *13*, 646, doi:10.3390/pharmaceutics13050646 . . . . . . . . . 15

**Ryo Kinoshita, Yu Ishima, Victor T. G. Chuang, Hiroshi Watanabe, Taro Shimizu and Hidenori Ando et al.**
The Therapeutic Effect of Human Serum Albumin Dimer-Doxorubicin Complex against Human Pancreatic Tumors
Reprinted from: *Pharmaceutics* **2021**, *13*, 1209, doi:10.3390/pharmaceutics13081209 . . . . . . . . 37

**Byungseop Yang and Inchan Kwon**
Thermostable and Long-Circulating Albumin-Conjugated *Arthrobacter globiformis* Urate Oxidase
Reprinted from: *Pharmaceutics* **2021**, *13*, 1298, doi:10.3390/pharmaceutics13081298 . . . . . . . . 49

**Meike-Kristin Abraham, Elena Jost, Jan David Hohmann, Amy Kate Searle, Viktoria Bongcaron and Yuyang Song et al.**
A Recombinant Fusion Construct between Human Serum Albumin and NTPDase CD39 Allows Anti-Inflammatory and Anti-Thrombotic Coating of Medical Devices
Reprinted from: *Pharmaceutics* **2021**, *13*, 1504, doi:10.3390/pharmaceutics13091504 . . . . . . . . 61

**Itzik Cooper, Orly Ravid, Daniel Rand, Dana Atrakchi, Chen Shemesh and Yael Bresler et al.**
Albumin-EDTA-Vanadium Is a Powerful Anti-Proliferative Agent, Following Entrance into Glioma Cells via Caveolae-Mediated Endocytosis
Reprinted from: *Pharmaceutics* **2021**, *13*, 1557, doi:10.3390/pharmaceutics13101557 . . . . . . . . 79

**Niuosha Sanaeifar, Karsten Mäder and Dariush Hinderberger**
Molecular-Level Release of Coumarin-3-Carboxylic Acid and Warfarin-Derivatives from BSA-Based Hydrogels
Reprinted from: *Pharmaceutics* **2021**, *13*, 1661, doi:10.3390/pharmaceutics13101661 . . . . . . . . 93

**Itzik Cooper, Michal Schnaider-Beeri, Mati Fridkin and Yoram Shechter**
Albumin–Methotrexate Prodrug Analogues That Undergo Intracellular Reactivation Following Entrance into Cancerous Glioma Cells
Reprinted from: *Pharmaceutics* **2021**, *14*, 71, doi:10.3390/pharmaceutics14010071 . . . . . . . . . . 113

**Ryan A. Davis, Sven H. Hausner, Rebecca Harris and Julie L. Sutcliffe**
A Comparison of Evans Blue and 4-(*p*-Iodophenyl)butyryl Albumin Binding Moieties on an Integrin $_{v6}$ Binding Peptide
Reprinted from: *Pharmaceutics* **2022**, *14*, 745, doi:10.3390/pharmaceutics14040745 . . . . . . . . . 129

# About the Editor

**Gábor Katona**

Dr. Gábor Katona currently works in an Assistant Professor position at the Institute of Pharmaceutical Technology and Regulatory Affairs of University of Szeged. His research field is the development of protein- and polymeric-based nanoparticles for alternative administration routes. Currently, his research focuses on the investigation of nose-to-brain transport routs of albumin-based drug delivery systems with the support of János Bolyai Research Scholarship of the Hungarian Academy of Sciences.

# Preface to "Albumin-Based Drug Delivery Systems"

Albumin is playing an increasing role as a versatile, biodegradable drug carrier in clinical theranostics. By applying different techniques, smart drug-delivery systems can be developed from albumin in order to improve drug delivery of different active pharmaceutical ingredients, even small-molecule drugs, peptides or enzymes. Principally, three drug delivery technologies can be distinguished for binding small-molecule or peptide drugs through the charged amino acids, carboxyl, and amino groups of albumin: physical or covalent binding of the drug to albumin through a ligand- or protein-binding group, the fusion of drugs with albumin or the encapsulation of drugs into albumin nanoparticles. The accumulation of albumin in inflamed tissues and solid tumours forms the rationale for developing albumin-based drug delivery systems for targeted drug delivery. Besides tumour therapy albumin-based drug delivery systems can be successfully applied as anti-inflammatory and anti-thrombotic coating for medical devices. The development and optimization of albumin nanoparticles may also be a rational and promising tool for conventional or alternative administration routes in order to improve therapy. This collection provides an overview of the significant scientific research works in this field, which may inspire researchers towards further development and utilization of these smart drug delivery systems. This topic is respectfully dedicated to Dr Piroska Szabó-Révész Professor Emerita for her scientific support and research motivation in the field of innovative drug formulation.

**Gábor Katona**
*Editor*

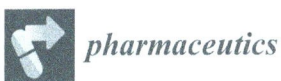

Article

# Effect of C-terminus Conjugation via Different Conjugation Chemistries on In Vivo Activity of Albumin-Conjugated Recombinant GLP-1

Junyong Park [1,†], Mijeong Bak [2,†], Kiyoon Min [2,†], Hyun-Woo Kim [3], Jeong-Haeng Cho [3], Giyoong Tae [2] and Inchan Kwon [1,2,3,*]

1. Department of Biomedical Science and Engineering, Gwangju Institute of Science and Technology (GIST), Gwangju 61005, Korea; happydragon@gist.ac.kr
2. Gwangju Institute of Science and Technology (GIST), School of Materials Science and Engineering, Gwangju 61005, Korea; al4527@gm.gist.ac.kr (M.B.); kymin324@gist.ac.kr (K.M.); gytae@gist.ac.kr (G.T.)
3. R&D Center, ProAbTech Co., Ltd., Gwangju 61005, Korea; kimhw@proabtech.com (H.-W.K.); nucleic@proabtech.com (J.-H.C.)
* Correspondence: inchan@gist.ac.kr; Tel.: +82-62-715-2312
† These authors contributed equally to this work.

**Abstract:** Glucagon-like peptide-1 (GLP-1) is a peptide hormone with tremendous therapeutic potential for treating type 2 diabetes mellitus. However, the short half-life of its native form is a significant drawback. We previously prolonged the plasma half-life of GLP-1 via site-specific conjugation of human serum albumin (HSA) at position 16 of recombinant GLP-1 using site-specific incorporation of p-azido-phenylalanine (AzF) and strain-promoted azide-alkyne cycloaddition (SPAAC). However, the resulting conjugate GLP1_8G16AzF-HSA showed only moderate in vivo glucose-lowering activity, probably due to perturbed interactions with GLP-1 receptor (GLP-1R) caused by the albumin-linker. To identify albumin-conjugated GLP-1 variants with enhanced in vivo glucose-lowering activity, we investigated the conjugation of HSA to a C-terminal region of GLP-1 to reduce steric hindrance by the albumin-linker using two different conjugation chemistries. GLP-1 variants GLP1_8G37AzF-HSA and GLP1_8G37C-HSA were prepared using SPAAC and Michael addition, respectively. GLP1_8G37C-HSA exhibited a higher glucose-lowering activity in vivo than GLP1_8G16AzF-HSA, while GLP1_8G37AzF-HSA did not. Another GLP-1 variant, GLP1_8A37C-HSA, had a glycine to alanine mutation at position 8 and albumin at its C-terminus and exhibited in vivo glucose-lowering activity comparable to that of GLP1_8G37C-HSA, despite a moderately shorter plasma half-life. These results showed that site-specific HSA conjugation to the C-terminus of GLP-1 via Michael addition could be used to generate GLP-1 variants with enhanced glucose-lowering activity and prolonged plasma half-life in vivo.

**Keywords:** plasma half-life extension; albumin conjugation; in vivo glucose-lowering activity; glucagon-like peptide-1

## 1. Introduction

Diabetes mellitus is one of the most common chronic diseases worldwide, involving the loss of control of blood glucose levels, which results in a continuously elevated glucose concentration. The global prevalence of diabetes mellitus among adults over 18 years of age increased from 4.7% in 1980 to 8.5% in 2014 [1]. In 2016, an estimated 1.6 million deaths were directly caused by diabetes [2]. To prevent these complications, controlling the blood glucose levels of patients with diabetes is of great importance. Glucagon-like peptide-1 (GLP-1) is an essential hormone that contributes to the regulation of blood glucose levels. After secretion from L-cells of the intestine [3], GLP-1 is directed toward many organs to reduce the blood glucose levels, including the pancreas, heart, muscles, kidneys, liver, and even the brain [4]. The activity of GLP-1 is mediated by its binding to the GLP-1 receptor

(GLP-1R) on the membrane of cells found in various organs, including pancreatic beta cells [5–7]. After GLP-1R is stimulated by GLP-1 binding, it activates the G-protein and upregulates cyclic adenosine monophosphate (cAMP) inside the cell and causes other synergistic effects, which leads to proliferation of pancreatic beta cells, enhanced insulin production inside the pancreatic beta cells, and insulin secretion to control the blood glucose levels [8–11].

Because of its rapid renal clearance due to its small size (~3 kDa) and its vulnerability to proteolytic cleavage by dipeptidyl peptidase-IV (DPP-IV), GLP-1 is reported to have an extremely short half-life in the body (~2–3 min). Although GLP-1 exerts significant effects in an individual's body, its short half-life is a significant drawback. Many studies have been conducted in effort to overcome the hurdles of GLP-1 and to develop it as a medication. Traditional efforts to increase the size of small therapeutic proteins have included polyethylene glycol (PEG) conjugation. However, PEG conjugation has been reported to cause several complications, including renal accumulation and potential immunogenicity [12–17]. Recently, serum albumin has been proposed as a good half-life extender, as it is a naturally abundant protein that is amenable to chemical conjugation via the free thiol on cysteine 34. Furthermore, albumin can bind to the neonatal Fc receptor (FcRn) in an acidic environment, which protects it from intracellular degradation and allows it to be recycled into the extracellular space. Accordingly, we and other researchers have attempted to use direct chemical conjugation or indirect binding of proteins to albumin via albumin-binding ligands to prolong the plasma half-life of the proteins [18,19]. To address the short half-life of GLP-1 resulting from its cleavage by DPP-IV, the GLP-1 backbone of GLP-1R agonists has been changed. For instance, the alanine at position 8 of GLP-1 is cleaved by DPP-IV [20] and the cleaved GLP-1 fragment (residues 9-39) is known for its low biological activity as the N-terminal moiety of GLP-1 is important for receptor activation [21]. Therefore, substitution of the alanine with glycine, or any other amino acid including non-natural amino acids (NNAAs), has been used in attempt to confer resistance to DPP-IV-induced cleavage [22,23].

We previously reported the site-specific HSA conjugation to GLP-1 by expressing recombinant GLP-1 variants bearing an NNAA as an albumin conjugation site fused to superfolder green fluorescent protein (sfGFP) in genetically engineered *Escherichia coli* [24]. Two of the resulting GLP-1 variants with human serum albumin (HSA) conjugated at positions 16 and 28, respectively, exhibited significantly prolonged plasma half-lives in mice (~8 h) [24]. Although we carefully selected the albumin conjugation site on GLP-1 in order for it not to interfere with the interactions of position 16 of GLP-1 with GLP-1R (Figure 1A), in vitro and in vivo glucose-lowering activities of the resulting albumin conjugates were only moderate [24]. Enhancing the biological potency of a drug can help reduce the amount of injected drug needed for efficacy, thereby contributing to a reduction in production cost.

In the current study, we investigated the effects of albumin conjugation sites and conjugation chemistry on in vivo blood-lowering activities with the ultimate goal of designing albumin-GLP1 conjugates with enhanced therapeutic potency. Based on mutation studies, an albumin conjugate site at GLP1 position 16 was selected in a previous study to minimize the perturbation of interactions between the GLP-1 variant and GLP-1R [24]. However, considering the bulky structure of albumin, we hypothesize that the albumin conjugated to GLP-1 may to some extent block the binding of the conjugate to GLP-1R. The crystal structure of GLP-1 complexed with GLP-1R (PDB ID: 5VAI) indicates that albumin conjugated to the C-terminal region of GLP-1 causes less steric hindrance with GLP1-1R than that of albumin conjugated to the middle region of GLP-1. Therefore, we prepared GLP1_8G37AzF-HSA, a new GLP1-HSA conjugate generated by HSA conjugation to the C-terminal region of GLP-1 (Figure 1B), as well as GLP1_8G16AzF-HSA, a GLP1-HSA conjugate generated by HSA conjugation to position 16 of GLP-1 [24]. In addition to the albumin conjugate site, we hypothesized that the conjugation chemistry may also affect in vivo activity of GLP1-HSA conjugates. In a previous study, we used strain-promoted azide-alkyne cycloaddition (SPAAC) to couple azido groups to dibenzocyclooctyne (DBCO), which resulted in a very bulky four-ring structure. Such a bulky structure could reduce the binding affinity of the conjugate to GLP-1R by either direct or indirect interactions with GLP-1R. Therefore, we also prepared the GLP1-HSA conjugate GLP1_8G37C-HSA by conjugating HSA to a GLP-1 variant bearing a cysteine at position 34 (GLP1_8G37C) via a Michael addition reaction (Figure 1C). The cysteine at position 34 was often used for albumin modification, because it is away from FcRn binding site [24]. The effects of alanine and glycine at position 8 of GLP-1 were also investigated in the current study. Replacing the alanine at position 8 with glycine prevented DPP-IV-mediated cleavage of GLP-1. However, there are reports that this mutation results in a mild loss of biological activity in vitro (4-10-fold decrease) [23,25,26]. To further investigate this, we substituted glycine with alanine at position 8 on GLP1_8G37C, resulting in GLP1_8A37C (Figure 2A). All GLP-1 variants were expressed in *E. coli* using sfGFP as a fusion tag (Figure 2B,C), as previously reported [24]. After expression of each GLP-1 protein, albumin conjugation was completed, followed by proteolytic cleavage using factor Xa to dissociate the fusion tag from the desired conjugate (Figure 2B,C). We subsequently investigated the in vivo activities, in vivo half-life, and in vitro activities of each variant.

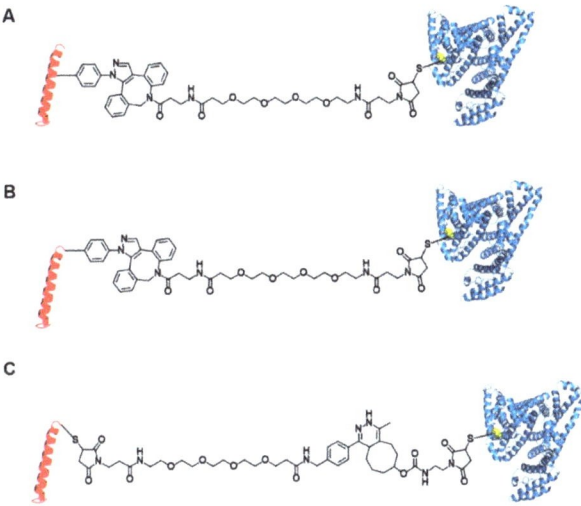

**Figure 1.** Structures of three glucagon-like peptide-1 (GLP-1)-human serum albumin (HSA) variants. GLP-1 variants conjugated to HSA at position 16 (**A**) and position 37 (**B**) using strain-promoted azide-alkyne cycloaddition and Michael addition. (**C**) GLP-1 variants conjugated to HSA at position 37 using inverse-electron demand Diels-Alder reaction and Michael addition.

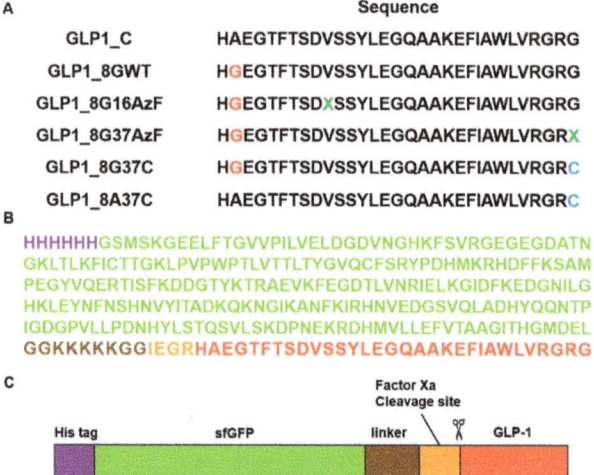

**Figure 2.** Construction of the GLP-1 and superfolder green fluorescent protein (sfGFP)-fused GLP-1 (sfGFP-GLP1) variants. (**A**) The amino acid sequences of six GLP-1 variants. The green-colored X notated at GLP1_8G16AzF and GLP1_8G37AzF was the incorporation site of the non-natural amino acid, AzF. (**B**) The amino acid sequence and (**C**) protein features of sfGFP-GLP1_C with the polyhistidine-tag (purple), sfGFP (green), linker (brown), factor Xa cleavage site (orange), and GLP1_C (red).

## 2. Materials and Methods

### 2.1. Materials

Polypropylene columns and nickel-nitrilotriacetic acid (Ni-NTA) agarose beads were purchased from Qiagen (Valencia, CA, USA). Trans-cyclooct-2-ene maleimide (TCO-MAL) and methyltetrazine-PEG4-maleimide (TET-PEG4-MAL) were obtained from Futurechem (Seoul, Korea). Dibenzocyclooctyne-PEG4-maleimide (DBCO-PEG4-MAL) was purchased from Click Chemistry Tools LLC (Scottsdale, AZ, USA). p-Azido-l-phenylalanine (AzF) was purchased from Chem-Impex International (Wood Dale, IL, USA). Disposable PD-10 desalting columns with Sephadex G-25 resin, Ion exchange chromatography columns (HiTrap Q HP and HiTrap SP HP) were obtained from GE Healthcare (Little Chalfont, Buckinghamshire, UK). Factor Xa was obtained from New England Biolabs (Ipswich, MA, USA). The GLP-1_WT and GLP-1_8GWT peptides were synthesized by GenScript (Piscataway, NJ, USA). Vivaspin 6 concentrator and 10,000 MWCO were purchased from Sartorius (Weender Landstraße, Göttingen, Germany). The mouse anti-GLP-1 monoclonal antibody was purchased from Thermo Fisher Scientific (Waltham, MA, USA). Rabbit anti-albumin polyclonal antibody was purchased from Sigma-Aldrich (St. Louis, MO, USA). The anti-mouse IgG, horseradish peroxidase (HRP)-linked antibody was purchased from Cell Signaling Technology (Beverly, MA, USA). Human embryonic kidney 293 (HEK293) cells were obtained from American Type Culture Collection (ATCC; Manassas, VA, USA). Fetal bovine serum and antibiotic-antimycotic for cell culture were purchased from Gibco (Gaithersburg, MD, USA). Iscove's modified Dulbecco's medium and the Transfection Reagent Kit for the in vitro assays were purchased from Sigma Aldrich. DNA transfection reagent (X-tremeGENE HP) was obtained from Roche Diagnostics GmbH (Mannheim, Germany). The cAMP assay kit was obtained from R&D Systems (Minneapolis, MN, USA). Unless otherwise noted, all other chemicals were obtained from Sigma-Aldrich.

### 2.2. Preparation of sfGFP and GLP-1 Fusion Protein

Construction of the pQE80-sfGFP-GLP1_C plasmid was described in a previous report [24]. This plasmid encodes a fusion protein of sfGFP and GLP1_C and was used as a template for mutagenesis. To confer resistance to proteolytic degradation by DPP-

IV, a PCR-based site-directed mutagenesis was used to replace the alanine at position 8 of GLP-1 with glycine by using primers A8G_F and A8G_R. For site-specific incorporation of AzF, the V16 and G37 sites of GLP-1 were mutated to an amber codon (TAG). The final plasmids generated were pQE80-sfGFP-GLP1_8G16Amb and pQE80-sfGFP-GLP1_8G37Amb, which were obtained by a PCR-based site-directed mutagenesis using primers V16AzF_F, V16AzF_R, G37AzF_F, and G37AzF_R (Table S1). To generate the 37C variants pQE80-sfGFP-GLP1_8A37C and pQE80-sfGFP-GLP1_8G37C, cysteine was substituted for glycine at position 37 of GLP-1 using primers G37C_F and G37C_R (Table S1). The pEvol-pAzFRS.1.t1 plasmid encoding the orthogonal pair MjTyrRS/MjtRNA$_{CUA}$ was obtained from Addgene (Addgene plasmid #73547, Watertown, MA, USA) [27]. To express the AzF-incorporated fusion protein, one of the amber codons-containing plasmids and pEvol-pAzFRS.1.t1 were co-transformed into C321ΔA.exp. E. coli cells (Addgene plasmid #49018) [28]. For the expression of variants 8A37C and 8G37C, each plasmid (pQE80-sfGFP-GLP1_8A37Cys and pQE80-sfGFP-GLP1_8G37Cys) was transformed into TOP10 E. coli cells.

The overnight cultures of C321ΔA.exp cells containing one of the amber codons-containing plasmids and pEvol-pAzFRS.1.t1 were inoculated into 200 mL of 2×YT media containing ampicillin (100 µg/mL) and chloramphenicol (35 µg/mL) and incubated at 37 °C with 210 rpm shaking. When the absorbance at 600 nm (OD$_{600}$) reached 0.4, AzF was supplemented to the culture to a final 1 mM concentration. When the OD$_{600}$ reached 0.5, sfGFP-GLP1 fusion protein expression was induced by the addition of isopropyl-β-D-thiogalactopyranoside (IPTG) and L-(+)-arabinose to the culture at final 1 mM and 0.2% (w/v) concentrations, respectively. The cells were cultured at 25 °C with 210 rpm shaking and collected after 15 h by centrifugation (6000 rpm, 15 min). The expression of sfGFP-GLP1_8G37C and sfGFP-GLP1_8A37C were performed as described above, except TOP10 E. coli was used for pQE80-sfGFP-GLP1_8G37Cys and TOP10 E. coli was used for pQE80-sfGFP-GLP1_8A37Cys, and chloramphenicol, AzF, and L-(+)-arabinose were not added.

The sfGFP-GLP1 fusion protein variants containing AzF were purified using Ni-NTA resin (QIAGEN, Hilden, Germany) and an N-terminal hexahistidine-tag according to the manufacturer's manual. The purified sfGFP-GLP1 was then exchanged with 20 mM Tris (pH 8.0), and then subjected to anion exchange chromatography using a HiTrap Q HP column. The sfGFP-GLP1_8G37C and sfGFP-GLP1_8A37C were purified by similar affinity purification steps except 5 mM tris(2-carboxyethyl)phosphine (TCEP) was added to all buffers. Subsequently, sfGFP-GLP1_8A37C and sfGFP-GLP1_8G37C were functionalized by the thiol-maleimide reaction using cysteine at position 37 of GLP-1. The purified proteins were buffer-exchanged with PBS (pH 7.3) and mixed with TET-PEG4-MAL (1:4 molar ratio). Unreacted linker was removed by desalting with 20 mM Tris (pH 8.0) using a PD-10 column after 3 h. The functionalization process ended with the production sfGFP-GLP1_8A37C-TET and sfGFP-GLP1_8G37C-TET, respectively.

*2.3. Preparation of GLP1_8G16AzF-HSA, GLP1_8G37AzF-HSA, GLP1_8G37C-HSA, and GLP1_8A37C-HSA Conjugates*

HSA-DBCO was prepared as described previously [24]. The prepared HSA-DBCO was conjugated with sfGFP-GLP1_8G16AzF and sfGFP-GLP1_8G37AzF and HSA-TCO was conjugated at room temperature (RT) overnight with sfGFP-GLP1_8G37C-TET and sfGFP-GLP1_8A37C-TET (1:2 molar ratio). Each mixture was buffer exchanged into 20 mM sodium phosphate buffer (pH 6.0). Then, cation exchange chromatography was performed to remove the unreacted HSA and sfGFP-GLP1 by using a HiTrap SP HP column with 20 mM sodium phosphate (pH 6.0).

The separated sfGFP-GLP1-HSA was buffer-exchanged into a buffer (2 mM CaCl$_2$, 10 mM NaCl, 20 mM Tris; pH 8) and then concentrated (final 10 µM concentration) using a Vivaspin 6 concentrator, 10,000 MWCO. The sfGFP-GLP1-HSA was incubated with 1/200 (w/w) Factor Xa protease for 18 h at room temperature. The Factor Xa reaction was terminated by the addition of dansyl-Glu-Gly Arg-chloromethyl ketone (0.1 mg/mL). The

Factor Xa-processed conjugate solution was further purified to obtain the GLP1-HSA by the buffer-exchange into 20 mM Bis-Tris (pH 6.0) and anion exchange chromatography using a HiTrap Q HP column.

*2.4. Labeling of Linker Conjugated sfGFP-GLP1_8G37C by Inverse Electron-Demand Diels-Alder Reaction (IEDDA)*

For labeling, 20 µM sfGFP-GLP1_8G37C or 20 µM sfGFP-GLP1_8G37C-TET in PBS (pH 7.4) was mixed with TCO-cy5.5 dye at a molar ratio of 1:5 for 2 h. As a control, sfGFP-GLP1_8G37C-TET without dye was prepared. Each mixture was subjected to sodium dodecyl sulfate-polyacrylamide gel electrophoresis (SDS-PAGE) and fluorescence imaging using a Bio-Rad ChemiDoc XRS + Imaging System (Bio-Rad, Hercules, CA, USA).

*2.5. Mass Spectrometric Analysis*

All analytes were prepared using a ZipTip C18 system in accordance with the manufacturer's manual. After ZipTip processing, GLP1_8G37AzF, GLP1_8G37C, and GLP1_8A37C were mixed 1:1 (*v:v*) with α-cyano-4-hydroxy cinnamic acid (HCCA)-saturated TA30, which was a solution (30% acetonitrile; 0.1% trifluoroacetic acid). The GLP1_8G37AzF-HSA, GLP1_8G37C-HSA, and GLP1_8A37C-HSA after ZipTip processing were mixed with 20 mg/mL 2,5-dihydroxybenzoic acid (DHB) in TA30. Each mixture placed on a polished steel plate and mass characterization was conducted using Autoflex matrix-assisted laser desorption-ionization/time-of-flight mass spectroscopy (MALDI-TOF MS) and the corresponding flexControl software (Bruker Daltonics, Bremen, Germany).

*2.6. Enzyme-Linked Immunosorbent Assay (ELISA) of GLP1-HSA Conjugate*

The immunoplate was coated with 5 µg/mL anti-albumin rabbit antibody in 0.1 M bicarbonate pH 9.6 at 4 °C overnight and then blocked with 5% skim milk. After removal of the solution from each well, the serum samples were diluted in 5% skim milk and incubated in each well for 2 h at room temperature. The GLP1-HSA variant was used as a calibration standard. After washing each well, 1 µg/mL anti-GLP-1 mouse antibody diluted in 5% skim milk was incubated at RT for 2 h. Each well of the plate was washed and then incubated with an anti-mouse HRP-conjugated IgG antibody diluted 1/3000 in 5% skim milk at RT for 1 h. Once again after washing, 3, 3′,5, 5-tetramethylbenzidine was applied and incubated at room temperature for a short time. The reaction was quenched using 100 µL of 2 M $H_2SO_4$. Then, the absorbance at 450 nm was monitored using a Synergy™ microplate reader (BioTek, Winooski, VT, USA).

*2.7. Pharmacokinetic Studies of GLP1-HSA Conjugates*

In vivo pharmacokinetic studies were conducted using eight-week-old female BALB/c mice (DBL, Korea). The mice were maintained in a 12-h light/12-h dark cycle and freely accessed to water and food. All animal protocols were approved by the Animal Ethics Committee of GIST (Approval number: GIST-2019-071 (4 October 2019)) in accordance with the Guidelines for Care and Use of Laboratory Animals proposed by the Gwangju Institute of Science and Technology (GIST). The mice were randomly divided into two groups (n = 4/group). Either GLP1_8G37C-HSA or GLP1_8A37C-HSA (10 nmol/kg dose) was intravenously administered to the respective groups of mice. Blood samples (<70 µL) were collected from the retroorbital venous sinus at 0.16, 1, 3, 6, 12, and 24 h after conjugate administration. The acquired blood samples were placed at RT for 30 min and then centrifuged at 4 °C (2500 rpm, for 10 min). The serum was collected, and the samples stored at −20 °C until analyzed. Plasma concentrations of the GLP1-HSA conjugate at each time point was measured in triplicate by ELISA.

*2.8. In Vivo Intraperitoneal Glucose Tolerance Test (IPGTT)*

Normal seven-week-old C57BL/6J male mice (DBL, Korea) were randomly divided into six groups (*n* = 6/group). The mice were fasted for 3–6 h prior to the experiment.

GLP1_C (30 nmol/kg), the GLP1-HSA variants (30 nmol/kg), or saline were subcutaneously administered 20 min before an intraperitoneal injection of glucose (1.5 g/kg). Blood samples were collected from the tail and glucose levels were determined using an Accu-Check Guide (Roche Diabetes Care, Indianapolis, IN, USA).

*2.9. In Vitro Activity Assay*

An in vitro activity assay for GLP1_C and its variants was performed as described in our previous study [24]. Briefly, 10,000 HEK293 cells were seeded per well onto a 48-well plate and incubated at 37 °C under 5% CO2 for 16 h. The plasmid pcDNA3.1-GLP-1R_tango (Addgene, Cambridge, MA, USA) [29] and transfection reagent were then mixed in serum-free medium for 20 min, in accordance with the manufacturer's recommendation. Then, 30 µL of the mixture was dropped into each well and the plate was incubated for 48 h at 37 °C. GLP1_C or variant peptides were diluted 10-fold with media and added to the transfected cells for 15 min. The levels of cAMP in the cell lysate were measured using the cAMP Parameter Assay Kit following the manufacturer's protocol. The synthetic GLP1_C peptide solutions at required concentrations were prepared using deionized water just prior to performing the assay. The values were normalized to the amount of cAMP secreted with GLP1_C of $10^{-6}$ M and converted to % activity. The half maximal effective concentrations ($EC_{50}$) of each curve were estimated from a dose–response curve using OriginPro software. Absorbance at 450 nm was monitored using a Varioskan Lux microplate reader (Thermo Fisher Scientific).

## 3. Results and Discussion

### 3.1. Preparation of C-terminus-Modified GLP-1 Varints

Preparation of sfGFP-GLP1_8G37C was representatively described in detail. Comparison of cell lysates before induction (BI) and after induction (AI) of sfGFP-GLP1_8G37C showed a prominent new band in the A.I. sample in a Coomassie blue-stained gel (Figure 3A). The protein band was shown between 25 kDa and 37 kDa molecular markers, consistent with the expected molecular weight of sfGFP-GLP-1_8G37C (~32 kDa). Purified sfGFP-GLP1_8G37C was obtained by Ni-NTA affinity chromatography (Figure 3B), and its size shown to be between 25 kDa and 37 kDa. However, two bands were observed for the purified sfGFP-GLP1_8G37C, which we speculated was a result of different oxidation status of sfGFP-GLP1_8G37C [30]. The preparation of sfGFP-GLP1_8A37C was performed in a similar manner to that of sfGFP-GLP1_8G37C and the preparation of sfGFP-GLP1_8G16AzF was performed as previously reported [24].

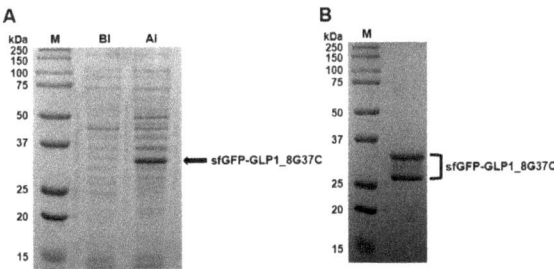

**Figure 3.** Expression, purification, and confirmation of C-terminal cysteine-substituted sfGFP-GLP-1_8G37C. (**A**) SDS-PAGE protein gel images of cell lysates before induction (BI) and after induction (AI). A prominent band expected to be sfGFP-GLP1_8G37C is observed (arrow). (**B**) Purified sfGFP-GLP1_8G37C in an SDS-PAGE gel after Ni-NTA affinity chromatography.

To append the sfGFP-GLP1_8G37C functional group for reaction with HSA, TET-PEG4-MAL was reacted with sfGFP-GLP1_8G37C to generate sfGFP-GLP1_8G37C-TET. We chose this linker in order to use the IEDDA, which is known for its high reactivity compared to that of the formerly used bioorthogonal SPAAC [31]. The reactivity of methyltetrazine was evaluated by conjugating the linker to a fluorescent dye. Briefly, the sfGFP-GLP1_8G37C-TET conjugate was reacted with TCO-Cy5.5 dye and the in-gel fluorescence of the reaction mixture analyzed (Figure S1). In the Coomassie-stained gel, the upper band showed a mild upward shift after conjugation with TET-PEG4-MAL. In contrast, migration of the lower band, which we speculated to be the oxidized form of sfGFP-GLP-1_8G37C, did not change after conjugation with the TET-PEG4-MAL linker. This was attributed to the absence of a reduced cysteine, which was required to undergo the reaction with maleimide. TCO-Cy5.5 dye-labeled sfGFP-GLP-1_8G37C-TET showed prominent fluorescence, whereas sfGFP-GLP-1_8G37C, which could not react with the TCO-Cy5.5, failed to show fluorescence after incubation with the dye. Labeling the conjugate with the dye confirmed the sfGFP-GLP1_8G37C-TET construct.

Meanwhile, the construction of GLP1_8G37AzF, GLP1_8G37C, and GLP1_8A37C were verified by MALDI-TOF MS. GLP1_8G37AzF, GLP1_8G37C, and GLP1_8A37C were obtained by processing the respective sfGFP_GLP1 fusion proteins by Factor Xa. The monoisotopic mass of GLP1_8G37AzF, GLP1_8G37C, and GLP1_8A37C were 3474.0, 3414.9, and 3428.7 m/z, respectively (Figure 4). This closely matched the expected values of 3473.6, 3414.7, and 3428.7 m/z, respectively, with less than a 0.1% difference being observed. These results were consistent with the successful construction of the GLP1 variants fused with sfGFP in *E. coli*.

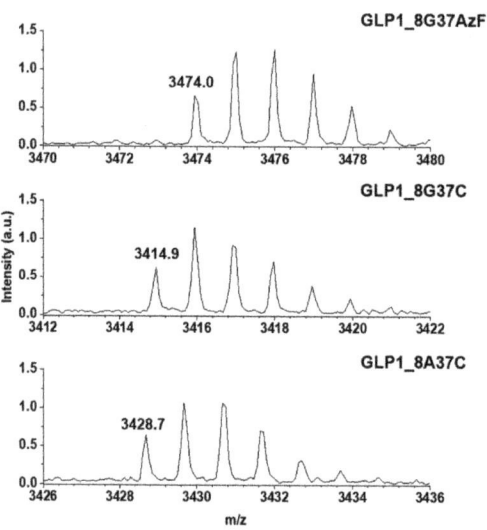

**Figure 4.** Monoisotopic mass confirmation of GLP1_8G37AzF, GLP1_8G37C, and GLP1_8A37C by matrix-assisted laser desorption/ionization time-of-light mass spectroscopy (MALDI-TOF MS). The monoisotopic mass to charge ratio for GLP1_8G37AzF, GLP1_8G37C, and GLP1_8A37C were 3474.0, 3414.9, and 3428.7 m/z, respectively.

*3.2. Preparation of Albumin-Conjugated GLP-1 Variants*

Preparation of the GLP1_8G37AzF-HSA variant was performed as previously reported [24], except for the use of sfGFP-GLP1_8G37AzF instead of sfGFP-GLP1_8G16AzF. Preparation of the HSA-conjugated GLP-1 cysteine variants was initiated by conjugation of a linker to HSA. To confer TCO functionality to HSA, a TCO-MAL linker was used to generate HSA-TCO as we wanted to match the distance between GLP-1 and HSA to the other GLP1-HSA conjugates (GLP1_8G16AzF-HSA and GLP1_8G37AzF-HSA). GLP1_8G16AzF-HSA and GLP1_8G37AzF-HSA have PEG4 and an azide-DBCO complex between GLP-1 and HSA. As TET-PEG4-MAL possesses PEG4, a linker conjugated to HSA does not need PEG. After the generation of HSA-TCO, HSA-TCO was reacted with sfGFP-GLP1_8G37C-TET, resulting in a mixture containing sfGFP-GLP1_8G37C-HSA (Figure 5A). Cation exchange chromatography was performed to isolate sfGFP-GLP1_8G37C-HSA from unreacted albumin (Figure S2). We collected fractions containing sfGFP-GLP1_8G37C-HSA and then proceeded to the next purification step. In the next step, the conjugate was processed by factor Xa, resulting in the GLP1_8G37C-HSA variant, which was purified from the cleaved sfGFP by anion exchange chromatography (Figure S3). The same procedures were used to generate and isolate the GLP1_8A37C-HSA variant. Bands of purified GLP1_8G37C-HSA and GLP1_8A37C-HSA were clearly observed between the 50 and 75 kDa molecular weight standard bands (Figure 5B), which was consistent with the expected molecular weight of ~70 kDa for the GLP1-HSA variants.

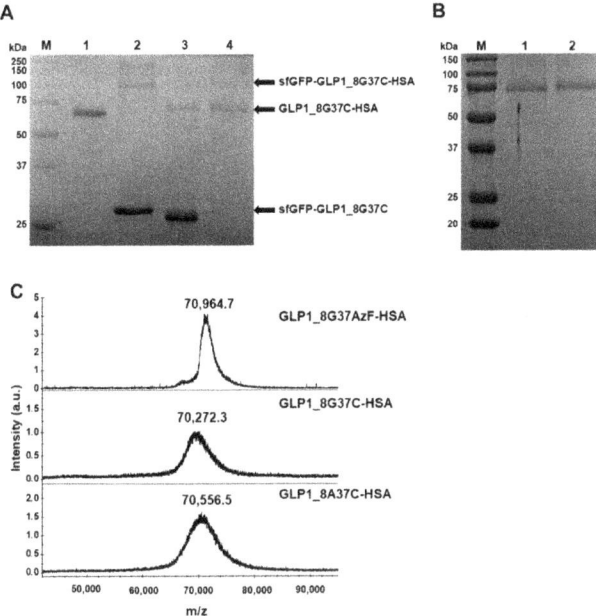

**Figure 5.** Purification and confirmation of GLP1_8G37C-HSA and their intermediates. (**A**) Protein gel image after Coomassie blue staining of the intermediates during GLP1_8G37C-HSA production. Molecular weight standards (lane M), purified HSA (lane 1), sfGFP-GLP1_8G37C-HSA purified with unreacted sfGFP-GLP1_8G37C (lane 2), GLP1_8G37C-HSA with sfGFP-GLP1_8G37C after factor Xa cleavage (lane 3), and purified GLP1_8G37C-HSA (lane 4). In lane 3, the band for sfGFP-GLP1_8G37C is observed at a lower position compared to the band in lane 2, which is expected to be the result of factor Xa cleavage. (**B**) Protein gel image after Coomassie blue staining of the final products of GLP1_8G37C-HSA (lane 1) and GLP1_8A37CHSA (lane 2). (**C**) MALDI-TOF MS spectrum of GLP1_8G37AzF-HSA, GLP1_8G37C-HSA, and GLP1_8A37C-HSA.

The purified GLP1_8G37AzF-HSA, GLP1_8A37C-HSA, and GLP1_8G37C-HSA were subjected to MALDI-TOF MS analysis (Figure 5C). The observed mass to charge ratios of GLP1_8G37AzF-HSA, GLP1_8G37C-HSA, and GLP1_8A37C-HSA were 70,964.7, 70,272.3, and 70,556.5 m/z, respectively, which were comparable to the expected values of 70,649, 70,782, and 70,796 m/z. The actual ratios compared to expected ratios demonstrated only minor differences (<0.5%). The results of protein gel electrophoresis and MALDI-TOF MS analysis confirmed the successful preparation of GLP1_8G37AzF-HSA, GLP1_8G37C-HSA, and GLP1-8A37C-HSA.

## 3.3. In Vivo Study

To investigate the plasma half-lives of GLP1_8G37C-HSA and GLP1_8A37C-HSA, we determined the pharmacokinetic profiles of these variants. Each variant was intravenously administered to BALB/c mice. The serum concentrations of the variants were then evaluated at multiple time points post administration. A sandwich ELISA was used to analyze the serum concentrations. The terminal plasma half-lives of GLP1_8G37C-HSA and GLP1_8A37C-HSA were determined to be 9.0 h and 7.1 h, respectively (Figure 6). The difference is significant (two-tailed student's $t$-test; $p < 0.01$). The half-lives of these variants were comparable with those of other GLP1-HSA conjugates as previously reported (8.4, 7.4, and 8.0 h for GLP1_8G16AzF-HSA, GLP1_8G19AzF-HSA, and GLP1_8G28AzF-HSA, respectively) [24]. As the site-specific HSA conjugation at positions 16, 19, and 28 of GLP1 led to very similar plasma half-lives [24], we speculated that the terminal plasma half-life of GLP1_8G37AzF-HSA would also be comparable. These results indicated the conjugation of HSA at the C-terminus of GLP-1 successfully extended the plasma half-life of GLP-1.

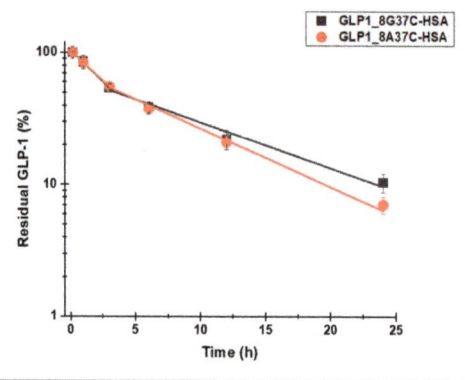

| | GLP1_8G37C-HSA | GLP1_8A37C-HSA |
|---|---|---|
| $t_{½ (α)}$ | 3.2 h | 3.3 h |
| $t_{½ (β)}$ | 9.0 h | 7.1 h |

**Figure 6.** Pharmacokinetic profiles of intravenously injected GLP1_8G37C-HSA and GLP1_8A37C-HSA conjugates in BALB/c mice. Data in the graph indicate the mean ± standard deviation ($n = 4$/group). The plasma concentrations of the samples were plotted using a logarithmic scale.

Notably, the capture antibody used in the sandwich ELISA to recognize GLP-1 (ABS 033-10-12, Thermo Fischer Scientific) is reported to recognize only the intact N-terminus of GLP-1 (residues 7–17) and does not bind to the DPP-IV-cleaved GLP-1 structure (residues 9-37). This property of the antibody may explain why the plasma half-life of GLP1_8G37C-HSA was slightly longer than that of GLP1_8A37C-HSA, as GLP1_8A37C-HSA is more vulnerable to DPP-IV cleavage than that of GLP1_8G37C-HSA.

To evaluate the glucose-lowering activity of the GLP1-HSA variants in vivo, an IPGTT was performed for each of the variants in C57/BL7 mice (Figure 7). In the negative control (PBS) group, blood glucose increased sharply following the glucose injection and slowly returned to normal levels by 120 min after the injection (Figure 7A). As expected, the injection of GLP1_C lowered the blood glucose level. Compared to GLP1_C, GLP1_8G16AzF-HSA was less effective at lowering blood glucose level up to 30 min after glucose injection, but then became more effective after 30 min. Therefore, the in vivo glucose-lowering activities of GLP1_C and GLP1_8G16AzF-HSA were comparable in terms of area under the curve (AUC) values (Figure 7B). Although GLP1_8G37AzF-HSA appeared to be less effective at lowering blood glucose levels than that of GLP1_C and GLP1_8G16AzF-HSA (Figure 7A), its AUC value was not substantially different from those of GLP1_C and

GLP1_8G16AzF-HSA (Figure 7B). Therefore, it is clear that a change in the HSA conjugation site from position 16 to position 37 of GLP-1 did not enhance in vivo activity. However, GLP1_8G37C-HSA more effectively lowered blood glucose levels at all times after the glucose injection than GLP1_8G16AzF-HSA and GLP1_8G37AzF-HSA (Figure 7A). Similarly, the AUC value of GLP1_8G37C-HSA was significantly smaller than those of GLP1_C, GLP1_8G16AzF-HSA, and GLP1_8G37AzF-HSA (Figure 7B). GLP1_8A37C-HSA showed very similar patterns regarding blood glucose levels and AUC value compared to that of GLP1_8G37C-HSA. Therefore, both GLP1_8G37C-HSA and GLP1_8A37C-HSA showed the greatest in vivo activities among GLP1_C and the four GLP1-HSA conjugates tested.

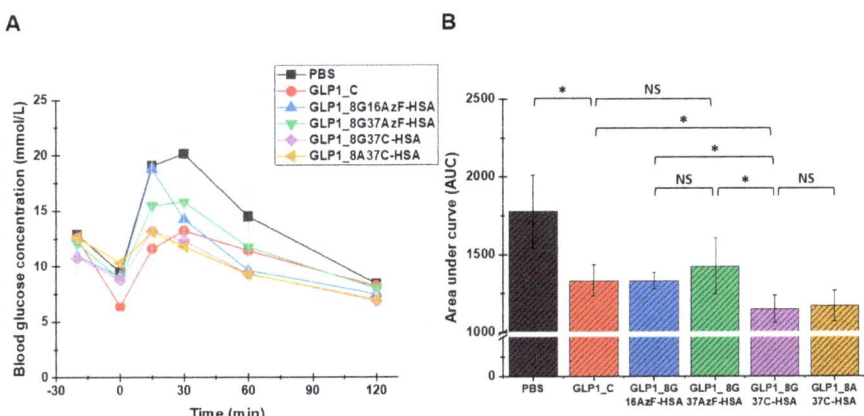

**Figure 7.** Blood glucose levels of PBS (negative control), GLP1_C (positive control), and the GLP1-HSA variants. (**A**) PBS or 30 nmol/kg doses of GLP1_C or the GLP1-HSA variants were subcutaneously injected into C57BL/6J mice ($n$ = 3/group) 20 min prior to the intraperitoneal injection of glucose (1.5 g/kg, 0 min). Data in the graph indicate the mean value ± standard deviation ($n$ = 3/group). (**B**) The area under curves (AUC) calculated from 0 to 120 min were compared. Mean value ± standard deviation is presented ($n$ = 3/group), * $p$-value < 0.01; NS: not significant.

As noted in the Introduction, we hypothesized that albumin conjugation to the C-terminus of GLP-1 would reduce the potential steric hindrance of HSA with GLP-1 binding to GLP-1R and enhance in vivo activity, compared to when albumin conjugation is done in the middle of GLP-1. However, when the same bioorthogonal chemistry (SPAAC) used to conjugate albumin to the middle of GLP-1 was used to conjugate it to the C-terminus, in vivo activity was not enhanced. Instead, the change from SPAAC to Michael addition using GLP1_37C variants led to significant enhancement of in vivo blood glucose-lowering activity. This was likely due to reduced steric hindrance caused by the structure obtained after the thiol-maleimide reaction. These results were consistent with previous results that showed even a minor change in the linker or spacer between GLP-1 and the half-life extender can cause considerable differences in biological activity [26].

*3.4. In Vitro Activity Assay*

GLP1-HSA variants were also subjected to in vitro activity assays to evaluate their biological activities. In vitro measurement of cAMP production by GLP-1R-overexpressing HEK-293 cells yielded $EC_{50}$ values of 1.6 nM, 13.2 nM, 1115 nM, 1340 nM, and 185 nM for GLP1_C, GLP1_8GWT, GLP1_8G16AzF-HSA, GLP1_8G37C-HSA, and GLP1_8A37C-HSA, respectively (Figure 8). The $EC_{50}$ value of GLP1_8G37AzF-HSA could not be determined as its activity was too low.

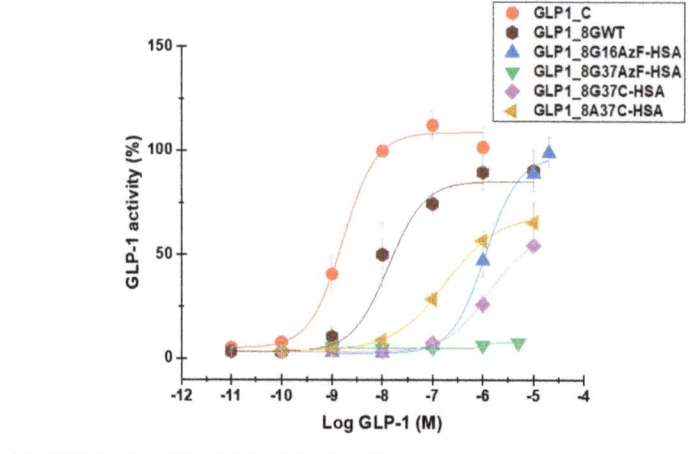

| | GLP1_C | GLP1_8GWT | GLP1_8G 16AzF-HSA | GLP1_8G 37AzF-HSA | GLP1_8G 37C-HSA | GLP1_8A 37C-HSA |
|---|---|---|---|---|---|---|
| $EC_{50}$ | 1.6 nM | 13.2 nM | 1115 nM | Not determined | 1340 nM | 185 nM |

**Figure 8.** In vitro biological activity of GLP1_C, GLP1_8GWT, GLP1_8G16AzF-HSA, GLP1_8G37AzF-HSA, GLP1_8G37C-HSA, and GLP1_8A37C-HSA evaluated in GLP-1R-expressing HEK-293 cells. The Y-axis denotes the percent activity calculated as a percentage of average cyclic adenosine monophosphate (cAMP) production by 1 µM GLP1_C. Each point in the graph indicates the mean value ± standard deviation ($n = 3$/group).

GLP1_8G37AzF-HSA exhibited very weak in vitro activity (Figure 8), which was consistent with its poor in vivo blood-lowering activity (Figure 7A). The in vitro activity of GLP1_8A37C-HSA was greater than that of GLP1_8G37C-HSA, probably due to the alanine to glycine change at position 8 (A8G) affecting the interactions with GLP-1R. Introduction of the A8G change to GLP1_C also resulted in a similar reduction in in vitro activity, consistent with previous findings [23,25]. The in vitro activity of GLP1-8G37C-HSA was comparable to that of GLP1-8G16AzF-HSA. Despite the low $EC_{50}$ value of GLP1_C, in vivo glucose lowering activity of GLP1_C was inferior to those GLP1-8G37C-HSA or GLP1-8A37C-HSA (Figure 7B) due to its very short plasma half-life (only a few minutes in animal) [32,33]. Some trend differences between the in vitro activities and in vivo activities suggested there are additional mechanisms for in vivo blood glucose level control by GLP-1 beyond the one related to cAMP production.

## 4. Conclusions

We report the successful preparation of GLP1-HSA conjugates GLP1_8G37C-HSA and GLP1_8A37C-HSA, which exhibited enhanced in vivo glucose-lowering activity by albumin conjugation to the C-terminus of GLP-1 via a thiol-maleimide reaction compared to that of a previously developed GLP1-HSA conjugate (GLP1_8G16AzF-HSA). Another GLP1-HSA conjugate, GLP1_8G37AzF-HSA, prepared by albumin conjugation to the C-terminus of GLP-1 via SPAAC did not exhibit enhanced in vivo glucose-lowering activity. These results indicated that both the albumin conjugation site and conjugation chemistry were important for preparing GLP1-HSA conjugates with enhanced in vivo glucose-lowering activity. Both GLP1_8G37C-HSA and GLP1_8A37C-HSA exhibited prolonged plasma half-lives, comparable to that of GLP1_8G16AzF-HSA, demonstrating the extension of the half-life by albumin conjugation was not significantly affected by albumin conjugate site.

**Supplementary Materials:** The following are available online at https://www.mdpi.com/1999-4923/13/2/263/s1, Table S1: Oligonucleotide primers used in this study, Figure S1: Protein gel image of sfGFP-GLP1_8G37C and sfGFP-GLP1_8G37C-TET incubated with or without TCO-Cy5.5, Figure S2: Purification of sfGFP-GLP1_8G37C-HSA after conjugation of sfGFP-GLP1_8G37C-TET to HSA-TCO using IEDDA, Figure S3: Purification of GLP1_8G37C-HSA after factor Xa treatment.

**Author Contributions:** Conceptualization, J.P., M.B., J.-H.C., and I.K.; formal analysis, J.P., M.B., K.M., H.-W.K., J.-H.C., G.T., and I.K.; investigation, J.P., M.B., K.M., and H.-W.K.; methodology, H.-W.K.; resources, J.-H.C., G.T., and I.K.; supervision, G.T. and I.K.; writing—original draft preparation, J.P., M.B., K.M., and I.K.; writing—review and editing, H.-W.K., J.-H.C., G.T., and I.K. All authors have read and agreed to the published version of the manuscript.

**Funding:** The authors acknowledge the financial support from the National Research Foundation of Korea (NRF), funded by the Ministry of Science and ICT (Grant No. 2019R1A2C1084910).

**Institutional Review Board Statement:** All animal studies were conducted according to the Guidelines for Care and Use of Laboratory Animals proposed by GIST and approved by the Animal Ethics Committee of GIST (Approval number: GIST-2019-071 (4 October 2019)).

**Informed Consent Statement:** Not applicable.

**Data Availability Statement:** The supporting data presented in this study are available in the Supplementary Material.

**Acknowledgments:** The authors are grateful to George Church at Harvard Medical School for a generous gift of 321.ΔA.exp (Addgene plasmid #49018). The authors also thank to Bryan Roth at the University of North Carolina for providing GLP1R-Tango (Addgene plasmid #66295). The authors acknowledge the insightful discussion of Jae Il Kim and Gyeong Min Kim at GIST on cAMP assays.

**Conflicts of Interest:** The authors declare no conflict of interest. ProAbtech Co., Ltd. was not involved in the design of the study, analyses or interpretation of data, writing of the manuscript, or decision to publish the results.

# References

1. Emerging Risk Factors Collaboration; Sarwar, N.; Gao, P.; Seshasai, S.R.K.; Gobin, R.; Kaptoge, S.; di Angelantonio, E.; Ingelsson, E.; Lawlor, D.A.; Selvin, E.; et al. The Emerging Risk Factors Collaboration Diabetes mellitus, fasting blood glucose concentration, and risk of vascular disease: A collaborative meta-analysis of 102 prospective studies. *Lancet* **2010**, *375*, 2215–2222. [CrossRef] [PubMed]
2. Nathan, D.M. For the DCCT/EDIC Research Group the Diabetes Control and Complications Trial/Epidemiology of Diabetes Interventions and Complications Study at 30 Years: Overview. *Diabetes Care* **2014**, *37*, 9–16. [CrossRef]
3. Kieffer, T.J.; Habener, J.F. The Glucagon-Like Peptides. *Endocr. Rev.* **1999**, *20*, 876–913. [CrossRef] [PubMed]
4. Sharma, D.; Verma, S.; Vaidya, S.; Kalia, K.; Tiwari, V. Recent updates on GLP-1 agonists: Current advancements & challenges. *Biomed. Pharmacother.* **2018**, *108*, 952–962. [CrossRef]
5. Alvarez, E.; Martínez, M.D.; Roncero, I.; Chowen, J.A.; Garcia-Cuartero, B.; Gispert, J.D.; Sanz, C.; Vazquez, P.; Maldonado, A.; De Cáceres, J.; et al. The expression of GLP-1 receptor mRNA and protein allows the effect of GLP-1 on glucose metabolism in the human hypothalamus and brainstem. *J. Neurochem.* **2005**, *92*, 798–806. [CrossRef]
6. Bullock, B.P. Tissue distribution of messenger ribonucleic acid encoding the rat glucagon-like peptide-1 receptor. *Endocrinol.* **1996**, *137*, 2968–2978. [CrossRef] [PubMed]
7. Campos, R.V.; Lee, Y.C.; Drucke, D.J. Divergent tissue-specific and developmental expression of receptors for glucagon and glucagon-like peptide-1 in the mouse. *Endocrinology* **1994**, *134*, 2156–2164. [CrossRef]
8. Holst, J.J. The Physiology of Glucagon-like Peptide 1. *Physiol. Rev.* **2007**, *87*, 1409–1439. [CrossRef] [PubMed]
9. Pabreja, K.A.; Mohd, M.; Koole, C.; Wootten, D.; Furness, S.G.B. Molecular mechanisms underlying physiological and receptor pleiotropic effects mediated by GLP-1R activation. *Br. J. Pharmacol.* **2014**, *171*, 1114–1128. [CrossRef] [PubMed]
10. Doyle, M.E.; Egan, J.M. Mechanisms of action of glucagon-like peptide 1 in the pancreas. *Pharmacol. Ther.* **2007**, *113*, 546–593. [CrossRef]
11. Buteau, J. GLP-1 receptor signaling: Effects on pancreatic β-cell proliferation and survival. *Diabetes Metab.* **2008**, *34* (Suppl. 2), S73–S77. [CrossRef]
12. Conover, C.; Lejeune, L.; Linberg, R.; Shum, K.; Shorr, R.G.L. Transitional Vacuole Formation Following a Bolus Infusion of Peg-Hemoglobin in the Rat. *Artif. Cells Blood Substit. Biotechnol.* **1996**, *24*, 599–611. [CrossRef] [PubMed]
13. Bendele, A.; Seely, J.; Richey, C.; Sennello, G.; Shopp, G. Short Communication: Renal Tubular Vacuolation in Animals Treated with Polyethylene-Glycol-Conjugated Proteins. *Toxicol. Sci.* **1998**, *42*, 152–157. [CrossRef] [PubMed]
14. Verhoef, J.J.F.; Anchordoquy, T.J. Questioning the use of PEGylation for drug delivery. *Drug Deliv. Transl. Res.* **2013**, *3*, 499–503. [CrossRef] [PubMed]

15. Thi, T.T.H.; Pilkington, E.H.; Nguyen, D.H.; Lee, J.S.; Park, K.D.; Truong, N.P. The Importance of Poly(ethylene glycol) Alternatives for Overcoming PEG Immunogenicity in Drug Delivery and Bioconjugation. *Polymers* **2020**, *12*, 298. [CrossRef]
16. Kozma, G.T.; Shimizu, T.; Ishida, T.; Szebeni, J. Anti-PEG antibodies: Properties, formation, testing and role in adverse immune reactions to PEGylated nano-biopharmaceuticals. *Adv. Drug Deliv. Rev.* **2020**, *154–155*, 163–175. [CrossRef]
17. Yang, Q.; Lai, S.K. Anti-PEG immunity: Emergence, characteristics, and unaddressed questions. *Wiley Interdiscip. Rev. Nanomed. Nanobiotechnol.* **2015**, *7*, 655–677. [CrossRef]
18. Yang, B.; Kim, J.C.; Seong, J.; Tae, G.; Kwon, I. Comparative studies of the serum half-life extension of a protein via site-specific conjugation to a species-matched or -mismatched albumin. *Biomater. Sci.* **2018**, *6*, 2092–2100. [CrossRef] [PubMed]
19. Cho, J.; Park, J.; Kim, S.; Kim, J.C.; Tae, G.; Jin, M.S.; Kwon, I. Intramolecular distance in the conjugate of urate oxidase and fatty acid governs FcRn binding and serum half-life in vivo. *J. Control. Release* **2020**, *321*, 49–58. [CrossRef]
20. Mentlein, R.; Gallwitz, B.; Schmidt, W.E. Dipeptidyl-peptidase IV hydrolyses gastric inhibitory polypeptide, glucagon-like peptide-1(7-36)amide, peptide histidine methionine and is responsible for their degradation in human serum. *Eur. J. Biochem.* **1993**, *214*, 829–835. [CrossRef] [PubMed]
21. Donnelly, D. The structure and function of the glucagon-like peptide-1 receptor and its ligands. *Br. J. Pharmacol.* **2012**, *166*, 27–41. [CrossRef]
22. Knudsen, L.B.; Lau, J. The Discovery and Development of Liraglutide and Semaglutide. *Front. Endocrinol.* **2019**, *10*, 155. [CrossRef] [PubMed]
23. Deacon, C.F.; Knudsen, L.B.; Madsen, K.; Wiberg, F.C.; Jacobsen, O.; Holst, J.J. Dipeptidyl peptidase IV resistant analogues of glucagon-like peptide-1 which have extended metabolic stability and improved biological activity. *Diabetologia* **1998**, *41*, 271–278. [CrossRef] [PubMed]
24. Bak, M.; Park, J.; Min, K.; Cho, J.; Seong, J.; Hahn, Y.S.; Tae, G.; Kwon, I. Recombinant Peptide Production Platform Coupled with Site-Specific Albumin Conjugation Enables a Convenient Production of Long-Acting Therapeutic Peptide. *Pharmaceutics* **2020**, *12*, 364. [CrossRef] [PubMed]
25. Alavi, S.E.; Cabot, P.J.; Yap, G.Y.; Moyle, P.M. Optimized Methods for the Production and Bioconjugation of Site-Specific, Alkyne-Modified Glucagon-like Peptide-1 (GLP-1) Analogs to Azide-Modified Delivery Platforms Using Copper-Catalyzed Alkyne–Azide Cycloaddition. *Bioconjugate Chem.* **2020**, *31*, 1820–1834. [CrossRef] [PubMed]
26. Knudsen, L.B.; Nielsen, P.F.; Huusfeldt, P.O.; Johansen, N.L.; Madsen, K.; Pedersen, F.Z.; Thøgersen, H.; Wilken, M.; Agersø, H. Potent Derivatives of Glucagon-like Peptide-1 with Pharmacokinetic Properties Suitable for Once Daily Administration. *J. Med. Chem.* **2000**, *43*, 1664–1669. [CrossRef] [PubMed]
27. Chin, J.W.; Santoro, S.W.; Martin, A.B.; King, D.S.; Wang, L.; Schultz, P.G. Addition ofp-Azido-l-phenylalanine to the Genetic Code ofEscherichiacoli. *J. Am. Chem. Soc.* **2002**, *124*, 9026–9027. [CrossRef] [PubMed]
28. Lajoie, M.J.; Rovner, A.J.; Goodman, D.B.; Aerni, H.; Haimovich, A.D.; Kuznetsov, G.; Mercer, J.A.; Wang, H.H.; Carr, P.A.; Mosberg, J.A.; et al. Genomically recoded organisms expand Biological Functions. *Science* **2013**, *342*, 357–360. [CrossRef]
29. Kroeze, W.K.; Sassano, M.F.; Huang, X.-P.; Lansu, K.; McCorvy, J.D.; Giguère, P.M.; Sciaky, N.; Roth, B.L. PRESTO-Tango as an open-source resource for interrogation of the druggable human GPCRome. *Nat. Struct. Mol. Biol.* **2015**, *22*, 362–369. [CrossRef]
30. Mørtz, E.; Sareneva, T.; Haebel, S.; Julkunen, I.; Roepstorff, P. Mass spectrometric characterization of glycosylated interferon-γ variants separated by gel electrophoresis. *Electrophoresis* **1996**, *17*, 925–931. [CrossRef]
31. Yang, B.; Kwon, K.; Jana, S.; Kim, S.; Avila-Crump, S.; Tae, G.; Mehl, R.A.; Kwon, I. Temporal Control of Efficient In Vivo Bioconjugation Using a Genetically Encoded Tetrazine-Mediated Inverse-Electron-Demand Diels–Alder Reaction. *Bioconjugate Chem.* **2020**, *31*, 2456–2464. [CrossRef] [PubMed]
32. Kieffer, T.J.; McIntosh, C.H.; Pederson, R.A. Degradation of glucose-dependent insulinotropic polypeptide and truncated glucagon-like peptide 1 in vitro and in vivo by dipeptidyl peptidase IV. *Endocrinology* **1995**, *136*, 3585–3596. [CrossRef] [PubMed]
33. Vilsbøll, T.; Agersø, H.; Krarup, T.; Holst, J.J. Similar Elimination Rates of Glucagon-Like Peptide-1 in Obese Type 2 Diabetic Patients and Healthy Subjects. *J. Clin. Endocrinol. Metab.* **2003**, *88*, 220–224. [CrossRef] [PubMed]

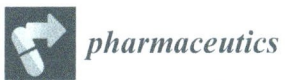 

Article

# Development of In Situ Gelling Meloxicam-Human Serum Albumin Nanoparticle Formulation for Nose-to-Brain Application

Gábor Katona [1,*], Bence Sipos [1], Mária Budai-Szűcs [1], György Tibor Balogh [2,3], Szilvia Veszelka [4], Ilona Gróf [4], Mária A. Deli [4], Balázs Volk [5], Piroska Szabó-Révész [1] and Ildikó Csóka [1]

1. Institute of Pharmaceutical Technology and Regulatory Affairs, Faculty of Pharmacy, University of Szeged, Eötvös Str. 6, H-6720 Szeged, Hungary; sipos.bence@szte.hu (B.S.); budai-szucs.maria@szte.hu (M.B.-S.); ReveszPiroska@szte.hu (P.S.-R.); csoka.ildiko@szte.hu (I.C.)
2. Department of Pharmacodynamics and Biopharmacy, Faculty of Pharmacy, University of Szeged, Eötvös Str. 6, H-6720 Szeged, Hungary; balogh.gyorgy.tibor@szte.hu
3. Department of Chemical and Environmental Process Engineering, Budapest University of Technology and Economics, Műegyetem Quay 3, H-1111 Budapest, Hungary
4. Biological Research Centre, Institute of Biophysics, Temesvári Blvd. 62, H-6726 Szeged, Hungary; veszelka.szilvia@brc.hu (S.V.); grof.ilona@brc.hu (I.G.); deli.maria@brc.hu (M.A.D.)
5. Egis Pharmaceuticals Plc., Keresztúri Str. 30–38, H-1106 Budapest, Hungary; volk.balazs@egis.hu
* Correspondence: katona.gabor@szte.hu; Tel.: +36-62-545-575

**Abstract:** The aim of this study was to develop an intranasal in situ thermo-gelling meloxicam-human serum albumin (MEL-HSA) nanoparticulate formulation applying poloxamer 407 (P407), which can be administered in liquid state into the nostril, and to increase the resistance of the formulation against mucociliary clearance by sol-gel transition on the nasal mucosa, as well as to improve drug absorption. Nanoparticle characterization showed that formulations containing 12–15% $w/w$ P407 met the requirements of intranasal administration. The Z-average (in the range of 180–304 nm), the narrow polydispersity index (PdI, from 0.193 to 0.328), the zeta potential (between −9.4 and −7.0 mV) and the hypotonic osmolality (200–278 mOsmol/L) of MEL-HSA nanoparticles predict enhanced drug absorption through the nasal mucosa. Based on the rheological, muco-adhesion, drug release and permeability studies, the 14% $w/w$ P407 containing formulation (MEL-HSA-P14%) was considered as the optimized formulation, which allows enhanced permeability of MEL through blood–brain barrier-specific lipid fraction. Cell line studies showed no cell damage after 1-h treatment with MEL-HSA-P14% on RPMI 2650 human endothelial cells' moreover, enhanced permeation (four-fold) of MEL from MEL-HSA-P14% was observed in comparison to pure MEL. Overall, MEL-HSA-P14% can be promising for overcoming the challenges of nasal drug delivery.

**Keywords:** quality by design; rapid equilibrium dialysis; muco-adhesion; brain PAMPA; RPMI 2650 nasal epithelial cell

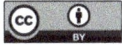

## 1. Introduction

Albumin is a versatile, biodegradable drug carrier for numerous therapeutic agents that have poor water solubility, unsatisfying pharmacokinetics with low circulation half-life, inefficient targetability and even instability in vivo. Strategies for applying albumin for drug delivery can be classified broadly into exogenous and in situ binding formulations that utilize covalent attachment, non-covalent association, or encapsulation of the drug in the form of albumin-based nanoparticles [1].

Neurodegenerative diseases are associated with neuroinflammation. The combination of albumin with non-steroid anti-inflammatory drugs (NSAID) can be promising in therapy, which depends on passing the blood–brain barrier (BBB). NSAIDs can have a protective effect in neurodegenerative diseases through different mechanisms. They can depolarize the mitochondria, therefore inhibiting calcium ion uptake, due to the ionizable carboxylic group [2,3]. Moreover, inhibition of cyclooxygenase (COX) enzymes can suppress glia activity and reduce amyloidosis [4]. COX-2 inhibitor NSAIDs such as meloxicam (MEL) can be advantageous in the treatment of neurodegenerative disorders as they have improved anti-amnesic activity through inhibiting lipid peroxidation and acetylcholinesterase activity in the brain [2] supplemented by additional antioxidant effect [3], but the therapeutic application is limited due to the poor BBB transport [5]. To overcome this obstacle, choosing the appropriate carrier system and route of administration has a prominent role [6].

Nasal administration can be a suitable means of transport route for that purpose; moreover, it has been reported that the initial formation of Alzheimer's disease begins in the entorhinal cortex, a region innervated by the olfactory nerves, then progresses according to the corresponding pattern [7]. Due to the high surface area and rich vascularization, drugs or drug-delivery systems can be easily absorbed from the nasal cavity; moreover, first-pass metabolism is negligible through this administration route, which can be advantageous in terms of preserving pharmacological activity [8–10]. Nano drug delivery systems (nanoDDSs) are able to transport drugs as cargo, bypassing the BBB through the trigeminal and olfactory nerves directly into the brain [11]. Moreover, they support intranasal NSAID administration, due to their poor water solubility at nasal pH (5.3–5.6) and low residence time (10–15 min) due to mucociliary clearance [12]. In our previous study was demonstrated that MEL-human serum albumin (HSA) nanoparticles could be successfully applied for nose-to-brain delivery, with improved in vivo brain targeting efficacy [13].

As mucociliary clearance is a limiting factor in nose-to-brain delivery, the application of viscosity enhancers or mucoadhesive polymers can be advantageous by increasing the residence time on the nasal mucosa, which supports drug absorption [14–16]. To satisfy these requirements formulation of in situ thermo-gelling systems can be efficacious. Poloxamer 407 (P407), a triblock copolymer consisting of a hydrophobic residue of poly-oxy-propylene (POP) between the two hydrophilic units of poly-oxyethylene (POE), can be applied for development of in situ thermo-reversible gelling systems, through temperature-controlled micelle forming [17–19]. Thermo-gelling occurs due to hydrophobic interactions between the P407 copolymer chains [20]. By optimization of P407 concentration in the formulation, a sol–gel transition can be reached at the temperature of the nasal cavity, while it remains in a liquid state below that temperature during storage and administration.

As continuous improvement is part of industrial manufacturing and research processes, the quality management of nanocarriers having higher potential, in the case of beneficial therapeutic applications and effects, should be of paramount importance. Quality by Design (QbD) offers a proper methodology based on knowledge and risk assessment, ensuring the quality, safety and efficacy of the desirable nanocarrier [21]. In the case of nose-to-brain applicable nanocarriers, many physiological and pharmaceutical aspects must be taken into account, which are adapted to the versatile biological and chemical aspects of this route. As part of the QbD assessment, a comparison study was performed between MEL-HSA and MEL-HSA-P407 formulations to evaluate the change of risk severity during a continuous development process [22].

Our aim was to optimize an in situ thermo-gelling MEL-HSA-P407 formulation, which can be administered in liquid state into the nostril and to increase resistance of formulation against mucociliarly clearance by sol–gel transition on the nasal mucosa, as well as to improve drug absorption.

## 2. Materials and Methods

### 2.1. Materials

Meloxicam (MEL, 4-hydroxy-2-methyl-$N$-(5-methyl-2-thiazolyl)-2$H$-benzothiazine-3-carboxamide-1,1-dioxide) was donated by EGIS Pharmaceuticals Plc. (Budapest, Hungary) for research work. Human serum albumin (HSA, lyophilized powder, purity > 97%), fluorescein isothiocyanate-labelled HSA (FITC-HSA), Tween 80 (Tween), P407, disodium hydrogen phosphate ($Na_2HPO_4$), sodium dihydrogen phosphate ($NaH_2PO_4$), polar brain lipid extract, cholesterol, mucin from porcine stomach (Type III), and all reagents for cell line studies were purchased from Sigma Aldrich Co. Ltd. (Budapest, Hungary) if not indicated otherwise. Analytical grade solvents such as methanol, dimethyl sulfoxide (DMSO) and dodecane were purchased from Molar Chemicals (Budapest, Hungary). Sodium hyaluronate (NaHA, Mw = 1400 kDa) was obtained from Gedeon Richter Plc. (Budapest, Hungary). In all experiments, water was purified by the Millipore Milli-Q® 140 Gradient Water Purification System.

### 2.2. Preparation of In Situ Gelling MEL-HSA Nanoparticle Formulations

MEL-HSA nanoparticles were produced by applying a modified coacervation method (Figure 1) according to the following steps [23]: first, Tween-80 was dispersed in 4 mL of HCl solution (0.1 M), whereas MEL was dissolved in 4 mL of NaOH solution (0.1 M) and HSA was dissolved in 8 mL of purified water. Then, the Tween 80 solution was added dropwise (0.5 mL/min) to the MEL solution at 4 °C under constant stirring (800 rpm). Next, this MEL–Tween 80 solution was added dropwise to the HSA solution at 4 °C under constant stirring (800 rpm). After complete homogenization, additional HCl was added dropwise to adjust pH to 5.6, and as a result the solution became turbid. Then, the formulation was incubated for 12 h under constant stirring (800 rpm) to obtain nanoparticle dispersion. P407 in various concentrations (based on preliminary experimental results 12, 13, 14, 15 and 16% $w/w$) was added to the formulation and kept in a cool place (5 ± 3 °C) overnight until complete hydration and dissolution of the polymer, before further investigations.

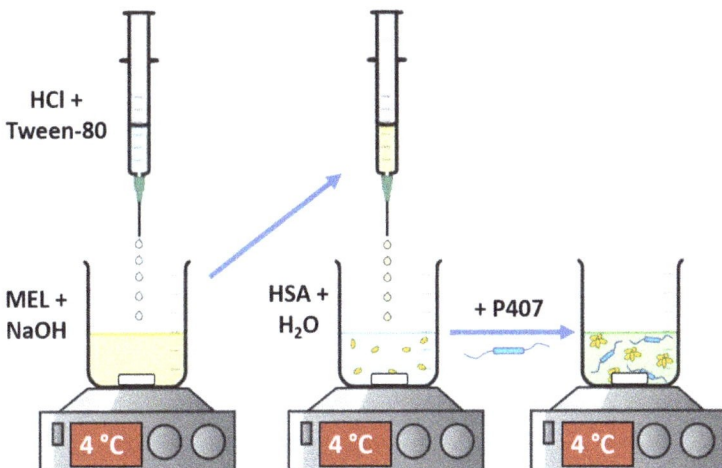

**Figure 1.** Preparation of MEL-HSA-P407.

### 2.3. QbD-Based Comparative Risk Assessment

As the in situ thermo-gelling carrier system is part of a continuous development process, it needs to be compared to the HSA nanoparticles, validating the product life cycle, and therefore ensuring quality. At first, the quality target product profile (QTPP) was determined based on the mandatory requirements of a nose-to-brain applicable nanocarrier. The critical quality attributes (CQAs) were also determined as they are physicochemical factors affecting product safety, efficacy and quality. Critical process parameters (CPPs) and critical material attributes (CMAs) were not taken into account during the risk assessment process as an extensive optimization of P407 concentration was performed. For the identified elements, risk levels were assigned for both the MEL-HSA and MEL-HSA-P407. A three-level scale was used to describe the relation between these parameters: each relation was assigned with a "high" (H), "medium" (M) or "low" (L) attributive. To quantify the risk values, LeanQbD® Software (QbD Works LLC, Fremont, CA, USA) was used. As the output of this comparative risk assessment, severity scores were compared and evaluated to determine the influence of the in situ thermo-gelling carrier system on product quality.

*2.4. Optimization of In Situ Thermogelling Carrier System*

2.4.1. Rheological Studies

The rheological measurements were carried out with a Physica MCR302 rheometer (Anton Paar, Graz, Austria). A cone and plate type measuring device with cone angle of 1° was applied; the diameter of the cone was 25 mm, and the gap height in the middle of the cone was 0.046 mm. The gelation temperature was measured while the temperature was increased from 20 to 40 °C, using 1 °C/min heating rate. The measurement was performed at a constant frequency of 1.0 rad/min and at a constant strain of 1%. The gelation time of the polymer solutions was followed at a constant frequency of 1.0 rad/min and at a constant strain of 1% at 37 °C. The samples were stored at $5 \pm 1$ °C and taken immediately before the measurement. Viscoelastic character was determined by frequency sweep tests immediately after the gelation measurement, with a strain of 1% at 37 °C. Storage modulus (G'), loss modulus (G") and loss factor were determined over the angular frequency range from 0.1 to 100 rad/s. The applied strain value (1%) was in the range of the linear viscoelasticity of the gels.

2.4.2. Muco-Adhesion Measurement

Muco-adhesion was analyzed by means of tensile tests (TA-XT Plus texture analyzer (Metron Kft, Budapest, Hungary)) equipped with a 5-kg load cell. As a simulated mucosal membrane, a filter paper (Whatman® qualitative filter paper, Sigma Aldrich Co. Ltd., Budapest, Hungary) with 25 mm diameter, impregnated with 50 µL of an 8% $w/w$ mucin dispersion, was used, prepared with a simulated nasal electrolyte solution (SNES) consisting of 8.77 g/L sodium chloride (NaCl), 2.98 g/L potassium chloride (KCl), 0.59 g/L anhydrous calcium chloride (CaCl$_2$) and dissolved in purified water; the pH was adjusted to 5.6 with 0.1 M HCl [12]. Five parallel measurements were performed. 20 mg of the sample was attached to the cylinder probe and placed in contact with the filter paper wetted with mucin. A 2500 mN preload was used for 3 min, then the cylinder probe was moved upwards to separate the sample from the substrate at a prefixed speed of 2.5 mm/min. The maximum detachment force (adhesive force) and the work of adhesion (A, mN/mm) were measured, the latter calculated as the area (AUC) under the "force versus distance" curve using the Exponent Connect software of the instrument. The formulations were thermostated at 37 °C for 30 min before measurement. As a reference system, 0.5% $w/w$ NaHA aqueous solution was applied.

2.4.3. Characterization of Nanoparticles

The formulations were characterized according to their average hydrodynamic diameter (Z-average), polydispersity index (PdI) and zeta potential using a Malvern Zeta sizer Nano ZS (Malvern Instruments, Worcestershire, UK) at 25 and 35 °C in folded capillary cells. The refractive index was set to 1.72. The pH of formulations was measured applying a WTW® inoLab® pH 7110 laboratory pH tester (Thermo Fisher Scientific, Budapest, Hungary). The osmolality of formulations was determined by osmometer (Knauer Semi-micro Osmometer, Berlin, Germany) based on the freezing point depression method. Each measurement was carried out in triplicate and data are shown as means ± SD. The encapsulation efficiency and loading capacity of gel-embedded nanoparticles were prepared with a Hermle Z323K high performance refrigerated centrifuge (Hermle AG, Gossheim, Germany) at 17.500 rpm, 4 °C for 30 min. The amount of free MEL in the supernatant was determined by high performance liquid chromatography (HPLC). Encapsulation efficiency (EE) and loading capacity (LC) of formulations were calculated according to the following equations [24]:

$$EE\ (\%) = \frac{Amount\ of\ drug\ applied - Amount\ of\ drug\ in\ the\ supernatant}{Amount\ of\ drug\ applied} \cdot 100 \quad (1)$$

$$LC\ (\%) = \frac{Mass\ of\ drug\ encapsulated}{Mass\ of\ nanoparticles} \cdot 100 \quad (2)$$

The distribution of FITC labelled HSA-MEL nanoparticles in gel structure was visualized by a Leica TCS SP5 confocal laser scanning microscope (Leica Microsystems GmbH, Wetzlar, Germany) and Visitron spinning disk confocal system (Visitron Systems GmbH, Puchheim, Germany). The P407 containing formulations and the FITC labelled HSA-MEL colloidal solution as reference were dropped onto slides and incubated for 10 min at 35 °C for thermo-gelling. Then, slides were excited with a 488 nm Argon laser, and fluorescence was detected with a 505 to 570 nm BP filter.

2.4.4. Rapid Equilibrium Dialysis (RED)

In order to investigate the in vitro dissolution kinetics and release profile of different MEL-HSA-P407 formulations at nasal conditions, the RED Device (Thermo Scientific™, Waltham, MA, USA) was used. A suspension of MEL was prepared in a phosphate buffer saline (PBS, pH 5.6) with a nominal concentration of 2 mg/mL as a control for the study. Both the control and in situ gelling MEL-HSA formulations were homogenized using an Eppendorf MixMate (Thermo Scientific™, Waltham, MA, USA) vortex mixer for 30 s and an ultrasonic bath (Sonorex Digiplus, Bandelin GmbH & Co. KG, Berlin, Germany) for 10 min. The RED Device inserts (8K MWCO) were fitted into the PTFE base plate, then 150 µL of samples was placed into the donor chambers, while 300 µL of PBS (pH 5.6) was added to the acceptor chambers. Thereafter, the RED unit was covered with a sealing tape and incubated above gelling temperature (37 °C) on an orbital shaker (at 350 rpm) for 4 h. 50 µL aliquots were withdrawn from the acceptor chamber at 5, 15, 30, 60, 120 and 240 min time points and immediately replaced with the same amount of fresh medium. 50 µL of acetonitrile was added to the withdrawn samples and the MEL content was determined using HPLC. Five parallel measurements were performed.

2.4.5. High Performance Liquid Chromatography (HPLC)

The determination of MEL concentration was performed with an Agilent 1260 HPLC (Agilent Technologies, Santa Clara, CA, USA). A Kinetex® C18 column (5 µm, 150 mm × 4.6 mm (Phenomenex, Torrance, CA, USA)) was used as stationary phase. The mobile phases consisted of 0.065 M $KH_2PO_4$ aqueous solution adjusted to pH = 2.8 with phosphoric acid (A), and methanol (B). A linear gradient from 50–50% to 25–75% (A-B eluent) was applied from 0 to 14 min. Then, from 14 to 20 min the phase composition was set back to 50–50% A-B. Separation was performed at 30 °C with 1 mL/min flow rate. 10 µL of the samples was injected to determine the MEL's concentration at 355 ± 4 nm using the UV-VIS diode array detector. Data were evaluated using ChemStation B.04.03. Software (Agilent Technologies, Santa Clara, CA, USA). The retention time of MEL was observed at 14.34 min. The regression coefficient ($R^2$) of the calibration curve was 0.999 in the concentration range 1–200 µg/mL. The determined limits of detection (LOD) and quantification (LOQ) of MEL were 16 ppm and 49 ppm, respectively.

2.4.6. In Vitro BBB Permeability Assay

Parallel artificial membrane permeability assay (PAMPA) was used to determine the brain specific effective permeability of MEL from the reference suspension and the MEL-HAS-P407 formulations [25]. The filter donor plate (Multiscreen™-IP, MAIPN4510, pore size 0.45 µm; Millipore, Merck Ltd., Budapest, Hungary) was coated with 5 µL of lipid solution containing 16 mg brain polar lipid extract (porcine) and 8 mg cholesterol dissolved in 600 µL dodecane. The Acceptor Plate (MSSACCEPTOR; Millipore, Merck Ltd., Budapest, Hungary) was filled with 300 µL of a PBS solution of pH 7.4. 150–150 µL of the formulation and the reference solutions were applied on the membrane of the donor plate. Then, this was covered with a plate lid in order to decrease the possible evaporation of the solvent. This sandwich system was incubated at 37 °C for 4 h (Heidolph Titramax 1000, Heidolph Instruments, Schwabach, Germany). The concentration of MEL permeated in the acceptor plate was determined using HPLC. The effective permeability and membrane retention of drugs were calculated using the following equation [25]:

$$P_e \text{ (cm/s)} = -\frac{2.303 \cdot V_A}{A(t - \tau_{SS})} \cdot \log\left[1 - \frac{c_A(t)}{S}\right] \quad (3)$$

where $P_e$ is the effective permeability coefficient (cm/s), $A$ is the filter area (0.24 cm$^2$), $V_A$ is the volume of the acceptor phase (0.3 mL), $t$ is the incubation time (s), $\tau_{SS}$ is the time to reach the steady state (s), $c_A(t)$ is the concentration of the compound in the acceptor phase at time point $t$ (mol/mL), and $S$ (mol/mL) is the solubility of MEL in the donor phase. The latter was determined after centrifugation (at 12000 rpm, 15 min, Eppendorf Centrifuge 5804 R) in Microcon Centrifugal Filter Devices (30,000 MWCO) and 50-times dilution of the formulations, using the same HPLC system. The flux of samples was calculated using the following equation [26]:

$$Flux \text{ (mol/cm}^2 \cdot \text{s)} = P_e \cdot S \quad (4)$$

*2.5. Cell Line Studies with Optimized Formulation*

2.5.1. Cell Cultures

Human RPMI 2650 (ATCC cat. no. CCL 30) nasal epithelial cells were grown in Dulbecco's Modified Eagle's Medium (DMEM, Gibco, Life Technologies, Gaithersburg, MD, USA) supplemented with 10% $v/v$ fetal bovine serum (FBS, Pan-Biotech GmbH, Aidenbach, Germany) and 50 µg/mL gentamicin in a humidified 37 °C incubator with 5% $CO_2$. The surfaces were coated with 0.05% rat tail collagen in sterile distilled water before cell seeding in culture dishes and the medium was changed every 2 days. When RPMI 2650 cells reached approximately 80–90% confluence in the dish, they were trypsinized with 0.05% trypsin-0.02% EDTA solution. One day before the experiment, retinoic acid (10 µM) and hydrocortisone (500 nM) were added to the cells to form a tighter barrier [27].

For permeability measurements epithelial cells were co-cultured with human vascular endothelial cells [28,29] to create a more physiological barrier, representing both the nasal epithelium and the submucosal vascular endothelium. The endothelial cells were grown in endothelial culture medium (ECM-NG, Sciencell Research Laboratories, Carlsbad, CA, USA) supplemented with 5% FBS, 1% endothelial growth supplement (ECGS, Sciencell Research Laboratories, Carlsbad, CA, USA) and 0.5% gentamicin on 0.2% gelatin-coated culture dishes (10 cm). For the permeability experiments, cells were used at passage 8.

2.5.2. Cell Viability Measurements

Real-time cell electronic sensing is a non-invasive, label-free, impedance-based technique to quantify the kinetics of proliferation and viability of adherent cells. Our group has successfully used this method to study cell damage and/or protection in living cells [30,31]. The RTCA-SP instrument (ACEA Biosciences, San Diego, CA, USA) monitored the impedance of cell layers every 10 min. Cell index was defined as $R_n$-$R_b$ at each time point of measurement, where $R_n$ is the cell-electrode impedance of the well when it contains cells, and $R_b$ is the background impedance of the well with the medium alone. Cell index values reflect cell number and viability.

The 96-well E-plates with integrated gold electrodes (E-plate 96, ACEA Biosciences, USA) were coated with 0.2% gelatin and incubated for 20 min in the incubator. Then gelatin was removed, and culture medium (50 µL) was added to each well for background readings. RPMI 2650 cell suspension was dispensed at the density of $2 \times 10^4$ cells/well in 50 µL volume and the plate was kept in a humidified incubator with 5% $CO_2$ at 37 °C. When cells reached a steady growth phase, they were treated with the nano-formulations and their components.

2.5.3. Permeability Study on the Co-Cultured Model

The tightness of the BBB co-culture model was verified by transepithelial electric resistance (TEER) measurement, which reflects the tightness of cell layers of biological barriers. TEER was measured by an EVOM volt-ohm meter (World Precision Instruments, Sarasota, FL, USA) combined with STX-2 electrodes, and it was expressed relative to the surface area of the monolayers as $\Omega \times cm^2$. TEER of coated, but cell-free, filters were subtracted from measured TEER values. Cells were treated with the nano-formulations when the cell layer reached steady TEER values.

For the permeability studies we used a co-culture model, in which RPMI 2650 cells were cultured together with endothelial cells on inserts of a 12-well trans-well system (Transwell, polycarbonate membrane, 3 µm pore size, 1.12 $cm^2$, Corning Costar Co., Lowell, MA, USA) for 5 days. In this model, endothelial cells were seeded ($1 \times 10^5$ cells/$cm^2$) to the bottom side of culture inserts coated with Matrigel (growth factor reduced, BD Biosciences, San Jose, CA, USA) and nasal epithelial cells were passaged ($2 \times 10^5$ cells/$cm^2$) to the upper side of the membranes coated with rat tail collagen.

During the permeability experiments, the inserts were placed on 12-well plates containing 1.5 mL Ringer-HEPES buffer in the acceptor (lower/basal) compartments. In the donor (upper/apical) compartments, the culture medium was changed and 0.5 mL buffer containing different formulations and meloxicam as reference were added. To avoid an unstirred water layer effect, the plates were kept on a horizontal shaker (120 rpm) during the assay in a humidified incubator with 5% $CO_2$ at 37 °C for 1 h. After incubation, samples were collected from the donor and acceptor compartments and the meloxicam concentration was measured by HPLC.

To test the function of our co-culture model, the flux of permeability marker molecules FITC-labeled dextran (FD10, Mw: 10 kDa) and Evans blue labeled albumin (EBA; MW: 67.5 kDa) was determined across the cell layers [31]. In the donor compartments of the inserts, 0.5 mL buffer containing FD10 (100 µg/mL) and EBA (167.5 µg/mL Evans blue dye and 10 mg/mL bovine serum albumin) was added and 12-well plates were placed on a horizontal shaker (120 rpm) for 30 min. After treatments, samples from the lower compartments were collected and the markers were measured with a fluorescence multi-well plate reader (Fluostar Optima, BMG Labtech, Ortenberg, Germany; FITC: excitation wavelength: 485 nm, emission wavelength: 520 nm; Evans-blue labeled albumin: excitation wavelength: 584 nm, emission wavelength: 680 nm).

The apparent permeability coefficients ($P_{app}$) were calculated as described previously [31] by the following equation:

$$P_{app}(cm/s) = \frac{\Delta[C]_A \times V_A}{A \times [C]_D \times \Delta t} \quad (5)$$

Briefly, $P_{app}$ was calculated from the concentration difference of the tracer in the acceptor compartment ($\Delta[C]_A$) after 60 min, initial donor compartments' concentration ($[C]_D$), $V_A$ is the volume of the acceptor compartment (1.5 mL) and $A$ is the surface area available for permeability (1.1 $cm^2$).

2.5.4. Treatments of Cultured Cells

For cell viability measurements, 10, 30 and 100 times dilutions from optimized MEL-HSA P407 formulation (14% $w/w$ P407), 2 mg/mL meloxicam, 3 mg/mL Tween 80 and 160 mg/mL P407 solutions were prepared in cell culture medium. For permeability measurements, 2 mg/mL meloxicam and 10× times dilution of MEL-HSA-P407 were prepared in Ringer-HEPES buffer and added to the donor compartments.

### 2.5.5. Immunohistochemistry

To evaluate morphological changes in RPMI 2650 cells caused by the MEL-HAS-P407 formulation and MEL, immunostaining for junctional proteins zonula occludens protein-1 (ZO-1) and β-catenin was made. After the permeability experiments, cells on culture inserts were washed with phosphate buffer (PBS) and fixed with ice cold methanol–acetone (1:1) solution for 2 min then washed with PBS 3 times. The nonspecific binding sites were blocked with 3% bovine serum albumin in PBS. Primary antibodies rabbit anti-ZO-1 (AB_138452, 1:400; Life Technologies, Carlsbad, CA, USA) and rabbit anti-β-catenin (AB_476831, 1:400) were applied as overnight treatment at 4 °C. Incubation with anti-rabbit IgG Cy3 conjugated (AB_258792, 1:400) secondary antibodies lasted for 1 h and Hoechst dye 33342 was used to stain cell nuclei. After mounting the samples (Fluoromount-G; Southern Biotech, Birmingham, AL, USA) staining was visualized by Leica TCS SP5 confocal laser scanning microscope (Leica Microsystems GmbH, Wetzlar, Germany).

### 2.6. Statistical Analysis

All data presented are means ± SD. In the case of mucoadhesive study, an unpaired $t$-test was applied. The values in the cell line studies were compared using the analysis of variance followed by Dunett or Bonferroni tests using GraphPad Prism 5.0 software (GraphPad Software Inc., San Diego, CA, USA). Changes were considered statistically significant at $p < 0.05$. The significance of differences of RED and PAMPA data was calculated with one-way ANOVA with post hoc test (Tukey's multiple comparisons test, $\alpha = 0.05$).

## 3. Results

### 3.1. Comparative Risk Assessment of MEL-HSA and MEL-HSA-P407

In addition to CQAs, well-defined goals must be set for the product to fit the nose-to-brain route of administration. This route has many obstacles and challenges to overcome, starting from the formulation process and the patient's administration until the developed effect in the central nervous system. Due to the physiological and chemical variety through this pathway, a number of formulation aspects must be taken into consideration ensuring the desired product quality and performance. This is determined by the QTPP of the product, the elements of which can be seen in Table 1.

**Table 1.** QTPP elements of the nose-to-brain applicable HSA nanoparticle- and poloxamer-based in situ thermogelling system.

| QTPP Element | Target |
| --- | --- |
| Carrier integrity | Nanosized particle size and distribution with uniform API content after gelation at gelation temperature. |
| Drug release in the nasal cavity | The formulation should release more MEL in the dissolution medium compared to initial MEL at pH 5.6. |
| Mucoadhesive properties | The mucoadhesive force and work should be high enough to meet the requirements of the nasal delivery. |
| Residence time on nasal mucosa | Increased residence time compared to non-gel formulations. |
| Nasal epithelial cellular uptake | The formulation should have higher permeability on nasal epithelial cells without damaging the cells forming the nasal barrier compared to raw MEL. |
| Transport in the central nervous system | The flux and permeability value of the gel formulation should be increased across BBB lipids compared to initial MEL |

The next step was to assign risk relations to MEL-HSA and MEL-HSA-P407 formulations which were first prepared by interdependence rating on a three-level scale. Quantifying these risks was interpreted using severity scores which were compared to each other. The tables of the interdependence rating and the severity scores are shown in Figure 2.

| A QTPP element | MEL-HSA | MEL-HSA-P407 |
|---|---|---|
| Carrier integrity | M | L |
| Drug release in the nasal cavity | M | M |
| Mucoadhesive properties | H | M |
| Residence time on nasal mucosa | H | L |
| Nasal epithelial cellular uptake | M | L |
| Transport in the CNS | M | M |

| C CQA element | MEL-HSA | MEL-HSA-P407 |
|---|---|---|
| Particle size | H | H |
| Particle size distribution | M | M |
| Zeta potential | M | M |
| Permeability rate | M | H |
| Dissolution rate | H | M |
| Drug loading | M | L |
| Mucoadhesivity | H | M |
| Cellular uptake rate | H | M |
| Osmolality | M | L |

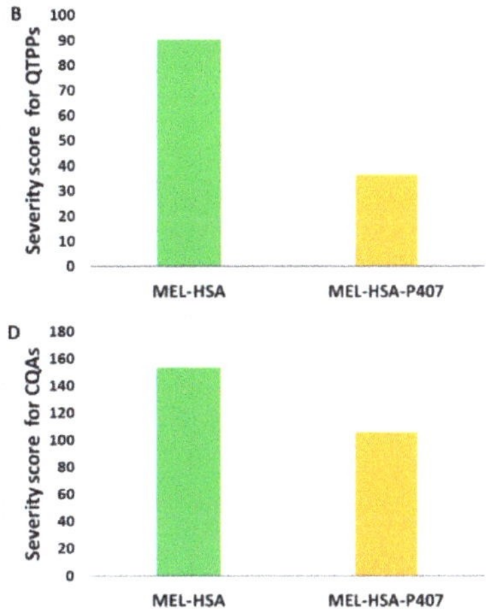

**Figure 2.** Interdependence rating amongst QTPPs (**A**), CQAs (**C**) and MEL-HSA, MEL-HSA-P407 formulations with the corresponding severity scores for QTPPs (**B**) and CQAs (**D**). Abbreviations: H: high, L: low, M: medium.

Based on the calculated severity scores, it can be claimed that, by incorporating HSA nanoparticles as a part of an in situ thermo-gelling system, the severity of risk can be heavily reduced. As desired for the nose-to-brain pathway, in theory, with increased muco-adhesion properties, an increased residence time can be observed. The particle characteristics are always of paramount importance and cannot be left out of the design space development. These parameters are closely related to the dissolution and absorption profile of the nanocarrier. The reduction in the added-up severity score means that the product quality can be improved and is the reason for the continuous manufacturing improvement. With optimal P407 concentration, the increased residence time and muco-adhesivity along with the penetration-enhancement also contribute to the possibly increased drug release and permeability. However, individual risks must be investigated, as seen from the structure of this article. The risk of decrease in permeability due to the more structured gel system, with less API exposed to the dissolution media per time, is always there, which is why it is of the utmost importance and can be characterized as a high-risk relation. This possible unbeneficial risk can be countered by the improved residence behavior in the nasal cavity, providing the pharmacokinetics to an adequate extent. P407 itself has also a solubilizing effect which also opposes some of the unbeneficial possibilities. The determination of gelling properties also helps to evaluate the success of the development, so these factors are also investigated; however, this cannot be part of a comparative risk assessment, as MEL-HSA nanoparticles themselves do not contain any gelling material.

*3.2. Optimization of P407 Concentration in the Formulation*

3.2.1. Investigation of In Situ Thermo-Gelling Properties

During the optimization process, the effect of the P407 concentration on the gelation and rheological properties was analyzed. In the first part of our rheological investigation, the effect of the P407 concentration on the lower critical solution temperature (LCST) was measured. LCST was defined as the temperature at the crossover point of the storage modulus ($G'$) and loss modulus ($G''$), and primary data can be seen in Figure S1. Based on our results, we can conclude that a minimum of 13% $w/w$ P407 concentration is needed for gelling at body temperature (Figure 3A). However, considering possible dilution in vivo, it is preferable to use a slightly higher concentration (at least 14% $w/w$ or above).

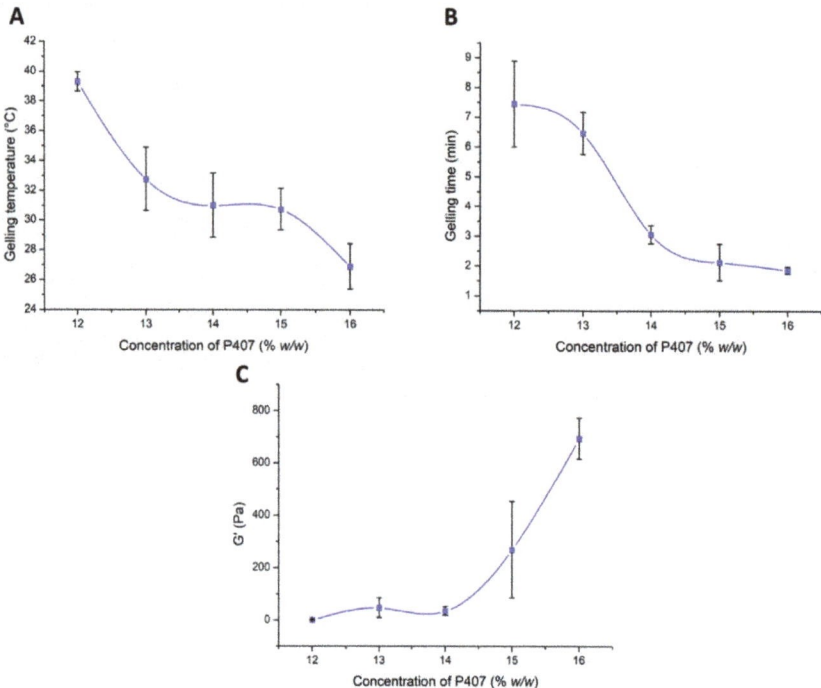

**Figure 3.** Effect of the P407 concentration on the gelling temperature (**A**), gelling time at 37 °C (**B**), and gel strength (**C**). Data is presented as means ± SD, $n = 5$.

The gelling time significantly affects the bioavailability of the nasal preparation. If gelation is too slow, the mucosal concentration of the product is significantly reduced due to the elimination mechanisms, and dilution with a liquid layer covering the mucosa prevents subsequent gelation. On the other hand, too fast a gelation can make it difficult to distribute the composition on the mucosa, therefore a reduced absorption surface can be expected. It can be clearly seen from our results that in case of 12–13% $w/w$ P407 gelation time was too slow (6–7 min), but with the increasing polymer concentration (14–16% $w/w$) gel formation occurs within 2–3 min at 37 °C (Figure 3B), which seems to be optimal for nasal application.

The rheological properties of gels at body temperature may also affect the bioavailability of the formulations. The stronger the gel structure, the more resistant it is against the mucosal elimination mechanisms. The nasal mucosa is characterized by the phenomenon of mucociliary clearance caused by the beating of the cilia. The effect of ciliary beating can usually be simulated by oscillatory rheological measurements at low oscillation frequency [32]. In our case, we compared our formulations at the angular frequency of 1 rad/s using frequency sweep tests.

As can be seen in Figure 3C an elastic characteristic can be measured with only higher P407 concentrations, i.e., only samples containing 15–16% $w/w$ P407 can be characterized with considerable elasticity at body temperature. Although gelation begins at body temperature in the case of the 13–14% $w/w$ systems, this results in only a very weak gel structure, which may not hinder drug release. As was also described in the literature [33], the poloxamer forms weak gels.

3.2.2. Muco-Adhesion Measurement

Gelling at body temperature results in the micellar arrangement of P407 molecules, which may affect the muco-adhesiveness of the formulation. During the tensile test, the contact of the two surfaces can generate the change in the gel structure and the formation of the mucoadhesive interaction simultaneously. As a result of the two processes, we can observe high variability in the adhesive work and force values.

In the case of our systems, adhesive forces of about 1000 mN were measured in almost all cases (Figure 4A), and it was found that the mucoadhesive force did not change remarkably with increasing P407 concentration. Only a slightly increasing tendency can be observed at higher polymer concentration (1100 mN). This can mean that the number of functional groups forming mucoadhesive bonds at the interface slightly increases. Comparing the muco-adhesivity of the in situ gelling systems with that of the NaHA, we can see a higher adhesive force value in the case of NaHA, but the difference cannot be considered as significant ($p > 0.05$ in each cases).

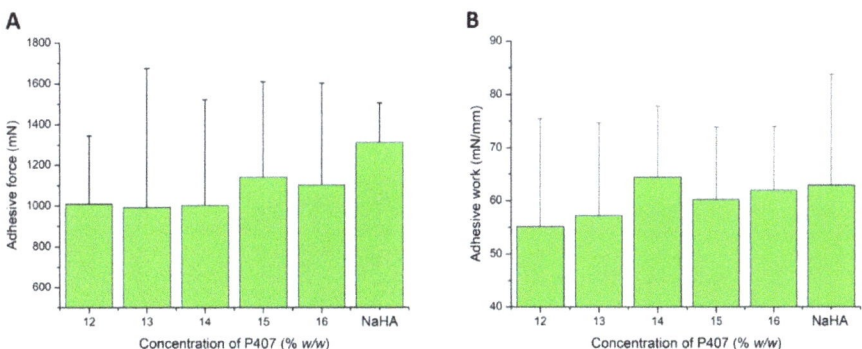

**Figure 4.** Adhesive force (**A**) and adhesive work (**B**) of the compositions in various P407 concentrations. Data is presented as means ± SD, $n = 5$.

In contrast, there is a slight increase in mucoadhesive work, and higher values of adhesive work can be measured in those compositions (14–16% $w/w$ P407) where a gel structure is already formed at near body temperature (Figure 4B). In this case, with the formation of the gel structure, the formation of mucoadhesive physical bonds is more significant. Comparing the formulated systems with the reference mucoadhesive, we could not detect significant differences ($p > 0.05$ in each cases), which could be the result of the large SD.

3.2.3. Characterization of Carrier Systems

Nanoparticle properties such as particle size, PdI, zeta potential, encapsulation efficacy, loading capacity, pH and osmolality are key parameters for characterization of the therapeutic applicability of nasal formulations. These nasal administration-related parameters of the P407-containing formulation in different concentrations are presented in Table 2.

The Z-average, PdI and zeta potential value of formulations was measured both in sol and gel state. Formulations containing 12–14% $w/w$ P407 meet the requirements of intranasally administered nanoparticles (<200 nm) even after thermo-gelling, but in case of 15–16% $w/w$ P407 these parameters are out of the acceptance criteria. Moreover, the Z-average (in the range of 180–193 nm) of gel embedded MEL-HSA nanoparticle suggests increased drug release. The narrow PdI (from 0.193 to 0.328) indicates monodispersed size distribution, which ensures the homogeneity of nanoparticles in the gel structure. The distribution of FITC labelled MEL-HSA nanoparticles was visualized in the gel structure using fluorescent microscopy (Figure 5).

Table 2. Physico-chemical parameters of in situ thermogelling nasal formulations.

| Notation of Formulation | Content of P407 (% w/w) | 25 °C | | 35 °C | | | EE (%) | LC (%) | pH | Osmolality (mOsmol/kg) |
|---|---|---|---|---|---|---|---|---|---|---|
| | | Z-Average (nm) | PdI | Z-Average (nm) | PdI | ZP (mV) | | | | |
| MEL–HSA-P12% | 12 | 172 ± 2 | 0.189 ± 0.02 | 180.7 ± 3 | 0.193 ± 0.03 | −9.4 ± 0.7 | 82.34 ± 0.12 | 1.26 ± 0.01 | 5.85 ± 0.08 | 200 ± 2 |
| MEL–HSA-P13% | 13 | 175 ± 2 | 0.211 ± 0.01 | 188.7 ± 2 | 0.282 ± 0.02 | −8.5 ± 0.5 | 82.01 ± 0.19 | 1.17 ± 0.02 | 5.81 ± 0.04 | 220 ± 3 |
| MEL–HSA-P14% | 14 | 176 ± 3 | 0.205 ± 0.02 | 193.7 ± 2 | 0.211 ± 0.02 | −7.9 ± 0.3 | 81.64 ± 0.21 | 1.09 ± 0.02 | 5.61 ± 0.05 | 242 ± 3 |
| MEL–HSA-P15% | 15 | 182 ± 3 | 0.234 ± 0.03 | 262.4 ± 3 | 0.306 ± 0.03 | −7.1 ± 0.4 | 81.19 ± 0.23 | 1.03 ± 0.01 | 5.60 ± 0.02 | 278 ± 2 |
| MEL–HSA-P16% | 16 | 231 ± 3 | 0.268 ± 0.02 | 304.3 ± 5 | 0.328 ± 0.04 | −7.0 ± 0.2 | 79.46 ± 0.24 | 0.97 ± 0.01 | 5.52 ± 0.07 | 311 ± 4 |

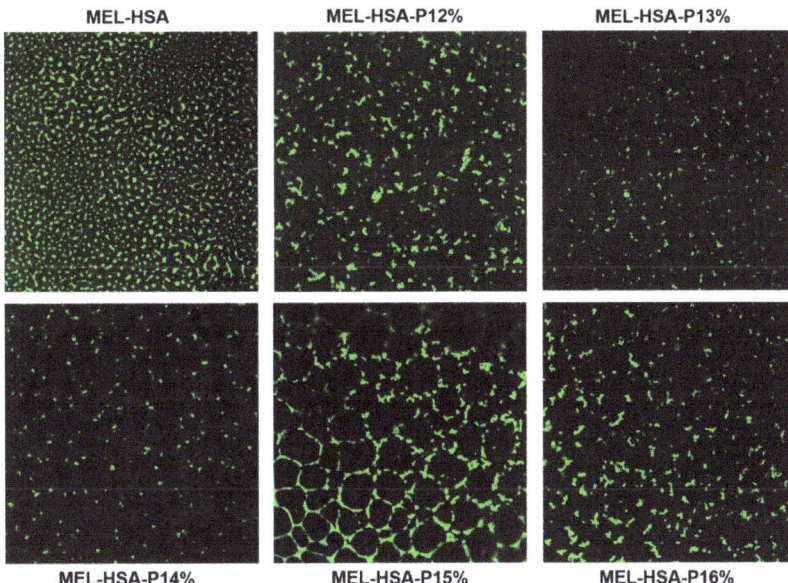

**Figure 5.** FITC-labelled MEL-HSA nanoparticles and their distribution in gel structure containing various concentrations of P407 at 60× magnification.

The fluorescent, microscopic images prove the homogenous distribution of MEL-HSA nanoparticles and narrow PdI, and gelling of the formulations did not show an aggregation tendency of the nanoparticles. There was no remarkable difference in zeta potential (between −9.4 and −7.0 mV) of formulations and these values indicate that repulsion of nanoparticles is not significant enough to avoid aggregation in sol form. Both encapsulation efficacy and loading capacity of formulations were slightly decreased with increasing P407 concentration, but even so this difference was not remarkable, therefore from this point of view each formulation can be suitable for application. The osmolality of formulations containing 12–15% $w/w$ P407 was hypotonic (200–278 mOsmol/L), which predicts enhanced drug absorption, offsetting the retention of gel structure. In case of 16% $w/w$ P407 the formulation was hypertonic (311 mOsmol/L), which can result in significant dehydration of nasal mucosa; therefore, from a therapeutic point of view the application of MEL-HSA-P16% is not recommended.

3.2.4. In Vitro Dissolution Profiles (RED)

The drug release kinetic of in situ gelling formulations is a critical part of rational drug design as it is a major determinant of the efficacy of delivery of the carrier in vivo and the subsequent release of the free drug. The in vitro release profile reveals important information on the structure and behavior of the formulation, on possible interactions between the drug and carrier composition, and on their influence on the rate and mechanism of drug release. The dialysis-based release method is a well-established and useful technique to study in vitro release from nano-particulate delivery systems. RED device was developed in order to reduce the time to equilibrium, and to provide results faster than other dialysis methods [34]. In this system, MEL conjugated HSA nanoparticles are physically separated from the acceptor media by a dialysis membrane with 8 kDa cutoff which allows only the passive diffusion of free MEL into the acceptor media. The time-dependent in vitro release profiles of MEL and formulations were determined with RED (Figure 6).

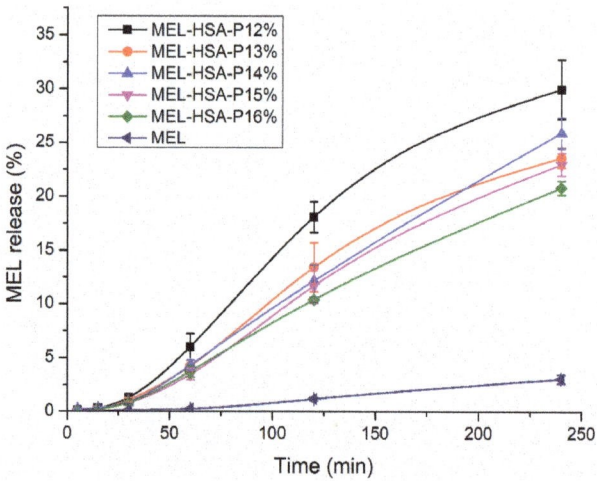

**Figure 6.** In vitro dissolution profiles of MEL-HSA-P407 formulations in comparison to starting MEL. Data is presented as means ± SD, $n = 5$.

The in vitro dissolution profiles of MEL-HSA-P407 and starting MEL were investigated in intranasal conditions (pH = 5.6). Due to the weak acidic character of MEL ($pK_a$ = 3.43 [26]) it can be found in fully ionized form in dissolution medium ($2 < \Delta pH = |pH - pK_a|$), although the dissolution profile of pure MEL shows only a slight increase. In the case of formulations, a significantly increased dissolution was observed compared to pure MEL (**, $p < 0.01$), due to the nano size and increased specific surface area of MEL-HSA nanoparticles and the solubilizing effect of Tween. The dissolution profiles of the formulations clearly demonstrate the effect of polymer on drug release. When increasing the concentration of P407 in the formulation, the dissolution of MEL was slower, which can be explained by the hindered liberation of MEL through the more viscous gel structure. Interestingly, formulations containing P407 in a lower concentration (12–13% $w/w$) followed Hixon-Crowell kinetics, which is presumably the less effective anti-aggregation effect due to the reduced polymer concentration; but in higher concentrations (14–16% $w/w$) zero-order kinetics dominated (Table 3) [35]. The best fit of kinetic data is presented in Figure S2. Similar types of effect of P407 gel on the release behavior of insulin [36], paclitaxel [37], ceftiofur [38] and recombinant hirudin [39] have also been observed, in which the mode of drug release followed zero order.

### 3.2.5. In Vitro BBB Permeability

In the case of nasal administration, it should be taken into account that a fraction of the drug can be absorbed into the systemic circulation, from where it can only reach the brain if it is able to pass the BBB. It has been reported that NSAIDs have low disposition in the CNS via systemic circulation [40]. To investigate this formulation ability, the brain lipid-specific PAMPA permeability assay (PAMPA-BBB) is suitable. The PAMPA-BBB results of MEL-HSA formulations containing P407 in various concentrations in comparison to pure MEL are shown in Figure 7. Each P407 containing formulation showed significantly higher flux compared to pure MEL (**, $p < 0.01$), which can be explained by the enhanced solubility of MEL due to the solubilizing effect of HSA and P407. Moreover, in the case of 14% $w/w$ P407 the flux was by far the highest among all of the formulations (**, $p < 0.01$). This phenomenon can be explained by the adequate balance of the resultant effect of nanoparticle characteristics and drug release kinetics. Formulations containing P407 in lower concentrations (12–13%) followed Hixon-Crowell kinetics, assuming a lower sustained saturation of drug, whereas the formulations containing P407 in higher concentrations (14–16%) followed zero order kinetics, indicating a faster drug release. From these zero-order kinetics, the following compositions MEL-HSA-P14% had the highest rate constant (0.368 µg min$^{-1}$), which can be rationalized as the smaller Z-average resulting in a higher specific surface area; therefore, the higher dissolution rate ensures an increased gradient between donor and acceptor phases promoting permeation. In case of lower polymer concentration (12–13%) the effect of different drug release kinetics is negligible, as the remarkable Z-average difference of gel-embedded nanoparticles has a dominant influence on concentration in the donor phase.

Table 3. Obtained kinetic parameters of in situ thermogelling nasal formulations.

| Kinetic Model | Kinetic Parameters | MEL-HSA-P12% | MEL-HSA-P13% | MEL-HSA-P14% | MEL-HSA-P15% | MEL-HSA-P16% |
|---|---|---|---|---|---|---|
| Zero order | $k_0$ (µg min$^{-1}$) | 0.342 | 0.293 | 0.368 | 0.31 | 0.258 |
|  | $R^2$ | 0.9265 | 0.9251 | 0.9904 | 0.9968 | 0.9976 |
|  | $t_{0.5}$ (min) | 342.31 | 292.61 | 357.98 | 310.02 | 257.76 |
| First order | $k_1 \times 10^{-3}$ (min$^{-1}$) | 1.487 | 1.126 | 1.254 | 1.092 | 0.974 |
|  | $R^2$ | 0.9584 | 0.9586 | 0.9927 | 0.9723 | 0.9972 |
|  | $t_{0.5}$ (min) | 466.15 | 615.43 | 552.71 | 634.49 | 711.49 |
| Higuchi model | $k_H$ (µg min$^{-1/2}$) | 30.58 | 84.75 | 81.47 | 90.67 | 62.43 |
|  | $R^2$ | 0.7954 | 0.7855 | 0.8708 | 0.8883 | 0.8684 |
|  | $t_{0.5}$ (min) | 427.58 | 718.23 | 663.67 | 822.44 | 389.75 |
| Korshmeyer-Peppas model | $k_{K-P} \times 10^{-2}$ (min$^{-n}$) | 9.427 | 5.684 | 2.998 | 3.118 | 3.292 |
|  | n | 1.05 | 1.11 | 1.23 | 1.21 | 1.17 |
|  | $R^2$ | 0.6105 | 0.5516 | 0.7221 | 0.8396 | 0.7453 |
|  | $t_{0.5}$ (min) | 1043.99 | 1618.39 | 2047.18 | 1740.98 | 1848.54 |
| Hixon-Crowell model | $k_{H-C}$ (µg$^{1/3}$ min$^{-1}$) | 0.01 | 0.0046 | 0.0062 | 0.0043 | 0.0029 |
|  | $R^2$ | 0.9838 | 0.987 | 0.9877 | 0.9863 | 0.9974 |
|  | $t_{0.5}$ (min) | 1610.35 | 2055.94 | 1950.68 | 2178.88 | 2466.87 |
| Best fit |  | Hixon-Crowell model | Hixon-Crowell model | Zero order | Zero order | Zero order |

Summing up, and based on the rheological, muco-adhesion, drug release and permeability studies, the 14% $w/w$ P407 containing formulation (MEL-HSA-P14%) was considered as the optimized formulation from a therapeutic point of view. MEL-HSA-P14% forms a weak but mucoadhesive gel structure at 32 °C within 3 min which allows enhanced permeability of MEL through blood–brain barrier-specific lipids. Therefore, in the cell line studies, we decided to investigate that composition further.

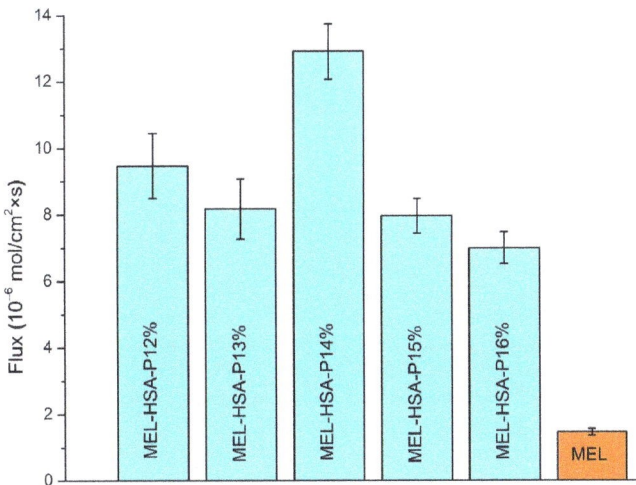

Figure 7. Fluxes in PAMPA-BBB permeability study of MEL-HSA-P407 formulations compared to starting MEL. Data is presented as means ± SD, $n = 6$.

## 3.3. Evaluation of Cell Line Studies

### 3.3.1. Cell Viability Assay

Impedance measurement as a sensitive method to detect alteration in cellular viability did not show cell damage after a 1-h treatment with MEL-HSA-P14% formulation or its components (Figure 8). As a comparison, the reference compound Triton X-100 detergent caused cell death, as reflected by the decrease in impedance.

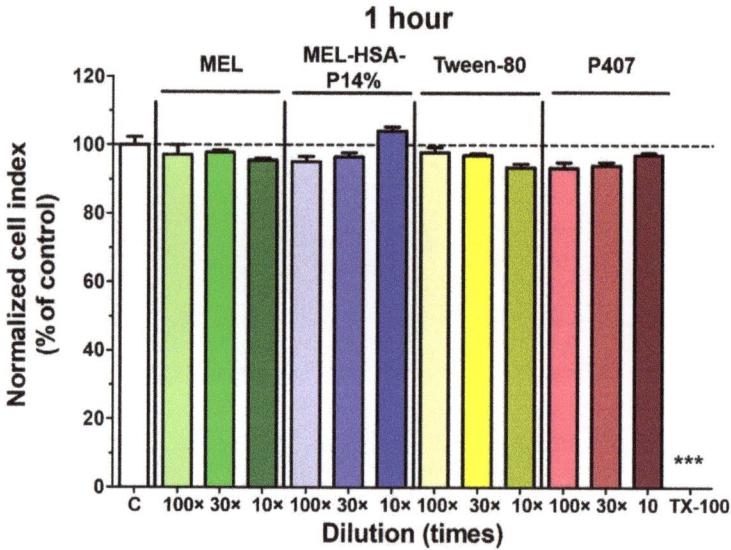

**Figure 8.** Cell viability of RPMI 2650 nasal epithelial cells after a 1-h treatment with MEL, MEL-HSA-P14% formulation, or with their components, measured by impedance. The values are presented as a percentage of the control group (means ± SD, $n$ = 6–12). Statistical analysis: ANOVA and Dunett's test. *** $p < 0.01$, compared to the control group. TX-100, Triton X-100 detergent.

### 3.3.2. MEL Permeability across the Culture Model of the Nasal Mucosa Barrier

The permeability of MEL was tested on the nasal epithelial and vascular endothelial cell co-culture model (Figure 9). After a 1-h treatment MEL in MEL-HSA-P14% showed significantly higher (four-fold) $P_{app}$ value compared with MEL suspension (MEL) (Figure 9). This result is in agreement with our previous finding using nanonized MEL in nasal formulation in the human RPMI 2650 nasal epithelial cell model [27] and also with results of PAMPA-BBB in the present study.

We found adequate TEER and low permeability values for paracellular markers indicating a good barrier property of the nasal mucosa co-culture model (Figure 10). Both the TEER and $P_{app}$ values were better than in the mono-culture model we described earlier [27]. The TEER values of the co-culture model remained at the level of the control group after a 1-h treatment with MEL-HSA-P14%, indicating that it did not damage the barrier function of the model (Figure 10A). MEL increased TEER and both treatments decreased $P_{app}$ values for the two hydrophilic paracellular marker molecules, dextran and albumin (Figure 10B). This result suggests that the anti-inflammatory MEL may have a beneficial effect on the nasal barrier either alone or in formulation.

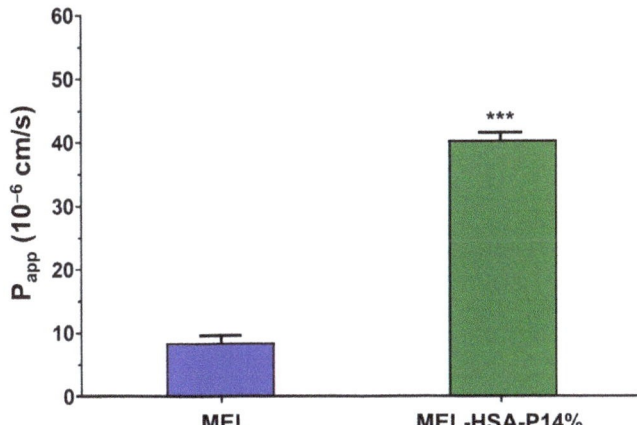

**Figure 9.** Permeability of MEL (2 mg/mL in all samples) and MEL-HSA-P14% nano-formulation across a co-culture model of human RPMI 2650 nasal epithelial cells and vascular endothelial cells (1-h assay). Values are presented as means ± SD, $n$ = 3. *** $p < 0.001$ significantly different from MEL control.

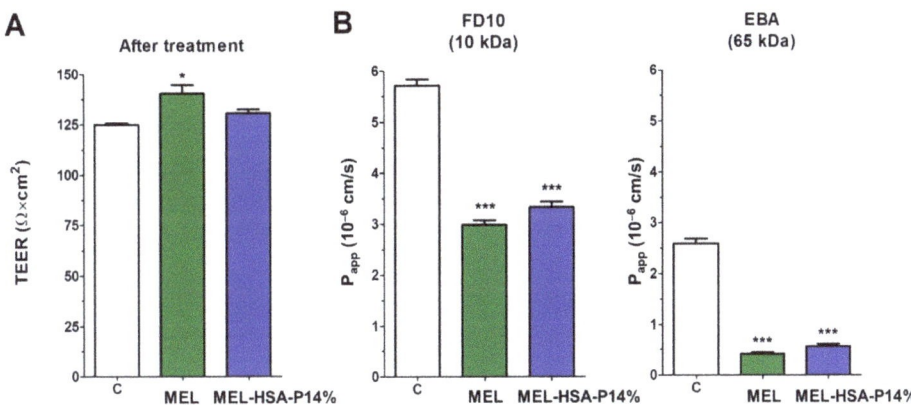

**Figure 10.** Transepithelial electrical resistance (TEER) of the co-culture model after a 1-h treatment with MEL and MEL-HSA-P14% (**A**). Values for paracellular permeability markers fluorescein-labeled dextran (FD10) and Evans blue-labeled albumin (EBA) after a 1-h treatment with MEL and the nano-formulation (**B**). Values are presented as means ± SD, $n$ = 3. C: control; MEL; MEL-HSA-P14%. * $p < 0.05$; *** $p < 0.001$ significantly different from control.

### 3.3.3. Immunohistochemistry

The staining pattern of the junctional linker proteins ZO-1 and β-catenin on human RPMI 2650 nasal epithelial cells in the co-culture model was typical for epithelial barriers. The cell shape was cobblestone, and the junctional proteins were visible in a belt-like manner at the cell borders (Figure 11), in concordance with our previous results [27]. We found no change in the staining pattern after the 1-h treatments as compared to the control group (Figure 11) indicating that the formulation did not damage the barrier model.

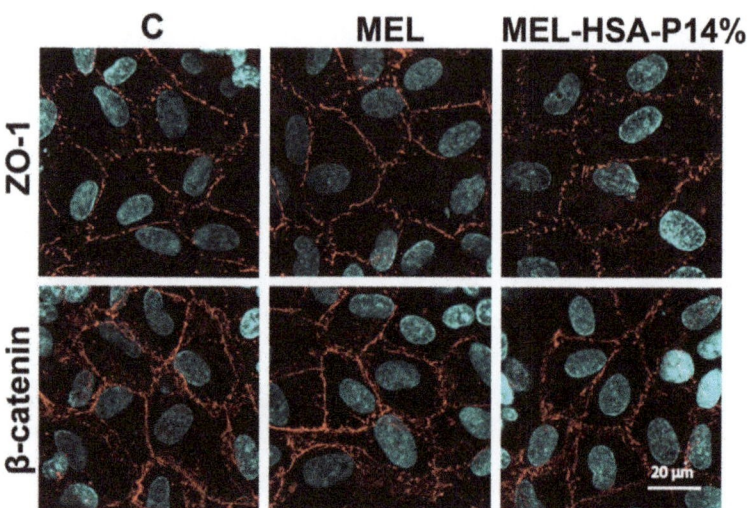

**Figure 11.** Immunostaining for junctional linker proteins ZO-1 and β-catenin on human RPMI 2650 nasal epithelial cell layers following a 1-h treatment with MEL and MEL-HSA-P14%. The control group (C) received only medium. Red: junctional proteins; blue: cell nuclei. Scale bar: 20 μm.

## 4. Discussion

A series of NSAIDs, including MEL, show significant potential in Alzheimer's disease although their administration through conventional routes results in low deposition in the CNS due to severe elimination mechanisms and low capability of by-passing the BBB. Therefore, the application of a suitable nano carrier can be promising in increasing, their bioavailability [40]. HSA, as a versatile, biodegradable nano-carrier is an auspicious tool for intranasal delivery of NSAIDs, as several studies have already proved the successful nose-to-brain delivery of candidates like flurbiprofen [41] or MEL [13] itself. Although the exact pathway of HSA through nose-to-brain delivery is still not clearly demonstrated, experimental results showed that isotope labelled albumin could reach the brain after nasal administration [42].

The intranasal applicability of MEL-HSA nanoparticles is limited by mucociliary clearance, therefore application of the in situ gelling mucoadhesive polymer P407 can be advantageous, since the above mentioned LCST, PPO chains become less soluble resulting in micelle formation and entanglements followed by gelation of the sol form [43,44]. Several studies have demonstrated that poloxamer-based in situ gelling formulations have been successfully applied in numerous therapeutic fields especially among neurological diseases such as in the therapy of migraine [45], Parkinson's syndrome [46], Alzheimer's disease [47–49] and depression [50]. The basic ingredient of the therapeutic effectiveness of in situ thermo-gelling nasal formulations is their advantageous nature, which besides improving the pharmacokinetic profile of the administered drug also increases patients' compliance [51]. Their sol form allows accurate dosing e.g., by the use of a metered dose nasal actuator system and after gelling, post-nasal drip into the throat can be reduced, therefore minimizing any undesired taste problem and loss of drug from the nasal cavity. The gel form ensures increased residence time of the formulation on nasal mucosa, exhibiting sustained release and supporting drug absorption. Moreover, gels can be used alongside demulcents or emollients which may not be suitable for solutions, suspensions or even powder dosage forms, in order to reduce the irritation potential.

Besides these mucoadhesive properties, particle characteristics play an important role in the applicability of formulations through the nasal administration route. It has been reported that nanoparticles with an average hydrodynamic diameter of 20–200 nm are the most suitable for nose-to-brain transport [52]. The PdI also plays a very important role in drug pharmacokinetics since a lower value indicates an enhanced probability of a more uniform absorption through the nasal mucosa, while a higher value may lead to pharmacokinetic irregularity and variability in the therapeutic outcome [53]. It is usually recommended that the PdI should be below 0.5. The zeta potential, which is dependent on both the surface charge of the particles and the ionic strength of the medium used for particle dispersion, is recommended to have a slightly negative or even positive surface charge, as this enhances nasal absorption as the nasal mucosa itself is negatively charged. Moreover, increased encapsulation efficacy and drug loading of nanoparticles is required to ensure proper dosing restricted by lower administration volume, up to a maximum of 200 µL. Our albumin nanoparticle gelling formulations containing 12–14% $w/w$ P407 met these requirements and became suitable for intranasal administration after thermo-gelling; moreover, these parameters were more promising than in case of flurbiprofen-albumin nanoparticles, which were already successfully administered intranasally, directly to the brain, by Wong et al. [41].

Besides the particle characteristics of albumin nano-particles, the physiological properties of the nasal cavity should be also taken into account. The pH of the formulations was in the range of the human nasal mucosa's physiologic pH range (4.62 to 7.00) supporting normal ciliary function and reducing the chance of damaging the barrier integrity of the nasal epithelial cells [54]. In this slightly acidic environment, lysozyme, the natural antimicrobial agent in the nose, is effective in the prevention of the growth of pathogenic bacteria in the nasal passage; therefore, preservative agents are negligible, which is usually incompatible with the applied polymer. Nasal preparations are normally isotonic (about 290 mOsmol/L), which is also best tolerated, but sometimes a deviation from isotonicity may be advantageous. Especially, hypotonic solutions can facilitate drug absorption through interfering with cilia movement [55]. Based on these perspectives, our optimized formulation MEL-HSA-P14% met all the listed requirements, which suggests suitable therapeutic applicability, which can be corroborated with the experimental results of Giuliano et al., according to which prolonged delivery of the drug for up to 5 h from P407 hydrogel was achieved via increasing the permeation profile of the compound, as measured through ex vivo porcine nasal mucosa [56].

## 5. Conclusions

In summary we optimized an in situ thermo-gelling MEL-HSA-P407 formulation, which can be administered in liquid state into the nostril. Temperature dependent sol-gel transition on the mucosa, resulting in increased resistance against mucoliciary clearance, can estimate improved drug absorption. Based on rheological, muco-adhesion, drug release and permeability studies, MEL-HSA-P14% was considered as the optimized formulation. Cell line studies showed no cell damage after a 1-h treatment with MEL-HSA-P14% on RPMI 2650 human endothelial cells; moreover, enhanced permeation (four-fold) of MEL from MEL-HSA-P14% was observed in comparison to MEL suspension. Overall, MEL-HSA-P14% is promising in terms of overcoming the challenges of nasal drug delivery by increasing resistance against mucociliary clearance, and therefore can improve nasal drug absorption.

**Supplementary Materials:** The following are available online at https://www.mdpi.com/article/10.3390/pharmaceutics13050646/s1, Figure S1: Primary data for the LCST and gelling time measurements, Figure S2. Drug release kinetics of in situ gelling formulations.

**Author Contributions:** Conceptualization, G.K., P.S.-R. and I.C.; methodology, G.K., B.S., M.B.-S., S.V., M.A.D. and I.C.; software, G.K., B.S., M.B.-S., G.T.B., S.V. and I.G.; validation, P.S.-R., G.T.B., M.A.D. and I.C.; formal analysis, P.S.-R., M.A.D. and I.C.; investigation, G.K., B.S., M.B.-S., G.T.B., S.V. and I.G.; resources, B.V. and I.C.; data curation, G.K. and B.S.; writing—original draft preparation, G.K., B.S., M.B.-S. and S.V.; writing—review and editing, P.S.-R., M.A.D. and I.C.; visualization, G.K., B.S. and I.G.; supervision, P.S.-R. and I.C.; project administration, G.K.; funding acquisition, G.K. and B.V. All authors have read and agreed to the published version of the manuscript.

**Funding:** This research received no external funding.

**Institutional Review Board Statement:** Not applicable.

**Informed Consent Statement:** Not applicable.

**Data Availability Statement:** The data presented in this study are available on request from the corresponding author.

**Acknowledgments:** The authors want to express their acknowledgment to the supporter. This work was supported by the ÚNKP-20-4-SZTE-327 the New National Excellence Program of the Ministry of Innovation and Technology from the source of the National Research, Development.

**Conflicts of Interest:** Egis Pharmaceuticals Plc. had no role in the design of the study; in the collection, analyses, or interpretation of data; in the writing of the manuscript, or in the decision to publish the results.

## References

1. Hoogenboezem, E.N.; Duvall, C.L. Harnessing albumin as a carrier for cancer therapies. *Adv. Drug Deliv. Rev.* **2018**, *130*, 73–89. [CrossRef] [PubMed]
2. Goverdhan, P.; Sravanthi, A.; Mamatha, T. Neuroprotective effects of Meloxicam and Selegiline in scopolamine-induced cognitive impairment and oxidative stress. *Int. J. Alzheimers Dis.* **2012**, *2012*. [CrossRef] [PubMed]
3. Cimen, M.Y.B.; Cimen, Ö.B.; Eskandari, G.; Sahin, G.; Erdoğan, C.; Atik, U. In vivo effects of meloxicam, celecoxib, and ibuprofen on free radical metabolism in human erythrocytes. *Drug Chem. Toxicol.* **2003**, *26*, 169–176. [CrossRef]
4. Ianiski, F.R.; Alves, C.B.; Ferreira, C.F.; Rech, V.C.; Savegnago, L.; Wilhelm, E.A.; Luchese, C. Meloxicam-loaded nanocapsules as an alternative to improve memory decline in an Alzheimer's disease model in mice: Involvement of Na+, K+-ATPase. *Metab. Brain Dis.* **2016**, *31*, 793–802. [CrossRef]
5. Szabó-Révész, P. Modifying the physicochemical properties of NSAIDs for nasal and pulmonary administration. *Drug Discov. Today Technol.* **2018**, *27*, 87–93. [CrossRef] [PubMed]
6. Merkus, F.W.H.M.; van den Berg, M.P. Can nasal drug delivery bypass the blood-brain barrier? *Drugs R D* **2007**, *8*, 133–144. [CrossRef]
7. van Hoesen, G.W.; Hyman, B.T.; Damasio, A.R. Entorhinal cortex pathology in Alzheimer's disease. *Hippocampus* **1991**, *1*, 1–8. [CrossRef]
8. Mistry, A.; Stolnik, S.; Illum, L. Nanoparticles for direct nose-to-brain delivery of drugs. *Int. J. Pharm.* **2009**, *379*, 146–157. [CrossRef]
9. Agrawal, M.; Saraf, S.; Saraf, S.; Antimisiaris, S.G.; Chougule, M.B.; Shoyele, S.A.; Alexander, A. Nose-to-brain drug delivery: An update on clinical challenges and progress towards approval of anti-Alzheimer drugs. *J. Control. Release* **2018**, *281*, 139–177. [CrossRef]
10. Lalatsa, A.; Schatzlein, A.G.; Uchegbu, I.F. Strategies to deliver peptide drugs to the brain. *Mol. Pharm.* **2014**, *11*, 1081–1093. [CrossRef]
11. Novakova, I.; Subileau, E.A.; Toegel, S.; Gruber, D.; Lachmann, B.; Urban, E.; Chesne, C.; Noe, C.R.; Neuhaus, W. Transport rankings of non-steroidal antiinflammatory drugs across blood-brain barrier in vitro models. *PLoS ONE* **2014**, *9*, 1–14. [CrossRef]
12. Sipos, B.; Szabó-Révész, P.; Csóka, I.; Pallagi, E.; Dobó, D.G.; Bélteky, P.; Kónya, Z.; Deák, Á.; Janovák, L.; Katona, G. Quality by design based formulation study of meloxicam-loaded polymeric micelles for intranasal administration. *Pharmaceutics* **2020**, *12*, 697. [CrossRef] [PubMed]
13. Katona, G.; Balogh, G.T.; Dargó, G.; Gáspár, R.; Márki, Á.; Ducza, E.; Sztojkov-Ivanov, A.; Tömösi, F.; Kecskeméti, G.; Janáky, T.; et al. Development of meloxicam-human serum albumin nanoparticles for nose-to-brain delivery via application of a quality by design approach. *Pharmaceutics* **2020**, *12*, 97. [CrossRef] [PubMed]
14. Tas, Ç.; Ozkan, C.K.; Savaser, A.; Ozkan, Y.; Tasdemir, U.; Altunay, H. Nasal absorption of metoclopramide from different Carbopol®981 based formulations: In vitro, ex vivo and in vivo evaluation. *Eur. J. Pharm. Biopharm.* **2006**, *64*, 246–254. [CrossRef] [PubMed]
15. Casettari, L.; Illum, L. Chitosan in nasal delivery systems for therapeutic drugs. *J. Control. Release* **2014**, *190*, 189–200. [CrossRef]
16. Mahajan, H.S.; Tyagi, V.K.; Patil, R.R.; Dusunge, S.B. Thiolated xyloglucan: Synthesis, characterization and evaluation as mucoadhesive in situ gelling agent. *Carbohydr. Polym.* **2013**, *91*, 618–625. [CrossRef]
17. Dumortier, G.; Grossiord, J.L.; Zuber, M.; Couarraze, G.; Chaumeil, J.C. Rheological study of a thermoreversible morphine gel. *Drug Dev. Ind. Pharm.* **1991**, *17*, 1255–1265. [CrossRef]
18. Dumortier, G.; Grossiord, J.L.; Agnely, F.; Chaumeil, J.C. A review of poloxamer 407 pharmaceutical and pharmacological characteristics. *Pharm. Res.* **2006**, *23*, 2709–2728. [CrossRef] [PubMed]
19. Balakrishnan, P.; Park, E.K.; Song, C.K.; Ko, H.J.; Hahn, T.W.; Song, K.W.; Cho, H.J. Carbopol-Incorporated thermoreversible gel for intranasal drug delivery. *Molecules* **2015**, *20*, 4124–4135. [CrossRef]
20. Fakhari, A.; Corcoran, M.; Schwarz, A. Thermogelling properties of purified poloxamer 407. *Heliyon* **2017**, *3*, e00390. [CrossRef]

21. Csóka, I.; Pallagi, E.; Paál, T.L. Extension of quality-by-design concept to the early development phase of pharmaceutical R&D processes. *Drug Discov. Today* **2018**, *23*, 1340–1343. [CrossRef]
22. Javed, M.N.; Alam, M.S.; Waziri, A.; Pottoo, F.H.; Yadav, A.K.; Hasnain, M.S.; Almalki, F.A. QbD Applications for the Development of Nanopharmaceutical Products. *Pharm. Qual. Des.* **2019**, 229–253. [CrossRef]
23. Li, Q.; Chen, F.; Liu, Y.; Yu, S.; Gai, X.; Ye, M.; Yang, X.; Pan, W. A novel albumin wrapped nanosuspension of meloxicam to improve inflammation-targeting effects. *Int. J. Nanomed.* **2018**, *13*, 4711–4725. [CrossRef]
24. Rather, M.A.; Amin, S.; Maqbool, M.; Bhat, Z.S.; Gupta, P.N.; Ahmad, Z. Preparation and in vitro characterization of albumin nanoparticles encapsulating an anti-tuberculosis drug-levofloxacin. *Adv. Sci. Eng. Med.* **2016**, *8*, 912–917. [CrossRef]
25. Müller, J.; Martins, A.; Csábi, J.; Fenyvesi, F.; Könczöl, Á.; Hunyadi, A.; Balogh, G.T. BBB penetration-targeting physicochemical lead selection: Ecdysteroids as chemo-sensitizers against CNS tumors. *Eur. J. Pharm. Sci.* **2017**, *96*, 571–577. [CrossRef]
26. Avdeef, A. Permeability-PAMPA. In *Absorption and Drug Development*; John Wiley & Sons: Hoboken, NJ, USA, 2012; pp. 319–498.
27. Kürti, L.; Veszelka, S.; Bocsik, A.; Ózsvári, B.; Puskás, L.G.; Kittel, Á.; Szabó-Révész, P.; Deli, M.A. Retinoic acid and hydrocortisone strengthen the barrier function of human RPMI 2650 cells, a model for nasal epithelial permeability. *Cytotechnology* **2013**, *65*, 395–406. [CrossRef] [PubMed]
28. Pedroso, D.C.S.; Tellechea, A.; Moura, L.; Fidalgo-Carvalho, I.; Duarte, J.; Carvalho, E.; Ferreira, L. Improved survival, vascular differentiation and wound healing potential of stem cells co-cultured with endothelial cells. *PLoS ONE* **2011**, *6*, 1–12. [CrossRef]
29. Cecchelli, R.; Aday, S.; Sevin, E.; Almeida, C.; Culot, M.; Dehouck, L.; Coisne, C.; Engelhardt, B.; Dehouck, M.P.; Ferreira, L. A stable and reproducible human blood-brain barrier model derived from hematopoietic stem cells. *PLoS ONE* **2014**, *9*. [CrossRef]
30. Harazin, A.; Bocsik, A.; Barna, L.; Kincses, A.; Váradi, J.; Fenyvesi, F.; Tubak, V.; Deli, M.A.; Vecsernyés, M. Protection of cultured brain endothelial cells from cytokine-induced damage by α-melanocyte stimulating hormone. *PeerJ* **2018**, *2018*, 1–22. [CrossRef] [PubMed]
31. Bocsik, A.; Gróf, I.; Kiss, L.; Ötvös, F.; Zsíros, O.; Daruka, L.; Fülöp, L.; Vastag, M.; Kittel, Á.; Imre, N.; et al. Dual action of the PN159/KLAL/MAP peptide: Increase of drug penetration across caco-2 intestinal barrier model by modulation of tight junctions and plasma membrane permeability. *Pharmaceutics* **2019**, *11*, 73. [CrossRef]
32. King, M. The role of mucus viscoelasticity in cough clearance. *Biorheology* **1987**, *24*, 589–597. [CrossRef]
33. Mayol, L.; Biondi, M.; Quaglia, F.; La Rotonda, M.I.; Fusco, S.; Borzacchiello, A.; Ambrosio, L. Injectable thermally responsive mucoadhesive gel for sustained protein delivery. In Proceedings of the 24th European Conference on Biomaterials—Annual Conference of the European Society for Biomaterials, Dublin, Ireland, 4–9 September 2011; pp. 28–33.
34. Gao, L.; Zhang, D.; Chen, M. Drug nanocrystals for the formulation of poorly soluble drugs and its application as a potential drug delivery system. *J. Nanoparticle Res.* **2008**, *10*, 845–862. [CrossRef]
35. Wójcik-Pastuszka, D.; Krzak, J.; Macikowski, B.; Berkowski, R.; Osiński, B.; Musiał, W. Evaluation of the release kinetics of a pharmacologically active substance from model intra-articular implants replacing the cruciate ligaments of the knee. *Materials* **2019**, *12*, 1202. [CrossRef] [PubMed]
36. Barichello, J.M.; Morishita, M.; Takayama, K.; Nagai, T. Absorption of insulin from Pluronic F-127 gels following subcutaneous administration in rats. *Int. J. Pharm.* **1999**, *184*, 189–198. [CrossRef]
37. Nie, S.; Hsiao, W.W.; Pan, W.; Yang, Z. Thermoreversible pluronic® F127-based hydrogel containing liposomes for the controlled delivery of paclitaxel: In vitro drug release, cell cytotoxicity, and uptake studies. *Int. J. Nanomed.* **2011**, *6*, 151–166. [CrossRef]
38. Zhang, L.; Parsons, D.L.; Navarre, C.; Kompella, U.B. Development and in-vitro evaluation of sustained release Poloxamer 407 (P407) gel formulations of ceftiofur. *J. Control. Release* **2002**, *85*, 73–81. [CrossRef]
39. Liu, Y.; Lu, W.L.; Wang, J.C.; Zhang, X.; Zhang, H.; Wang, X.Q.; Zhou, T.Y.; Zhang, Q. Controlled delivery of recombinant hirudin based on thermo-sensitive Pluronic®F127 hydrogel for subcutaneous administration: In vitro and in vivo characterization. *J. Control. Release* **2007**, *117*, 387–395. [CrossRef]
40. Biswas, G.; Kim, W.; Kim, K.T.; Cho, J.; Jeong, D.; Song, K.H.; Im, J. Synthesis of Ibuprofen Conjugated Molecular Transporter Capable of Enhanced Brain Penetration. *J. Chem.* **2017**, *2017*. [CrossRef]
41. Wong, L.R.; Ho, P.C. Role of serum albumin as a nanoparticulate carrier for nose-to-brain delivery of R-flurbiprofen: Implications for the treatment of Alzheimer's disease. *J. Pharm. Pharmacol.* **2018**, *70*, 59–69. [CrossRef] [PubMed]
42. Falcone, J.A.; Salameh, T.S.; Yi, X.; Cordy, B.J.; Mortell, W.G.; Kabanov, A.V.; Banks, W.A. Intranasal administration as a route for drug delivery to the brain: Evidence for a unique pathway for albumin. *J. Pharmacol. Exp. Ther.* **2014**, *351*, 54–60. [CrossRef]
43. Taylor, M.; Tomlins, P.; Sahota, T. Thermoresponsive Gels. *Gels* **2017**, *3*, 4. [CrossRef]
44. Zahir-Jouzdani, F.; Wolf, J.D.; Atyabi, F.; Bernkop-Schnürch, A. In situ gelling and mucoadhesive polymers: Why do they need each other? *Expert Opin. Drug Deliv.* **2018**, *15*, 1007–1019. [CrossRef]
45. Shelke, S.; Shahi, S.; Jalalpure, S.; Dhamecha, D.; Shengule, S. Formulation and evaluation of thermoreversible mucoadhesive in-situ gel for intranasal delivery of naratriptan hydrochloride. *J. Drug Deliv. Sci. Technol.* **2015**, *29*, 238–244. [CrossRef]
46. Ravi, P.R.; Aditya, N.; Patil, S.; Cherian, L. Nasal in-situ gels for delivery of rasagiline mesylate: Improvement in bioavailability and brain localization. *Drug Deliv.* **2015**, *22*, 903–910. [CrossRef]
47. Chen, X.; Zhi, F.; Jia, X.; Zhang, X.; Ambardekar, R.; Meng, Z.; Paradkar, A.R.; Hu, Y.; Yang, Y. Enhanced brain targeting of curcumin by intranasal administration of a thermosensitive poloxamer hydrogel. *J. Pharm. Pharmacol.* **2013**, *65*, 807–816. [CrossRef] [PubMed]

48. Wang, Y.; Jiang, S.; Wang, H.; Bie, H. A mucoadhesive, thermoreversible in situ nasal gel of geniposide for neurodegenerative diseases. *PLoS ONE* **2017**, *12*, e0189478. [CrossRef]
49. Salatin, S.; Barar, J.; Barzegar-Jalali, M.; Adibkia, K.; Jelvehgari, M. Thermosensitive in situ nanocomposite of rivastigmine hydrogen tartrate as an intranasal delivery system: Development, characterization, ex vivo permeation and cellular studies. *Colloids Surf. B* **2017**, *159*, 629–638. [CrossRef]
50. Pathan, I.B.; More, B. Formulation and characterization of intra nasal delivery of nortriptyline hydrochloride thermoreversible gelling system in treatment of depression. *Acta Pharm. Sci.* **2017**, *55*, 35–44. [CrossRef]
51. Singh, K.; HariKumar, S.L. Injectable in-situ gelling controlled release drug delivery system. *Int. J. Drug Dev. Res.* **2012**, *4*, 56–69.
52. Mistry, A.; Stolnik, S.; Illum, L. Nose-to-Brain Delivery: Investigation of the Transport of Nanoparticles with Different Surface Characteristics and Sizes in Excised Porcine Olfactory Epithelium. *Mol. Pharm.* **2015**, *12*, 2755–2766. [CrossRef]
53. Patel, R.B.; Patel, M.R.; Bhatt, K.K.; Patel, B.G.; Gaikwad, R.V. Evaluation of brain targeting efficiency of intranasal microemulsion containing olanzapine: Pharmacodynamic and pharmacokinetic consideration. *Drug Deliv.* **2016**, *23*, 307–315. [CrossRef] [PubMed]
54. Kapoor, M.; Cloyd, J.C.; Siegel, R.A. A review of intranasal formulations for the treatment of seizure emergencies. *J. Control. Release* **2016**, *237*, 147–159. [CrossRef] [PubMed]
55. Hong, S.S.; Oh, K.T.; Choi, H.G.; Lim, S.J. Liposomal formulations for nose-to-brain delivery: Recent advances and future perspectives. *Pharmaceutics* **2019**, *11*, 540. [CrossRef] [PubMed]
56. Giuliano, E.; Paolino, D.; Fresta, M.; Cosco, D. Mucosal applications of poloxamer 407-based hydrogels: An overview. *Pharmaceutics* **2018**, *10*, 159. [CrossRef] [PubMed]

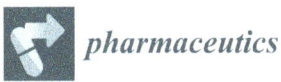

Article

# The Therapeutic Effect of Human Serum Albumin Dimer-Doxorubicin Complex against Human Pancreatic Tumors

Ryo Kinoshita [1,2], Yu Ishima [1,*], Victor T. G. Chuang [3], Hiroshi Watanabe [2], Taro Shimizu [1], Hidenori Ando [1], Keiichiro Okuhira [4], Masaki Otagiri [5], Tatsuhiro Ishida [1] and Toru Maruyama [2,*]

[1] Department of Pharmacokinetics and Biopharmaceutics, Institute of Biomedical Sciences, Tokushima University, 1-78-1 Sho-machi, Tokushima 770-8505, Japan; kinoshita.ryo.xu@daiichisankyo.co.jp (R.K.); shimizu.tarou@tokushima-u.ac.jp (T.S.); h.ando@tokushima-u.ac.jp (H.A.); ishida@tokushima-u.ac.jp (T.I.)
[2] Department of Biopharmaceutics, Graduate School of Pharmaceutical Sciences, Kumamoto University, 5-1 Oe-honmachi, Kumamoto 862-0973, Japan; hnabe@kumamoto-u.ac.jp
[3] Faculty of Health Sciences, Curtin Medical School, Curtin University, Perth 6845, Australia; victorchuang@hotmail.com
[4] Department of Environment and Health Sciences, Osaka Medical and Pharmaceutical University, 4-20-1 Nasahara, Takatsuki 569-1094, Japan; okuhira@gly.oups.ac.jp
[5] Faculty of Pharmaceutical Sciences, Sojo University, 4-22-1 Ikeda, Kumamoto 860-0082, Japan; otagirim@ph.sojo-u.ac.jp
* Correspondence: ishima.yuu@tokushima-u.ac.jp (Y.I.); tomaru@gpo.kumamoto-u.ac.jp (T.M.); Tel.: +81-88-633-7259 (Y.I.); +81-96-371-4153 (T.M.)

**Abstract:** Human serum albumin (HSA) is a versatile drug carrier with active tumor targeting capacity for an antitumor drug delivery system. Nanoparticle albumin-bound (nab)-technology, such as nab-paclitaxel (Abraxane®), has attracted significant interest in drug delivery research. Recently, we demonstrated that HSA dimer (HSA-d) possesses a higher tumor distribution than HSA monomer (HSA-m). Therefore, HSA-d is more suitable as a drug carrier for antitumor therapy and can improve nab technology. This study investigated the efficacy of HSA-d-doxorubicin (HSA-d-DOX) as next-generation nab technology for tumor treatment. DOX conjugated to HSA-d via a tunable pH-sensitive linker for the controlled release of DOX. Lyophilization did not affect the particle size of HSA-d-DOX or the release of DOX. HSA-d-DOX showed significantly higher cytotoxicity than HSA-m-DOX in vitro. In the SUIzo Tumor-2 (SUIT2) human pancreatic tumor subcutaneous inoculation model, HSA-d-DOX could significantly inhibit tumor growth without causing serious side effects, as compared to the HSA binding DOX prodrug, which utilized endogenous HSA as a nano-drug delivery system (DDS) carrier. These results indicate that HSA-d could function as a natural solubilizer of insoluble drugs and an active targeting carrier in intractable tumors with low vascular permeability, such as pancreatic tumors. In conclusion, HSA-d can be an effective drug carrier for the antitumor drug delivery system against human pancreatic tumors.

**Keywords:** human serum albumin; dimerization; doxorubicin; enhanced permeability and retention effect; antitumor

## 1. Introduction

Pancreatic tumors remain one of the most difficult human malignancies to be treated, having the worst mortality rate and the lowest overall survival rate among all tumors. The overall survival rate for pancreatic tumors is extremely low despite rapid advances in tumor diagnosis and treatment. The prognosis of pancreatic tumors is abysmal, with 5-year survival less than 5%. Less than 10% of pancreatic tumor patients are presented with resectable disease or are suitable for potentially curative surgery. Aggressive metastasis often occurs after the operation, which is highly resistant to conventional chemotherapy and radiation therapy. Chemotherapy is the only option in metastatic pancreatic tumor treatment, but sadly, most of the time, chemotherapy is purely palliative. Despite gemcitabine being the standard first-line treatment, gemcitabine-based combination chemotherapy showed either marginal or no improvement in survival for advanced pancreatic tumors. Pancreatic tumor patients with locally advanced disease have 6–10 months of median survival, and patients with metastatic disease only have 3–6 months of median survival. Hence, novel strategies to treat pancreatic tumors are urgently needed.

Effective drug delivery in pancreatic tumor treatment remains a major challenge. Improving the specificity and stability of the delivered chemotherapeutic agent using ligand or antibody-directed delivery represents a significant problem. Recent advances in antibody-drug conjugate (ADC) technology have led to the development of cancer-stroma targeting (CAST) therapy as a novel antitumor drug delivery system, especially for refractory, stromal-rich tumors, such as pancreatic tumors [1]. This CAST strategy is developed based on the aggressiveness of the tumor; the more aggressive, the greater the deposition of insoluble fibrin in tumor tissue. Peptide–drug conjugates (PDC) have recently gained significant attention as tools for developing specific delivery systems for pancreatic tumors [2]. Using a human pancreatic ductal adenocarcinoma cell line, PDC was sufficiently incorporated by the cells within 2 h, whereas ADC was not visible in the cell after 2 h. In addition, an in vivo study using tumor-bearing mice indicated that PDCs incorporating this peptide might exert potent antitumor effects without missing the target cells. PDC was efficiently and selectively incorporated into target pancreatic tumor lesions, including primary and metastatic sites. Conversely, current ADCs, such as anti-HER2 and anti-EGFR antibodies, are limited to targeting specific antigen-positive tumor cells.

Doxorubicin (DOX) is an anthracycline antibiotic used as a chemotherapeutic agent to treat a wide variety of tumors, including lymphoma, lung tumor, stomach tumor, breast tumor, and osteosarcoma [3,4]. Cardiotoxicity is a major clinical adverse reaction of DOX upon cumulative dosing. Liposome-based drug delivery systems are known to facilitate targeting of specific tumor treatment agents, improve pharmacokinetics, reduce side effects, and potentially increase tumor uptake for pancreatic tumor therapy. Liposomal DOX has been reported to alleviate cardiotoxicity with improved antitumor activity. In particular, pegylated liposomal DOX has shown significant pharmacologic advantages and an added clinical value over DOX. Doxil®, a PEGylated liposome preparation for passive targeting aimed at reducing the side effects of DOX, and various DOX-loaded nano-drug delivery system (DDS) preparations [5,6], including the micellar preparation NK911, have been developed [7].

Human serum albumin (HSA) has gained popularity as a nano-drug delivery carrier. Aldoxorubicin (INNO-206), an HSA binding prodrug of DOX, has been developed to increase tumor targeting efficiency. INNO-206 binds to the SH group of Cys-34 of endogenous HSA via the maleimide group in the linker structure attached to DOX [8,9]. Consequently, HSA-conjugated INNO-206 exhibits improved blood retention compared with free DOX. Recent clinical trials examined the efficacy of INNO-206 in treating soft tissue sarcoma and AIDS-related Kaposi's sarcoma and preclinical trials for solid tumors, such as pancreatic tumors [10]. Administered at the equivalent dose, INNO-206 is safer than free DOX due to its improved kinetics and antitumor activity [9]. This evidence highlights the need for further attempts to increase DOX potency, exploring the potential of a novel drug carrier with higher drug accumulation in pancreatic tumors.

The current nanoparticle albumin-bound (nab)-technology, such as nab-paclitaxel, uses HSA as a natural solubilizer of insoluble drugs, not as a tumor-targeting carrier [11]. After intravenous administration, nab-paclitaxel (Abraxane®) dispersed rapidly and behaved similarly to HSA monomer in the general circulation. Consequently, nab-paclitaxel almost lost its tumor-targeting ability via the enhanced permeability and retention (EPR) effect [12]. Kim's group developed anti-PD-L1 antibody conjugated nab technology as a novel combination of chemotherapeutic and immune-therapeutic antitumor approaches to improve its tumor-targeting ability. This approach demonstrated that the pH-responsive drug release and PD-L1 targeting does enhance the tumor selectivity [13]. Furthermore, insulin-like growth factor 1 receptor inhibitors enhance uptake and efficacy of nab-PTX by mimicking glucose deprivation and promoting macropinocytosis via AMPK, a nutrient sensor in cells. This suggests that nanoparticulate albumin-bound drug efficacy can be therapeutically improved by reprogramming nutrient signaling and enhancing macropinocytosis in tumor cells [14].

Previously, we demonstrated that HSA dimers (HSA-d) have higher blood circulation activity and lower vascular permeability than HSA monomers (HSA-m) [15]. Interestingly, HSA-d possesses a higher tumor distribution than HSA-m [16,17], so S-nitrosated HSA-d could enhance the EPR effect via an endogenous albumin transport (EAT) system [18]. Tumor cells actively "EAT" (consume) endogenous HSA as a source of amino acids to continue cell proliferation via several HSA receptors, such as gp60 or SPARC [19]. In particular, the EAT system should be activated in order to survive in a hypoxic region with inferior blood vessel density [20]. Therefore, EAT system targeting is a promising DDS strategy using HSA-d for refractory tumor therapy.

Herein, we designed the HSA-d-doxorubicin (HSA-d-DOX) as a next-generation nab technology therapeutic agent with both properties: as a natural solubilizer of insoluble drugs and active targeting capacity. DOX was conjugated to HSA-d via a tunable pH-sensitive linker for the controlled release of DOX. pH-responsive hydrazone bonds between DOX and the linker maintain the binding in normal tissues and blood circulation (pH 7.4–7.6). The bond is cleaved only in an acidic environment, such as tumor tissues, so it becomes possible to release DOX selectively. The antitumor activity of HSA-d-DOX was evaluated in vitro and in vivo using the SUIzo Tumor-2 (SUIT2) human pancreatic tumor model as a refractory tumor.

## 2. Materials and Methods

### 2.1. Materials

DOX was purchased from Wako Pure Chemical Industries, Ltd. (Osaka, Japan). 2-Iminothiolane hydrochloride and Amicon Ultra (4 and 15) 10 kDa were purchased from Merck KGaA (Darmstadt, Germany). INNO-206 was purchased from ChemScene (Monmouth Junction, NJ, USA). Cell Counting Kit-8 (CCK-8) was obtained from Dojindo Molecular Technologies (Kumamoto, Japan). Other chemicals were of the best commercially available grades, and all solutions were made using deionized water.

### 2.2. Expression and Purification of HSA-m and HSA-d

Recombinant HSA-m and HSA-d were expressed by *Pichia pastoris* (*P. pastoris*) [21] and defatted [22]. Briefly, these constructed plasmids (pPIC9-HSA-m and pPIC9-HSA-d) were transferred to XL10-Gold *Escherichia coli* (*E. coli*). *P. pastoris* GS115 his4 was transformed with SalI-digested pPIC9-HSA-m or pPIC9-HSA-d by electroporation. The protocol used to express the HSAs was a modification of a previously published protocol [23]. Single colonies of *P. pastoris* were grown for 48 h at 30 °C in buffered minimal glycerol-complex medium until an $A_{600}$ value of 2–4 was obtained. Cells were then harvested by centrifugation at 3000× g, and cell pellets were washed extensively and resuspended in buffered minimal methanol-complex medium to an approximate $A_{600}$ value of 10–15. Then, the baffled flasks were shaken for 96 h at 30 °C, with a daily addition of methanol at a final concentration of 1% to maintain the induction conditions. The recombinant HSAs were purified after 96 h of induction [24]. Preparation of the HSAs was first subjected to chromatography with the Blue Sepharose 6 Fast Flow column (Cytiva, Tokyo, Japan) equilibrated with 200 mM sodium acetate buffer (pH 5.5) after dialysis with the same buffer. The eluted HSAs were deionized and defatted via charcoal treatment, freeze-dried, and then stored at −80 °C until used.

### 2.3. Cells and Animals

Human pancreatic tumor transferred luciferase gene SUIzo Tumor-2 (SUIT2) cells were cultured in DMEM + 10% fetal bovine serum with antibiotics (100 units penicillin/mL, and

100 µg streptomycin/mL). The cells were passaged when approximately 90% confluence was reached. BALB/c nu/nu mice (male, 5 to 6 weeks old, Japan SLC Inc., Shizuoka, Japan) was used as SUIT2-bearing mice. SUIT2 bearing mice were prepared by subcutaneous transplantation with $1 \times 10^6$ cells into the back of the mice [17]. All animal experiments were carried out according to the Laboratory Protocol for Animal Handling T2019-47 (1 August 2019) of Tokushima University.

### 2.4. Preparation of HSA-DOX

HSA-m or HSA-d (150 µM) in 100 mM KPB + 0.5 mM DTPA (pH 7.8) incubated with 2-iminothiolane (final concentration 3.6 mM) and mixed gently for 1 h at 25 °C [25]. INNO-206 (final concentration 1.8 mM) was added to the solution under dark conditions and mixed at 25 °C for 3 h. Then, the unreacted 2-iminothiolane and INNO-206 were removed by ultrafiltration using Amicon Ultra 4 (NMWL: 10 kDa). Next, HSA-m-DOX or HSA-d-DOX was dialyzed against deionized water and lyophilized. These samples were stored at −20 °C until used. The particle sizes and polydispersity index (PDI) of HSA-DOX under PBS (pH 7.4) condition were recorded using a Malvern zetasizer Nano ZS (Malvern Instruments, Worcestershire, UK).

### 2.5. Quantification of DOX Loaded to HSA

To quantify DOX loaded to HSA, the absorbance (490 nm) of HSA-DOX was measured using 96-well plate by the iMark microplate reader (Bio-Rad, Hercules, CA, USA). Free DOX solutions (6.25, 12.5, 25, 50 µg/mL) were used as standard. The same protein concentration without DOX was also measured to adjust for background absorption. The protein concentration of HSA-DOX was determined by the Bradford method. DOX loading efficiency (DOX/HSA) was calculated using this concentration of HSA.

### 2.6. In Vitro Release Profile of DOX from HSA-m-DOX or HSA-d-DOX

To evaluate the stability of HSA-m-DOX or HSA-d-DOX in acidic and neutral pH conditions, HSA-m-DOX or HSA-d-DOX was dissolved with PBS (pH 7.4) and acetic acid buffer (pH 5.5), respectively, and adjusted to 2.0 µg (DOX)/mL. Then, HSA-m-DOX or HSA-d-DOX was incubated at 37 °C in each pH condition, and fluorescence intensity (Ex/Em = 488 nm/585 nm) was measured using a spectrofluorimeter FP-8200ST (JASCO) at 0, 3, 6, 12, 24, 36, 48 h. The % release of DOX was calculated as follows.

$$\% \text{ release of DOX} = (A - B)/(C - B) \times 100$$

A: Fluorescence intensity of sample;
B: Fluorescence intensity at 0% release condition (pH 7.4, 25 °C);
C: Fluorescence intensity at 100% release condition (pH 1.0, 37 °C, 2 h).

### 2.7. In Vitro Antitumor Activity of HSA-DOX

SUIT2 cells ($1 \times 10^4$ cells/well) were seeded in a 96-well plate. After being left overnight, free-DOX, HSA-m-DOX or HSA-d-DOX (10–5000 ng (DOX)/mL) was added to the cells and reacted for 48 h. HSA-m and HSA-d were used as a negative control. Cell viability was assessed by CCK-8.

### 2.8. Quantification of Intracellular DOX

SUIT2 cells ($1 \times 10^5$ cells/well) were seeded in a 12-well plate. After being left overnight, the medium was replaced with a serum-free medium, then incubated for 2 h. After serum starvation, free-DOX, HSA-m-DOX or HSA-d-DOX (10 nmol (DOX)/mL) was added, and the cells were harvested 2 h later. The collected cell suspension was centrifuged ($1500\times g$, 5 min, 4 °C), and the supernatant was removed. Then, 2 N HCl (500 µL) was added to the cell pellet to lyse the cells. Subsequently, deproteinization was performed by adding methanol (500 µL) and centrifugation ($1500\times g$, 5 min, 4 °C), and the fluorescence intensity of the supernatant (Ex/Em = 488 nm/585 nm) was spectrophotometrically determined using FP-8200ST (JASCO).

### 2.9. Pharmacokinetic Analysis of HSA-DOX

INNO-206, HSA-m-DOX or HSA-d-DOX (8.0 mg (DOX)/kg) was intravenously administered in SUIT2 human pancreatic tumors and subcutaneously implanted in mice with a tumor size of 100 mm$^3$. Then, some main organs (heart, lung, liver, spleen, and kidney) and the tumor were extirpated at 6 h after administration, and ex vivo imaging was performed using an IVIS imaging system. The DOX fluorescence intensity of these tissues was measured at Ex/Em = 465 nm/600 nm.

### 2.10. In Vivo Antitumor Activity and Side Effects of HSA-DOX

When tumors reached 100 mm$^3$ in mice implanted subcutaneously with SUIT2 human pancreatic tumor, the mice were divided into cohorts ($n$ = 4) and treated intravenously with PBS (control), INNO-206 (8.0 mg (DOX)/kg), HSA-m-DOX (8.0 mg (DOX)/kg), or HSA-d-DOX (8.0 mg (DOX)/kg) on days 0 and 7, and then monitored for 21 days [17]. During treatment, tumor volume and body weight were measured daily, and blood was collected from the inferior vena cava on day 21 to measure various biochemical parameters. Specifically, after measuring blood cell parameters using a multi-item automatic blood cell counter KX-21N (Sysmex, Kobe, Japan), centrifugation (1500× $g$, 10 min) was performed. After the collection of serum, liver injury markers (AST, ALT) and kidney injury markers (BUN) were evaluated using the respective measurement kit (Wako Pure Chemical Industries, Ltd., Tokyo, Japan).

### 2.11. Statistical Analysis

The experimental data are presented as the means ± standard deviation. The statistical significance of differences between groups was analyzed with Student's $t$-test or ANOVA with Tukey's post hoc test. A probability value of $p < 0.05$ was considered to indicate statistical significance.

## 3. Results and Discussion

### 3.1. Preparation of HSA-d-DOX

First, HSA-m-DOX and HSA-d-DOX were synthesized using the method shown in Figure 1A. Specifically, the primary amine of the HSA molecule is chemically modified with an SH group using iminothiolane. Then, the maleimide group was reacted beforehand with the pH-responsive linker of INNO-206. As a result, the particle sizes of HSA-m-DOX and HSA-d-DOX were 3.98 nm and 7.52 nm, and amounts of DOX binding to HSA-m-DOX and HSA-d-DOX were 4.08 mol/mol HSA-m and 7.9 mol/mol HSA-d, respectively (Table 1). These results suggest that HSA-m-DOX and HSA-d-DOX exist as almost homogeneous molecules without aggregated proteins. In the previous report, $N$-succinimidyl $S$-acetylthioacetate (SATA) reagent was used to introduce SH to amino groups [26]. In the case of the SATA reagent, the terminal is thioester after reaction, so a deprotection procedure with hydroxylamine is needed. In contrast, the preparation process was successfully shortened by one step using iminothiolane, where a deprotection operation could be omitted. Fortunately, the DOX loading efficiency using iminothiolane was equivalent to the value in the reference using SATA [26]. The stability of HSA-m-DOX and HSA-d-DOX after lyophilization was assessed by evaluating the particle sizes and DOX-loading rates. These data showed that both HSA-m-DOX and HSA-d-DOX were suspendable after lyophilization, and no other change, such as aggregates, can be observed (Figure 1B). In addition, since the DOX-loading rates of both compounds before and after lyophilization were the same, this result indicated that storage of HSA-m-DOX and HSA-d-DOX as a lyophilisate was possible (Figure 1C).

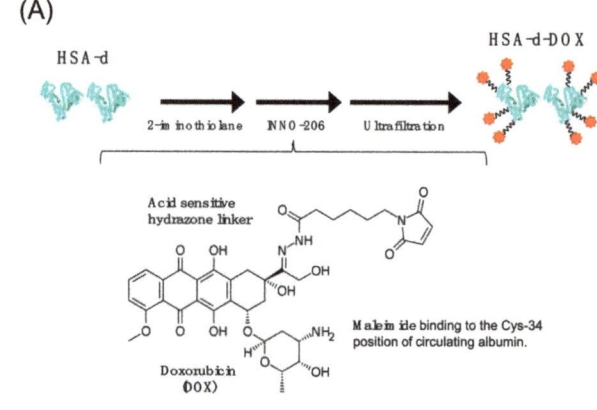
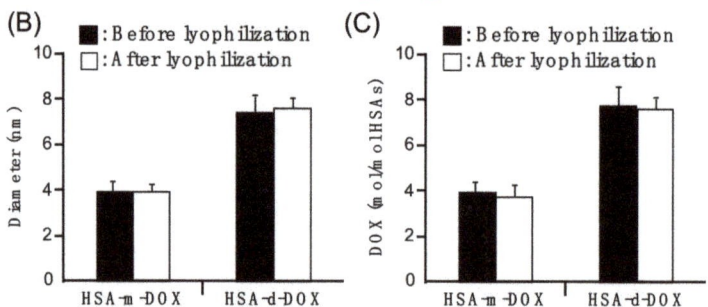

**Figure 1.** The preparation scheme of HSA-d-DOX, and the stability of HSA-m-DOX and HSA-d-DOX particles before and after lyophilization. (**A**) Preparation scheme of HSA-d-DOX. (**B**) The change of particle size and (**C**) DOX loading of HSA-DOX after lyophilization of HSA-m-DOX and HSA-d-DOX. Data are averages ± standard deviation (n = 4).

**Table 1.** Physicochemical characterization of HSA-m-DOX and HSA-d-DOX.

|  | Diameter (nm) | PDI | DOX/HSAs (Molar Ratio) |
|---|---|---|---|
| HSA-m-DOX | 3.98 ± 0.5 | 0.426 ± 0.01 | 4.08 ± 0.26 |
| HSA-d-DOX | 7.52 ± 0.7 | 0.297 ± 0.01 | 7.90 ± 0.46 |

Data are averages ± standard deviation (n = 4).

### 3.2. In Vitro Release Profile of DOX from HSA-m-DOX or HSA-d-DOX

Although DOX is a fluorescent substance, fluorescence self-quenching occurs when DOX is bound to HSA-m and HSA-d. The DOX release profile of HSA-m-DOX or HSA-d-DOX in buffers in different pH conditions was evaluated using this fluorescence self-quenching phenomenon. The release of DOX from HSA-m-DOX or HSA-d-DOX was not observed in the pH 7.4 buffer. In contrast, acidic conditions (pH 5.5) accelerated the release of DOX (Figure 2). These data suggest that the DOX release from HSA-m-DOX and HSA-d-DOX occurs in acidic conditions, like those in tumor tissues. In tumor tissues, malnutrition and hypoxia result from incomplete blood vessel construction and uncontrolled growth of the tumor cells. The release profile of HSA-m-DOX was very similar to HSA-d-DOX. The total release from HSA-d-DOX in pH 5.5 buffer at 48 h was around 80%, suggesting a result that is similar when compared with another published release assay for DOX [27]. As a result, glycolytic metabolism is enhanced, leading to the buildup of an acidic environment [28]. In particular, the acidic environment is more pronounced in pancreatic tumors. Therefore, after reaching the tumor tissue via the EPR effect, HSA-d-DOX is expected to release DOX more efficiently in pancreatic tumors.

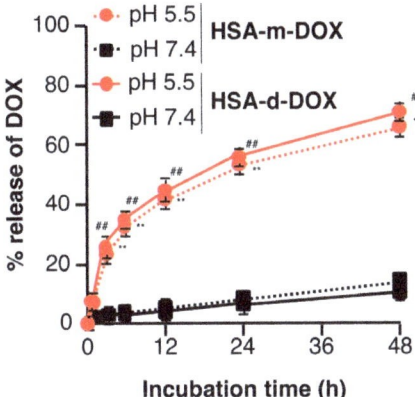

**Figure 2.** In vitro pH-dependent DOX release profile of HSA-m-DOX or HSA-d-DOX. HSA-m-DOX or HSA-d-DOX was diluted with PBS (pH 7.4) or acetate buffer (pH 5.5) to 2.0 mg (DOX)/mL. After incubation, the fluorescence intensity (Ex/Em: 488 nm/585 nm) was measured. Data are averages ± standard deviation ($n$ = 4). ** $p$ < 0.01 vs. HSA-m-DOX in pH 7.4 group. ## $p$ < 0.01 vs. HSA-d-DOX in pH 7.4 group.

### 3.3. In Vitro Antitumor Activity of HSA-d-DOX against Human Pancreatic Tumor Cells

To confirm the antitumor activity of HSA-d-DOX on SUIT2 human pancreatic tumor cells, an evaluation was performed. Free-DOX, HSA-m-DOX, and HSA-d-DOX were incubated with SUIT2 cells for 48 h, and the number of viable cells were quantified by CCK-8 assay. Figure 3A shows that free-DOX possessed the highest cytotoxicity against SUIT2 cells among all drugs, and HSA-d-DOX has significantly inhibited the survival rate compared with HSA-m-DOX (Figure 3A, Table 2). In addition, carriers alone, such as HSA-m or HSA-d, did not show any cytotoxicity (Table 2). To clarify the cytotoxic mechanism of HSA-d-DOX, the amount of intracellular DOX was analyzed. Free-DOX, HSA-m-DOX or HSA-d-DOX was incubated with SUIT2 cells for 2 h, and the amount of intracellular DOX was quantified by fluorescent spectroscopy. Figure 3B shows the amount of intracellular DOX in decreasing order, free-DOX > HSA-d-DOX > HSA-m-DOX. This result was highly consistent with the cytotoxicity results of these compounds. Previously, we reported that HSA-d-DOX is also taken into cells via caveolin-1-mediated macropinocytosis [17,29]. Additionally, pancreatic tumor cells are known to have increased expression of secreted protein acidic and are rich in cysteine (SPARC) for the EAT system [20]. This EAT System is activated at a region where the EPR effect must be enhanced, which is therefore considered a region where it is traditionally difficult to deliver a polymeric antitumor agent [18].

**Table 2.** IC$_{50}$ of DOX derives against pancreatic tumor cell.

| Treatment Groups | IC$_{50}$ (DOX ng/mL) |
|---|---|
| HSA-m | - |
| HSA-d | - |
| HSA-m-DOX | 676.7 ± 52.4 |
| HSA-d-DOX | 454.2 ± 66.7 * |
| free-DOX | 62.21 ± 24.5 ** |

Data are averages ± standard deviation ($n$ = 6). * $p$ < 0.05, ** $p$ < 0.01 vs. HSA-m-DOX.

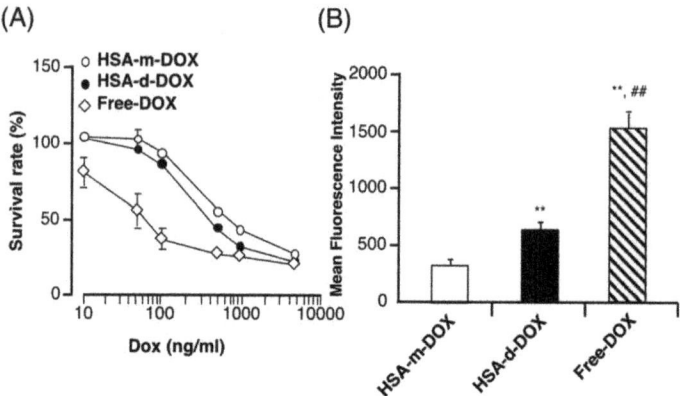

**Figure 3.** Cytotoxicity of HSA-d-DOX on pancreatic tumor cell. (**A**) SUIT-2 cells were treated with various concentration of HSA-m-DOX, HSA-d-DOX or free-DOX for 48 h. Survival cells were quantified by CCK-8 assay and expressed as percent survival to untreated control. (**B**) Cellular uptake of HSA-d-DOX by pancreatic tumor cells. SUIT2 cells were treated with HSA-m-DOX, HSA-d-DOX, free-DOX (150 μg/mL) in serum-free DMEM. Cellular uptake of DOX was analyzed by fluorescent spectroscopy (Ex/Em: 488 nm/585 nm; Data are averages ± standard deviation ($n = 6$). ** $p < 0.01$ vs. HSA-m-DOX, ## $p < 0.01$ vs. HSA-d-DOX.

### 3.4. Biodistribution of HSA-d-DOX

In order to confirm the tumor accumulation of HSA-d-DOX in tumor-bearing mice, the organ distribution of HSA-d-DOX in vivo was evaluated using a SUIT2 human pancreatic tumor subcutaneous transplantation model. INNO-206, HSA-m-DOX or HSA-d-DOX was intravenously administered in the SUIT2 subcutaneous transplantation model at a dose of 8 mg (DOX)/kg. The fluorescence intensity of DOX in each organ was measured by ex vivo imaging at 6 h after administration (Figure 4A). Intriguingly, HSA-d-DOX showed significantly higher tumor accumulation of DOX than other groups (Figure 4B). In addition, the liver distributions of HSA-m-DOX and HSA-d-DOX were higher than INNO-206, strongly suggesting that liver injury markers, such as AST and ALT, should be measured after the administration of HSA-m-DOX or HSA-d-DOX to clarify whether these administrations induce side effects related to liver injury. Previously, our collaborators demonstrated that modifications of basic amino acids on the surface of HSA have increased liver uptake of the HSA by 30-fold [30,31]. In general, modifications of basic amino acids led to the blockage of the positive charges of HSA. To conjugate DOX to HSA in this study, 2-iminothiolane reacted with lysine residues on the surface of HSA. This reaction induced the blockage of the positive charges. Therefore, this evidence suggested that this 2-iminothiolane reaction may induce the increase of liver uptake of HSA-m-DOX and HSA-d-DOX. To avoid this problem, the other method of DOX conjugation without the modification of basic amino acids would be necessary.

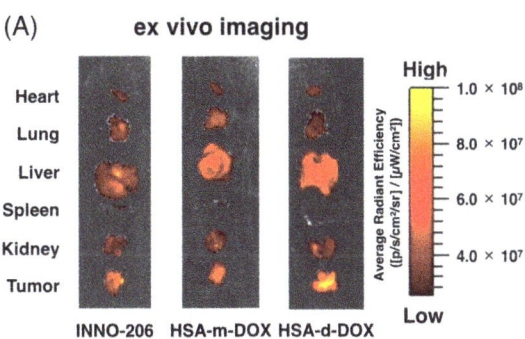
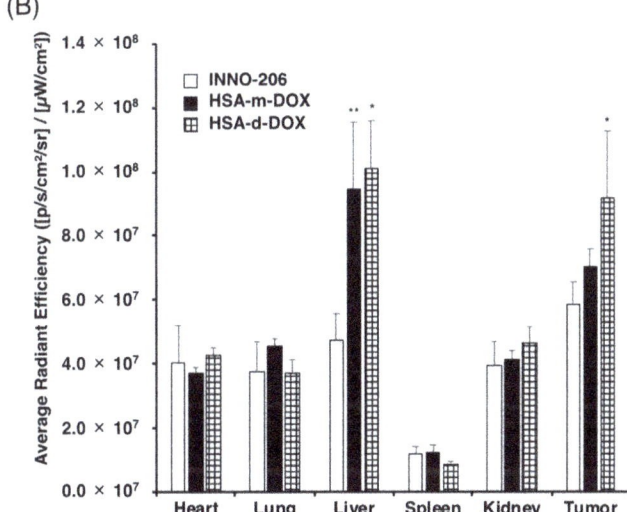

**Figure 4.** Organ distribution of HSA-DOX. (**A**) ex vivo imaging, (**B**) ex vivo radiant efficiency of the major organs from SUIT2 ectopic tumor bearing mice at 6 h after 8.0 mg (DOX)/kg of INNO-206, HSA-m-DOX and HSA-d-DOX were IV injected. The results obtained for the control group were used to correct for nonspecific background fluorescence. Data are averages ± standard deviation ($n$ = 3). * $p < 0.05$, ** $p < 0.01$ vs. INNO-206.

### 3.5. In Vivo Antitumor Activity of HSA-d-DOX

Finally, the therapeutic effect of HSA-d-DOX was evaluated using a SUIT2 human pancreatic tumor subcutaneous transplantation model to verify whether HSA-d-DOX exerts an antitumor effect in the SUIT2 human pancreatic tumor implantation model, which shows resistance to macromolecular antitumor drugs. SUIT2 tumor-bearing mice with a tumor volume of about 100 mm$^3$ were divided into Control, INNO-206, HSA-m-DOX, and HSA-d-DOX administration groups. The dose of INNO-206, HSA-m-DOX, and HSA-d-DOX was adjusted to 8.0 mg (DOX)/kg, which was intravenously administered to SUIT2 tumor-bearing mice on days 0 and 7. The data showed that HSA-d-DOX significantly suppressed tumor growth compared to INNO-206 and HSA-m-DOX (Figure 5A). Regarding body weight changes, although each group of INNO-206, HSA-m-DOX or HSA-d-DOX showed a slight weight loss after the second administration, there was no significant change overall (Figure 5B).

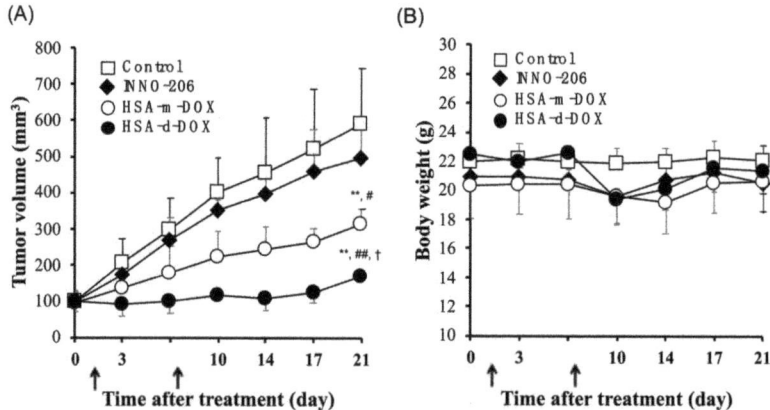

**Figure 5.** The antitumor activity of HSA-d-DOX in SUIT2 ectopic tumor bearing mice. (**A**) The tumor volume and (**B**) body weight were measured in SUIT2 ectopic tumor bearing mice at each of the selected time points. The mice were IV injected with PBS, INNO-206 (8.0 mg (DOX)/kg), HSA-m-DOX (8.0 mg (DOX)/kg) or HSA-d-DOX (8.0 mg (DOX)/kg) at each of the selected time points. The arrows indicate days of treatment. Data are averages ± standard deviation ($n$ = 4). ** $p < 0.01$ vs. control, # $p < 0.05$, ## $p < 0.01$ vs. INNO-206, † $p < 0.05$ vs. HSA-m-DOX.

The following dosing rates have been reported to be effective: on day 10, 17, and 24, dosings of DOX 24 mg/kg [9], and on day 10, 17, and 24, dosings of DOX 12 mg/kg [32], while the dosing rate used in the present study, on day 0 and 7, dosings of DOX 8.0 mg/kg, practically showed no antitumor efficacy. This 2 × DOX 8.0 mg/kg dosing rate explains why the antitumor activity of INNO-206 did not show a significant difference from that of the PBS treated group. In contrast, despite dosing at 2 × DOX 8.0 mg/kg, HSA-d-DOX showed antitumor activity.

To evaluate the onset of side effects, various biochemical parameters were measured at day 21. These biochemical parameters, including AST and ALT, showed no significant difference among all groups (Table 3). These data indicate that HSA-d-DOX possesses the highest therapeutic effect against human pancreatic tumors without severe side effects. Previously, we examined the antitumor effect of Abraxane® using the same SUIT2 human pancreatic tumor implantation model [17]. It is well-known that this model shows higher resistance to most antitumor drugs compared with C26 murine colon tumor and B16 murine melanoma subcutaneous inoculation models. The administration of Abraxane® (20 mg (paclitaxel)/kg) could not significantly inhibit the tumor growth like INNO-206. Although Table 2 shows that free DOX possesses higher cytotoxicity than HSA-d-DOX in vitro, HSA-d-DOX has the highest antitumor activity among other drugs. These data strongly suggest that the tumor accumulation and retention of HSA-d-DOX are significantly superior to other drugs. Taken together, HSA-d-DOX has the potential to be a promising macromolecular antitumor drug.

**Table 3.** Blood chemistry parameters after drugs treatment.

| | WBC ($\times 10^2/\mu L$) | RBC ($\times 10^4/\mu L$) | HGB (g/dL) | PLT ($\times 10^4/\mu L$) | AST (IU/L) | ALT (IU/L) | BUN (mg/dL) |
|---|---|---|---|---|---|---|---|
| Control | 24.3 ± 3.06 | 944.0 ± 32.5 | 114.4 ± 18.3 | 64.1 ± 12.4 | 19.6 ± 4.5 | 29.9 ± 3.2 | 78.8 ± 8.5 |
| INNO-206 | 20.5 ± 5.9 | 924.8 ± 47.8 | 106.5 ± 17.5 | 57.7 ± 11.1 | 16.6 ± 5.1 | 39.5 ± 4.4 | 78.3 ± 10.4 |
| HSA-m-DOX | 26.3 ± 8.3 | 934.8 ± 88.5 | 115.1 ± 13.2 | 62.8 ± 2.5 | 17.2 ± 5.1 | 33.7 ± 2.4 | 82.5 ± 19.3 |
| HSA-d-DOX | 17.8 ± 3.1 | 939.8 ± 79.0 | 102.6 ± 30.7 | 66.1 ± 7.5 | 20.4 ± 3.9 | 37.7 ± 2.6 | 78.8 ± 14.3 |

Parameters of blood cells (white blood cell (WBC) count, red blood cell (RBC) count, hemoglobin (HGB) count, platelet (PLT) count), aspartate transaminase (AST), alanine aminotransferase (ALT), blood urea nitrogen (BUN) in C26 ectopic tumor bearing mice at day 28. Data are averages ± standard deviation. ($n$ = 4).

## 4. Conclusions

In this study, HSA-d-DOX was developed as a novel antitumor drug nano-DDS loaded with DOX using next-generation nab technology. HSA-d exhibited excellent tumor migration and cellular uptake ability compared with HSA-m using conventional nab technology. HSA-d-DOX efficiently delivered DOX to pancreatic tumor cells, inducing a potent antitumor effect without severe side effects. Therefore, dimerization of HSA could function not only as a natural solubilizer of insoluble drugs, but also as the active targeting carrier in low vascular permeability or an intractable pancreatic tumor.

**Author Contributions:** Conceptualization, Y.I. and T.M.; methodology, R.K. and K.O.; validation, V.T.G.C., H.W. and T.S.; formal analysis, H.A.; investigation, R.K.; resources, Y.I.; writing—original draft preparation, Y.I.; writing—review and editing, M.O. and T.I.; supervision, Y.I. and T.M.; project administration, Y.I. and T.M.; funding acquisition, Y.I. All authors have read and agreed to the published version of the manuscript.

**Funding:** This work was supported, in part, by Grants-in-Aid from the Japan Society for the Promotion of Science (JSPS), a Grant-in-Aid from the Ministry of Education, Culture, Sports, Science and Technology (KAKENHI KIBAN (B) 21H02645) and (KAKENHI KIBAN (B) 18H02604), Japan. In part, the work was supported by grants from the Mishima Kaiun Memorial Foundation and the Takahashi Industrial and the Economic Research Foundation.

**Institutional Review Board Statement:** All animal experiments were carried out according to the Laboratory Protocol for Animal Handling of Tokushima University.

**Informed Consent Statement:** Not applicable.

**Conflicts of Interest:** The authors declare no conflict of interest.

## References

1. Matsumura, Y. Cancer stromal targeting therapy to overcome the pitfall of EPR effect. *Adv. Drug. Deliv. Rev.* **2020**, *154–155*, 142–150. [CrossRef]
2. Kondo, E.; Iioka, H.; Saito, K. Tumor-homing peptide and its utility for advanced cancer medicine. *Cancer Sci.* **2021**, *112*, 2118–2125. [CrossRef]
3. Blum, R.H.; Carter, S.K. Adriamycin. A new anticancer drug with significant clinical activity. *Ann. Intern. Med.* **1974**, *80*, 249–259. [CrossRef]
4. O'Bryan, R.M.; Luce, J.K.; Talley, R.W.; Gottlieb, J.A.; Baker, L.H.; Bonadonna, G. Phase II evaluation of adriamycin in human neoplasia. *Cancer* **1973**, *32*, 1–8. [CrossRef]
5. Safra, T.; Muggia, F.; Jeffers, S.; Tsao-Wei, D.D.; Groshen, S.; Lyass, O.; Henderson, R.; Berry, G.; Gabizon, A. Pegylated liposomal doxorubicin (doxil): Reduced clinical cardiotoxicity in patients reaching or exceeding cumulative doses of 500 mg/m$^2$. *Ann. Oncol.* **2000**, *11*, 1029–1034. [CrossRef] [PubMed]
6. Lyass, O.; Uziely, B.; Ben-Yosef, R.; Tzemach, D.; Heshing, N.I.; Lotem, M.; Brufman, G.; Gabizon, A. Correlation of toxicity with pharmacokinetics of pegylated liposomal doxorubicin (Doxil) in metastatic breast carcinoma. *Cancer* **2000**, *89*, 1037–1047. [CrossRef]
7. Matsumura, Y.; Hamaguchi, T.; Ura, T.; Muro, K.; Yamada, Y.; Shimada, Y.; Shirao, K.; Okusaka, T.; Ueno, H.; Ikeda, M.; et al. Phase I clinical trial and pharmacokinetic evaluation of NK911, a micelle-encapsulated doxorubicin. *Br. J. Cancer* **2004**, *91*, 1775–1781. [CrossRef]
8. Kratz, F. DOXO-EMCH (INNO-206): The first albumin-binding prodrug of doxorubicin to enter clinical trials. *Expert Opin. Investig. Drugs* **2007**, *16*, 855–866. [CrossRef] [PubMed]
9. Graeser, R.; Esser, N.; Unger, H.; Fichtner, I.; Zhu, A.; Unger, C.; Kratz, F. INNO-206, the (6-maleimidocaproyl hydrazone derivative of doxorubicin), shows superior antitumor efficacy compared to doxorubicin in different tumor xenograft models and in an orthotopic pancreas carcinoma model. *Investig. New Drugs* **2009**, *28*, 14–19. [CrossRef] [PubMed]
10. Kratz, F.; Warnecke, A. Finding the optimal balance: Challenges of improving conventional cancer chemotherapy using suitable combinations with nano-sized drug delivery systems. *J. Control. Release* **2012**, *164*, 221–235. [CrossRef]
11. Fu, Q.; Sun, J.; Zhang, W.; Sui, X.; Yan, Z.; He, Z. Nanoparticle Albumin—Bound (NAB) Technology is a Promising Method for Anti-Cancer Drug Delivery. *Recent Patents Anti-Cancer Drug Discov.* **2009**, *4*, 262–272. [CrossRef]
12. Kamaly, N.; Xiao, Z.; Valencia, P.M.; Radovic-Moreno, A.F.; Farokhzad, O.C. Targeted polymeric therapeutic nanoparticles: Design, development and clinical translation. *Chem. Soc. Rev.* **2012**, *41*, 2971–3010. [CrossRef] [PubMed]
13. Pham, L.M.; Poudel, K.; Ou, W.; Phung, C.D.; Nguyen, H.T.; Nguyen, B.L.; Karmacharya, P.; Pandit, M.; Chang, J.-H.; Jeong, J.-H.; et al. Combination chemotherapeutic and immune-therapeutic anticancer approach via anti-PD-L1 antibody conjugated albumin nanoparticles. *Int. J. Pharm.* **2021**, *605*, 120816. [CrossRef]

14. Li, R.; Ng, T.S.C.; Wang, S.J.; Prytyskach, M.; Rodell, C.B.; Mikula, H.; Kohler, R.H.; Garlin, M.A.; Lauffenburger, D.A.; Parangi, S.; et al. Therapeutically reprogrammed nutrient signalling enhances nanoparticulate albumin bound drug uptake and efficacy in KRAS-mutant cancer. *Nat. Nanotechnol.* **2021**, *16*, 830–839. [CrossRef] [PubMed]
15. Matsushita, S.; Chuang, V.T.G.; Kanazawa, M.; Tanase, S.; Kawai, K.; Maruyama, T.; Suenaga, A.; Otagiri, M. Recombinant Human Serum Albumin Dimer has High Blood Circulation Activity and Low Vascular Permeability in Comparison with Native Human Serum Albumin. *Pharm. Res.* **2006**, *23*, 882–891. [CrossRef]
16. Kinoshita, R.; Ishima, Y.; Ikeda, M.; Kragh-Hansen, U.; Fang, J.; Nakamura, H.; Chuang, V.T.G.; Tanaka, R.; Maeda, H.; Kodama, A.; et al. S-Nitrosated human serum albumin dimer as novel nano-EPR enhancer applied to macromolecular anti-tumor drugs such as micelles and liposomes. *J. Control. Release* **2015**, *217*, 1–9. [CrossRef] [PubMed]
17. Kinoshita, R.; Ishima, Y.; Chuang, V.T.G.; Nakamura, H.; Fang, J.; Watanabe, H.; Shimizu, T.; Okuhira, K.; Ishida, T.; Maeda, H.; et al. Improved anticancer effects of albumin-bound paclitaxel nanoparticle via augmentation of EPR effect and albumin-protein interactions using S-nitrosated human serum albumin dimer. *Biomater.* **2017**, *140*, 162–169. [CrossRef]
18. Ishima, Y.; Maruyama, T.; Otagiri, M.; Ishida, T. Drug Delivery System for Refractory Cancer Therapy via an Endogenous Albumin Transport System. *Chem. Pharm. Bull.* **2020**, *68*, 583–588. [CrossRef]
19. Desai, N.; Trieu, V.; Damascelli, B.; Soon-Shiong, P. SPARC Expression Correlates with Tumor Response to Albumin-Bound Paclitaxel in Head and Neck Cancer Patients. *Transl. Oncol.* **2009**, *2*, 59–64. [CrossRef] [PubMed]
20. Seno, T.; Harada, H.; Kohno, S.; Teraoka, M.; Inoue, A.; Ohnishi, T. Downregulation of SPARC expression inhibits cell migration and invasion in malignant gliomas. *Int. J. Oncol.* **2009**, *34*, 707–715. [CrossRef]
21. Ishima, Y.; Chen, D.; Fang, J.; Maeda, H.; Minomo, A.; Kragh-Hansen, U.; Kai, T.; Maruyama, T.; Otagiri, M. S-Nitrosated Human Serum Albumin Dimer is not only a Novel Anti-Tumor Drug but also a Potentiator for Anti-Tumor Drugs with Augmented EPR Effects. *Bioconjugate Chem.* **2012**, *23*, 264–271. [CrossRef]
22. Chen, R.F. Removal of Fatty Acids from Serum Albumin by Charcoal Treatment. *J. Biol. Chem.* **1967**, *242*, 173–181. [CrossRef]
23. Ishima, Y.; Sawa, T.; Kragh-Hansen, U.; Miyamoto, Y.; Matsushita, S.; Akaike, T.; Otagiri, M. S-Nitrosylation of Human Variant Albumin Liprizzi (R410C) Confers Potent Antibacterial and Cytoprotective Properties. *J. Pharmacol. Exp. Ther.* **2006**, *320*, 969–977. [CrossRef] [PubMed]
24. Matsushita, S.; Isima, Y.; Chuang, V.T.G.; Watanabe, H.; Tanase, S.; Maruyama, T.; Otagiri, M. Functional Analysis of Recombinant Human Serum Albumin Domains for Pharmaceutical Applications. *Pharm. Res.* **2004**, *21*, 1924–1932. [CrossRef]
25. Choi, S.H.; Byeon, H.J.; Choi, J.S.; Thao, L.; Kim, I.; Lee, E.S.; Shin, B.S.; Lee, K.C.; Youn, Y.S. Inhalable self-assembled albumin nanoparticles for treating drug-resistant lung cancer. *J. Control. Release* **2015**, *197*, 199–207. [CrossRef] [PubMed]
26. Ichimizu, S.; Watanabe, H.; Maeda, H.; Hamasaki, K.; Nakamura, Y.; Chuang, V.T.G.; Kinoshita, R.; Nishida, K.; Tanaka, R.; Enoki, Y.; et al. Design and tuning of a cell-penetrating albumin derivative as a versatile nanovehicle for intracellular drug delivery. *J. Control. Release* **2018**, *277*, 23–34. [CrossRef]
27. Sun, M.; Wang, J.; Lu, Q.; Xia, G.; Zhang, Y.; Song, L.; Fang, Y. Novel synthesizing method of pH-dependent doxorubicin-loaded anti-CD22-labelled drug delivery nanosystem. *Drug. Des. Dev. Ther.* **2015**, *9*, 5123–5133. [CrossRef]
28. Tian, L.; Bae, Y.H. Cancer nanomedicines targeting tumor extracellular pH. *Colloids Surf. B Biointerfaces* **2012**, *99*, 116–126. [CrossRef] [PubMed]
29. Chatterjee, M.; Ben-Josef, E.; Robb, R.; Vedaie, M.; Seum, S.; Thirumoorthy, K.; Palanichamy, K.; Harbrecht, M.; Chakravarti, A.; Williams, T.M. Caveolae-Mediated Endocytosis Is Critical for Albumin Cellular Uptake and Response to Albumin-Bound Chemotherapy. *Cancer Res.* **2017**, *77*, 5925–5937. [CrossRef]
30. Iwao, Y.; Anraku, M.; Yamasaki, K.; Kragh-Hansen, U.; Kawai, K.; Maruyama, T.; Otagiri, M. Oxidation of Arg-410 promotes the elimination of human serum albumin. *Biochim. Biophys. Acta (BBA) Proteins Proteom.* **2006**, *1764*, 743–749. [CrossRef]
31. Nakajou, K.; Watanabe, H.; Kragh-Hansen, U.; Maruyama, T.; Otagiri, M. The effect of glycation on the structure, function and biological fate of human serum albumin as revealed by recombinant mutants. *Biochim. Biophys. Acta (BBA) Gen. Subj.* **2003**, *1623*, 88–97. [CrossRef] [PubMed]
32. Kratz, F.; Azab, S.; Zeisig, R.; Fichtner, I.; Warnecke, A. Evaluation of combination therapy schedules of doxorubicin and an acid-sensitive albumin-binding prodrug of doxorubicin in the MIA PaCa-2 pancreatic xenograft model. *Int. J. Pharm.* **2013**, *441*, 499–506. [CrossRef] [PubMed]

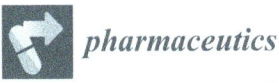 

*Article*

# Thermostable and Long-Circulating Albumin-Conjugated *Arthrobacter globiformis* Urate Oxidase

Byungseop Yang and Inchan Kwon *

School of Materials Science and Engineering, Gwangju Institute of Science and Technology (GIST), Gwangju 61005, Korea; yangbs@gist.ac.kr
* Correspondence: inchan@gist.ac.kr; Tel.: +82-62-715-2312

**Abstract:** Urate oxidase derived from *Aspergillus flavus* has been investigated as a treatment for tumor lysis syndrome, hyperuricemia, and gout. However, its long-term use is limited owing to potential immunogenicity, low thermostability, and short circulation time in vivo. Recently, urate oxidase isolated from *Arthrobacter globiformis* (AgUox) has been reported to be thermostable and less immunogenic than the *Aspergillus*-derived urate oxidase. Conjugation of human serum albumin (HSA) to therapeutic proteins has become a promising strategy to prolong circulation time in vivo. To develop a thermostable and long-circulating urate oxidase, we investigated the site-specific conjugation of HSA to AgUox based on site-specific incorporation of a clickable non-natural amino acid (frTet) and an inverse electron demand Diels–Alder reaction. We selected 14 sites for frTet incorporation using the ROSETTA design, a computational stability prediction program, among which AgUox containing frTet at position 196 (Ag12) exhibited enzymatic activity and thermostability comparable to those of wild-type AgUox. Furthermore, Ag12 exhibited a high HSA conjugation yield without compromising the enzymatic activity, generating well-defined HSA-conjugated AgUox (Ag12-HSA). In mice, the serum half-life of Ag12-HSA was approximately 29 h, which was roughly 17-fold longer than that of wild-type AgUox. Altogether, this novel formulated AgUox may hold enhanced therapeutic efficacy for several diseases.

**Keywords:** *Arthrobacter globiformis*; gout; half-life extension; inverse electron demand Diels-Alder reaction; site-specific albumin conjugation; thermostability; urate oxidase

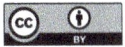

## 1. Introduction

A high level of uric acid followed by its crystallization is related to tumor lysis syndrome, hyperuricemia, and gout [1–3]. Gout is a common type of inflammatory arthritis in adults, resulting from the formation of uric acid crystals in the joints and other tissues [1–3]. Therefore, the treatment of gout has focused on reducing serum uric acid levels, which has been effectively achieved by the injection of urate oxidase [3,4]. Urate oxidase (Uox, Enzyme Commission number: 1.7.3.3) is a peroxisomal liver enzyme that catalyzes the conversion of insoluble uric acid (0.06 g/L) to the more water-soluble 5-hydroxyisourate (10.6 g/L; predicted using ALOGPS) [5–8]. In humans, intravenous administration of Uox has been used for enzymatic therapy of hyperuricemia, supplementing the enzyme activity lost during hominoid evolution [3]. Rasburicase [9,10] and pegloticase [11–13] have been approved for the treatment of tumor lysis syndrome and gout, respectively. Rasburicase is a recombinant version of Uox derived from *Aspergillus flavus* that was demonstrated to be therapeutically superior to allopurinol for the control of uric acid levels in adult patients [9–11]. Pegloticase (marketed under the name Krystexxa) is a PEG-conjugated chimeric porcine–baboon Uox, with an extended serum half-life in vivo [12–14]. However, several concerns have been raised regarding PEG-conjugated therapeutics, such as the potential immunogenicity and toxicity of accumulated PEG molecules [15]. Human serum albumin (HSA) has low to no immunogenicity and is biodegradable. Furthermore, HSA has an exceptionally long serum half-life in humans (>3 weeks) via neonatal Fc receptor (FcRn)-mediated recycling [16–20]. Therefore, in order to overcome the potential issues of PEG conjugation, we previously reported that direct conjugation or indirect binding of HSA to Uox isolated from *A. flavus* (AfUox) resulted in a prolonged circulation time in vivo [21,22], enhancing its potential use as a therapeutic agent for gout. Direct HSA conjugation leads to a greater extension of circulation time than that achieved with indirect HSA binding via fatty acid conjugation [21,22]. However, the clinical applications of HSA-conjugated AfUox may be limited by its intrinsic immunogenicity and low thermostability [23]. Recently, Uox derived from *Arthrobacter globiformis* (AgUox) was determined to hold desirable properties for therapeutic development, including soluble expression in *Escherichia coli*, good solubility at neutral pH, low immunogenicity, and good thermostability [4,24]. We confirmed that wild-type AgUox is more thermostable than wild-type AfUox (Figure S1). To develop HSA-conjugated Uox with promising potential for clinical applications, we investigated site-specific HSA conjugation to AgUox. We hypothesized that the conjugation of HSA to a permissive site of AgUox would lead to high thermostability, low immunogenicity, prolonged circulation time in vivo (particularly in mice), and retained enzymatic activity. It was reported that HSA interacts with mouse FcRn, resulting in the long serum half-life in mice [25]. Furthermore, the attachment of HSA to insulin and glucagon-like peptide 1 extended the circulation time in mice, likely due to the HSA interactions with mouse FcRn [26,27].

## 2. Materials and Methods

### 2.1. Materials

Bactotryptone and yeast extract were obtained from BD Biosciences (San Jose, CA, USA). Ni-nitrilotriacetic acid (NTA) agarose was obtained from Qiagen (Hilden, Germany), and frTet (4-(1,2,3,4-tetrazin-3-yl) phenylalanine) was purchased from Aldlab Chemicals (Woburn, MA, USA). TCO–Cy3 was purchased from AAT Bioquest (Sunnyvale, CA, USA). Axially substituted trans-cyclooctene maleimide (TCO-maleimide, A) was purchased from FutureChem (Seoul, Korea). Disposable PD-10 desalting columns, HiTrap Q HP anion exchange columns, and Superdex 200 10/300 GL Increase size exclusion columns were purchased from Cytiva (Uppsala, Sweden). All other chemical reagents were purchased from Sigma-Aldrich (St. Louis, MO, USA), unless otherwise indicated.

### 2.2. Computational Analysis of the frTet Incorporation Site in AgUox

Screening of the frTet incorporation site was performed using the molecular modeling software PyRosetta (Python-based Rosetta molecular modeling package, Pyrosetta4, the PyRosetta Team at Johns Hopkins University, Baltimore, MD, USA) [28,29], which performed point mutation and energy scoring functions based on the AgUox structure (PDB ID: 2YZE). The amino acid sequence in wild-type (WT) AgUox was replaced with the Y (tyrosine) or W (tryptophan) sequence, and then the energy of the full atoms in the protein was calculated. The energy function in PyRosetta is based on Anfinsen's hypothesis that native-like protein conformations represent a unique, low-energy, thermodynamically stable conformation. The score value represents the sum of the van der Waals force, attractive, repulsive energy, Gaussian exclusion implicit solvation, and hydrogen bonds (short, long range, backbone-side chain, and side chain) between atoms on different residues separated by distance.

### 2.3. Construction of Plasmids for Expression of AgUox-WT and AgUox-frTet Variants

AgUox was synthesized by Macrogen (Seoul, Korea) and cloned into pBAD for site-specific frTet incorporation, generating the pBAD_AgUox plasmid. To replace the site selected by PyRosetta scoring with amber codons, the site-directed mutagenesis polymerase chain reaction (PCR) was performed using the pBAD_AgUox vector as template. The primer pairs used are shown in Table S1.

*2.4. Expression and Purification of AgUox-WT and AgUox-frTet Variants*

To site-specifically incorporate frTet into AgUox, each mutant plasmid was transformed into C321ΔA.exp (pDule C11RS)-competent cells [30], generating C321ΔAexp (pDule C11RS) (pBAD_AgUox_Amb variants) *E. coli* cells. Transformants were cultured at 37 °C overnight in Luria broth medium containing ampicillin (100 μg/mL) and tetracycline (10 μg/mL). Pre-cultured *E. coli* cells were inoculated into identical fresh media. To induce protein expression, final concentrations of 1 mM and 0.4% of frTet and arabinose, respectively, were added to the medium, which reached an optical density of 0.5% (at 600 nm). The culture medium was incubated at 37 °C for 5 h with shaking, before being harvested via centrifugation at 5000 rpm for 10 min at 4 °C. AgUox-containing frTet variants were purified by immobilized metal affinity chromatography, using the interaction between Ni-NTA and His-tag, according to the manufacturer's protocols. The expression and purification of AgUox-WT was performed similarly to that of the AgUox-frTet variants, without the addition of tetracycline and frTet.

*2.5. Matrix-Assisted Laser Desorption Ionization Time-of-Flight Mass Spectrometry (MALDI-TOF MS) and Dye Labeling Analysis of AgUox Variants*

Purified AgUox-WT and AgUox-frTet variants (0.4 mg/mL) were digested with trypsin. The trypsin-digested mixture was desalted using ZipTip C18 (Millipore, Billerica, MA, USA). The desalted trypsin-digested protein sample was mixed with 2,5-dihydroxybenzoic acid (DHB) solution (20 mg/mL of DHB in 3:7, ($v/v$) acetonitrile: 0.1% trifluoroacetic acid in water) in a 1:1 ratio. Then, 0.5 μL of this mixture was loaded onto a ground steel target (Bruker Corporation, Billerica, MA, USA) and molecular weight analysis was performed by MALDI-TOF MS (Bruker Corporation, Billerica, MA, USA).

To identify the IEDDA reactivity of the AgUox-frTet variants, purified AgUox-WT and AgUox-frTet variants were desalted with phosphate-buffered saline (PBS, pH 7.4) and then mixed with TCO-Cy3 at a molar ratio of 1:2 for 2 h at room temperature. Afterwards, the mixture, with or without the addition of TCO-Cy3, was subjected to sodium dodecyl sulfate polyacrylamide gel electrophoresis (SDS-PAGE). The gel underwent fluorescence analysis (excitation: 302 nm, filter 510/610 nm) in a ChemiDoc XRS+ System (Bio-Rad Laboratories, Hercules, CA, USA), followed by visualization after Coomassie brilliant blue (CBB) staining.

*2.6. Enzymatic Activity Assay and Thermostability Assessment of AgUox-WT and AgUox-frTet Variants*

AgUox variants (100 μL at 120 nM in enzyme activity assay buffer (50 mM sodium borate with 150 mM NaCl)) were mixed with 100 μL of 200 μM uric acid in enzyme activity assay buffer. The degradation of uric acid was then measured using the absorbance of the mixture solution at 293 nm. Enzyme activities were expressed as specific activity (U/mg AgUox). One unit (U) of activity was defined as the amount of enzyme that catalyzed the oxidation of 1.0 μmol of uric acid per minute at 25 °C. The serum activity of the AgUox-WT and AgUox-frTet variants was measured by an enzymatic activity assay of diluted serum in the enzyme assay buffer containing uric acid. Briefly, 10 μL of serum separated from whole blood at different time points was diluted in 90 μL of enzyme activity assay buffer and then mixed with 100 μL of 200 μM uric acid solution, and absorbance was measured at 293 nm. To measure the thermostability of AgUox variants, each variant was incubated for 10 days in PBS (pH 7.4) and subjected to the enzyme activity assay described above at 0, 5, and 10 days.

*2.7. Generation of HSA-Conjugated AgUox-frTet Variants*

HSA was subjected to the elimination of high-molecular weight aggregates using anion exchange chromatography (Hitrap Q HP column) in 20 mM Tris buffer (pH 7.0), as previously reported [21,31]. Purified HSA was desalted with PBS (pH 7.0), and reacted with TCO-MAL heterobifunctional crosslinker at a molar ratio of 1:4 for 2 h at room temperature. Afterwards, the mixtures were desalted with PBS (pH 7.4), generating the HSA-TCO conjugate. Purified AgUox-frTet variants were mixed with HSA-TCO at a molar ratio of 1:4 for 5 h at room temperature, and then analyzed by SDS-PAGE to identify the site-specific albumin conjugation yield. For further activity and pharmacokinetic studies, the HSA-conjugated AgUox-196frTet (AgUox-196HSA) was separated from the reaction mixture using size-exclusion chromatography. The elution peak corresponding to the Uox-HSA conjugate was used for an enzyme activity assay and pharmacokinetic studies after measuring the molecular weight by SDS-PAGE analysis.

### 2.8. Pharmacokinetic Studies

Briefly, 4.4 nmol (monomeric AgUox basis) of AgUox-WT or AgUox-HSA4 in 200 μL PBS (pH 7.4) was intravenously injected into the tail of young female BALB/c mice ($n = 4$). To evaluate the serum half-life of AgUox variants in vivo, retro-orbital blood collection was performed at 15 min and 3, 6, and 12 h for AgUox-WT; and 15 min and 3, 6, 12, 24, 48, and 72 h post-injection for AgUox-HSA. Serum activity was measured in serum isolated from the different whole blood samples collected.

## 3. Results and Discussion

### 3.1. Preparation of AgUox-WT and AgUox Containing frTet (AgUox-frTet) Variants

As the first step for preparing HSA-conjugated AgUox variants, the optimal sites of AgUox for HSA conjugation were determined. In order to investigate the similarities between AfUox and AgUox, we performed amino acid sequence alignment and overlapped the crystal structures of AfUox and AgUox. The identity of the two amino acid sequences was only 38.5% (Figure S2). Due to the low identity, the crystal structures of AfUox and AgUox were poorly overlapped (Figure S3). Therefore, it was not straightforward to choose a site for frTet incorporation by comparing the amino acid sequence and crystal structures of the two Uox molecules. In the case of AfUox, the solvent accessibility and hydrophobicity of site were taken into consideration. However, a mutation often leads to misfolding or unfolding of a protein. Therefore, we performed a more systemic approach. Using PyRosetta, we calculated the energy score of AgUox variants containing a single mutation. Thus, the energy score of each variant was translated into its relative folding stability [29,32,33]. In order to mimic the mutation to frTet (a phenylalanine analog), the mutation to either Y or W was introduced to various sites of AgUox-WT. The top 14 sites for which the energy scores upon the mutation to both Y and W were greater than or comparable to that of AgUox-WT (Table S2), along with the 14 AgUox mutants containing frTet (AgUox-frTet) (named as Ag1–14, Figure 1), were identified. In order to prepare 14 AgUox-frTet variants, an amber codon was introduced to each of the 14 sites of AgUox-WT by PCR-mediated mutagenesis. Then, C321delAexp *E. coli* cells [34] were co-transformed into pDule C11RS plasmid [35] encoding the engineered MjtRNA$^{Tyr}$/MjTyrRS specific for ftTet as well as the vectors with each AgUox variant. The transformants were cultured to express each AgUox-frTet variant as described in 'Materials and Methods' (Section 2.3). In the CBB-stained protein gel, a molecular weight of 34 kDa, which corresponded to the monomeric AgUox, was detected in lanes of the cell lysate after induction and purified AgUox-frTet (Figure 2). Overall, these results demonstrate the successful expression and purification of AgUox-WT and AgUox-frTet variants.

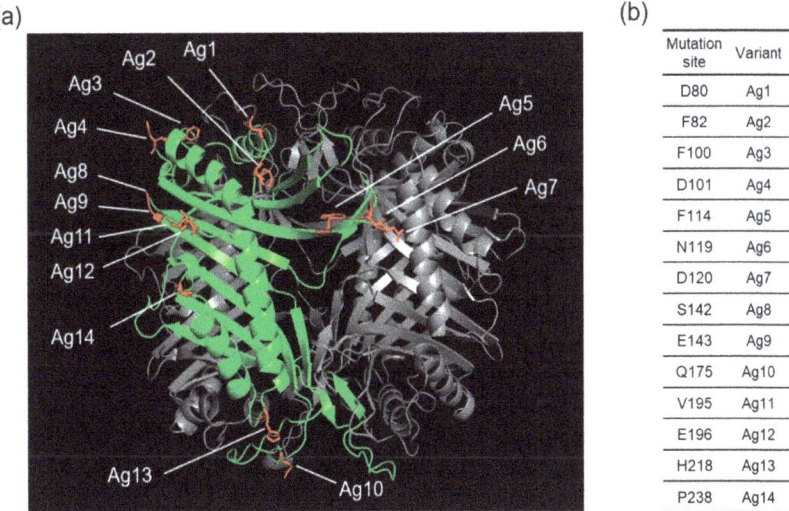

**Figure 1.** (a) Crystal structure of AgUox (PDB code: 2YZE) showing the selected sites for frTet incorporation. (b) The frTet incorporation sites and corresponding AgUox variants containing frTet are indicated in the table.

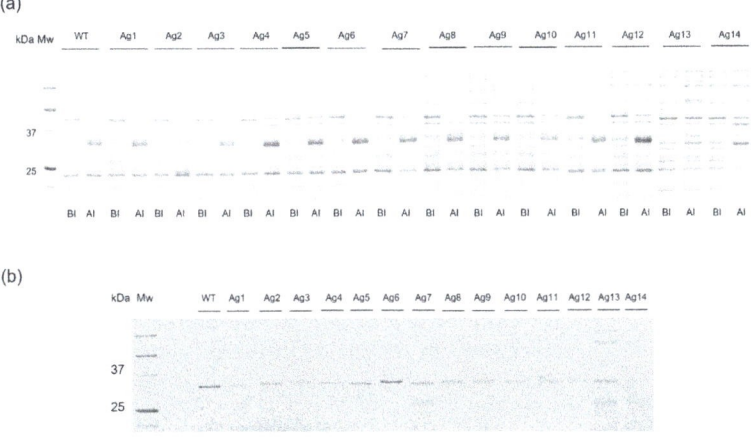

**Figure 2.** Expression and purification of AgUox-frTet variants. (a) Coomassie blue-stained protein gels of AgUox-WT and AgUox-frTet (Ag1–14) variants. Lanes: MW, molecular weight marker; BI, before induction; AI, after induction. (b) Image of Coomassie blue-stained protein gels of AgUox-WT and AgUox-frTet variants after purification.

## 3.2. Enzymatic Activity and Thermostability Assays of AgUox Variants

To investigate whether the site-specific incorporation of frTet into AgUox affected its biological function, the enzymatic activities of purified AgUox-WT and AgUox-frTet variants were compared. The enzymatic activities of the AgUox-frTet variants varied between 1 and 93% relative to that of AgUox-WT (Figure 3a), indicating that the frTet incorporation site significantly affects the function of AgUox. The AgUox-frTet variants Ag1, 6, 8, 10, and 12 exhibited relatively high enzymatic activity (Figure 3a). The active sites of AgUox are located at the interfaces between monomers [36]. Noteworthily, the frTet incorporation sites of those variants (Ag1, 6, 8, 10, and 12) were far away from the active sites and interfaces between monomers.

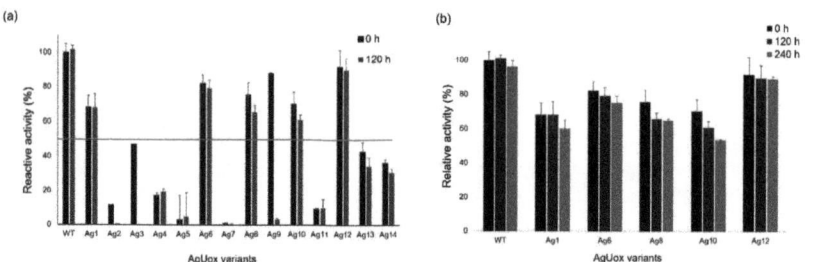

**Figure 3.** Thermostability assessment of AgUox-WT and AgUox-frTet variants. (**a**) Relative enzyme activity of AgUox-WT and AgUox-frTet (Ag1–14) variants in PBS monitored at 0 and 120 h. Red line indicates the 50% enzymatic activity of AgUox-WT. (**b**) Relative enzymatic activity of AgUox-WT and five AgUox-frTet variants (Ag1, 6, 8, 10, and 12) monitored at 0, 120, and 240 h. The relative activity of AgUox-frTet variants was normalized against the enzymatic activity of AgUox-WT.

AgUox-WT was reported to be thermostable [4]. In order to evaluate the thermostability of AgUox-frTet variants, the AgUox-frTet variants as well as AgUox-WT were incubated at 37 °C for five days, after which enzymatic activity assays were performed. As expected, no activity loss of AgUox-WT was observed after the 5-day incubation (Figure 3a). Among the 14 AgUox-frTet variants, Ag1, 6, 8, 10, and 12 exhibited more than 50% activity of AgUox-WT after the same period (Figure 3a). Those five variants were incubated for up to 10 days at 37 °C, after which Ag1, 6, 8, and 10 still showed an activity higher than 50% of AgUox-WT (Figure 3b). Although some activity loss was observed after the 10-day incubation, the Ag12 variant maintained an enzymatic activity similar to that of AgUox-WT (Figure 3b).

*3.3. Confirmation of the Site-Specific frTet Incorporation to AgUox*

To confirm the frTet incorporation into each site on AgUox, we performed the fluorescence dye labeling of intact AgUox-frTet variants. As representative cases, the five AgUox-frTet variants with a relatively high activity (Ag1, 6, 8, 10, and 12) were analyzed. First, we performed the fluorescence dye labeling using TCO-Cy3 to confirm the IEDDA reactivity of AgUox-frTet variants. Evaluation of the fluorescent image of the protein gel revealed no band in AgUox-WT samples, indicating no IEDDA reactivity of AgUox-WT (Figure 4). In contrast, the Ag1, 6, 8, 10, and 12 variants clearly exhibited the band in both the fluorescence image of protein gel and the CBB-stained protein gel, confirming the IEDDA reactivity of AgUox-frTet variants (Figure 4).

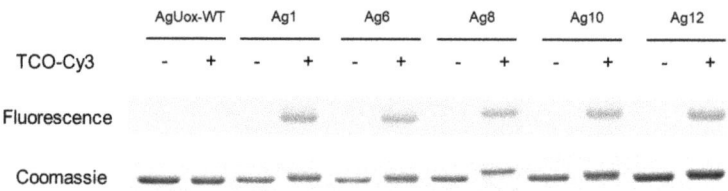

**Figure 4.** Incorporation of frTet into AgUox. Fluorescence (illumination λex = 302 nm, with wavelengths at 510 and 610 nm in Chemidoc XRS+ system) and Coomassie blue-stained protein gel for reaction mixture of TCO-Cy3 with AgUox-WT or AgUox-frTet (Ag) variants.

Next, frTet incorporation was further confirmed by MALDI-TOF MS of trypsin-digested AgUox-frTet (Ag1, 6, 8, 10, and 12) variants using AgUox-WT as control (Figure S4).

In the mass spectra of trypsin-digested AgUox-frTet variants, the observed masses of fragments containing frTet matched well with the respective theoretical values with a deviation of less than 0.05% (Table S3). These results confirm the site-specific incorporation of frTet into specific sites of AgUox-frTet variants.

### 3.4. Site-Specific HSA-Conjugation to AgUox-frTet

To prepare HSA-conjugated AgUox, we used the heterobifunctional crosslinker, TCO-MAL. First, TCO-MAL was conjugated to the free cysteine at position 34 (Cys34) of HSA via Michael addition. Since the only free cysteine (Cys34) on the HSA surface is located away from the FcRn binding domain, it has been frequently used for bioconjugation [37–40]. Then, TCO-HSA was conjugated to the purified AgUox-frTet variants via the IEDDA reaction to generate AgUox-HSA conjugates. The reaction mixtures were subjected to SDS-PAGE analysis (Figure 5). In the CBB-stained protein gel, the bands for HSA-conjugated AgUox-frTet (Ag1, 6, 8, 10, and 12) variants were clearly observed in the range of 100–120 kDa (Figure 5). In case of Ag1, 8, and 12 variants, no band of monomeric AgUox was observed, indicating the almost complete conjugation of AgUox to HSA. In the case of Ag6 and 10, the band of AgUox monomer was observed within 25–37 kDa, indicating poor AgUox conjugation to HSA. The trend in the HSA conjugation yield of Ag variants, except for Ag8, was similar to that of solvent accessibility (Ag1, 6, 8, 10, and 12: 0.93, 0.51, 0.9, 0.85, and 0.92, respectively). Since the Ag12 variant exhibited the highest HSA conjugation yield, as well as the highest enzymatic activity, it was selected for further characterization. To confirm the generation of Ag12-HSA, we performed MALDI-TOF MS analysis of the reaction mixture generating Ag12-HSA as well as AgUox-WT. The observed mass of intact AgUox-WT in the mass spectrum was 33,312 Da, which is quite consistent with its expected mass (33,305 Da) with a deviation of 0.03% (Figure S5a). In the mass spectrum of the conjugation mixture of Ag-HSA, three bands were observed. The band at 66,779 Da was expected to be that for HSA-TCO, as it matched well with its theoretical mass of 66,770 Da. The observed masses of Ag12 and Ag-HSA were 33,394, 66,779, and 100,378 Da, which are quite consistent with their expected masses (33,403, 66,770, and 100,363 Da), respectively (Figure S5b).

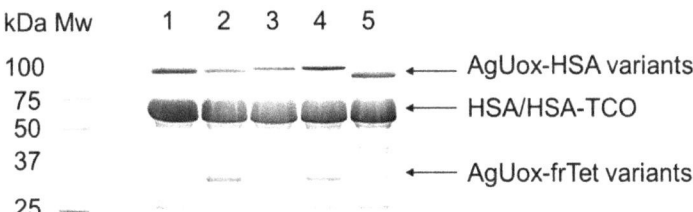

**Figure 5.** SDS-PAGE analysis of AgUox-HSA conjugate variants. The protein gel was visualized using Coomassie blue staining. Lanes: MW, molecular weight marker; 1, AgUox-HSA from Ag1 variant; 2, AgUox-HSA from Ag6 variant; 3, AgUox-HSA from Ag8 variant; 4, AgUox-HSA from Ag10 variant; 5, AgUox-HSA from Ag12 variant.

### 3.5. Enzymatic Activity of the AgUox-HSA Conjugate

We purified the HSA-conjugated Ag12 variant (Ag12-HSA) from the reaction mixture using size-exclusion chromatography. The eluted fractions in the chromatograms were analyzed by SDS-PAGE (Figure 6). The two major peaks indicate the Ag12-HSA and unreacted HSA-TCO, respectively, whereas the peak for Ag12 monomer was not detected, indicating that the HSA conjugation yield was high. The specific activities of Ag12 and Ag12-HSA were 51.7 and 52.3 U/mg AgUox, respectively, which were approximately 93%

of that of AgUox-WT (Figure 7). The specific activity of AgUox variants was calculated based on the weight of AgUox in order to avoid the underestimation of the specific activity of AgUox-HSA conjugates due to the weight of HSA molecules. These results indicate that the Ag12 variant is suitable for site-specific HSA conjugation with the retained enzymatic activity.

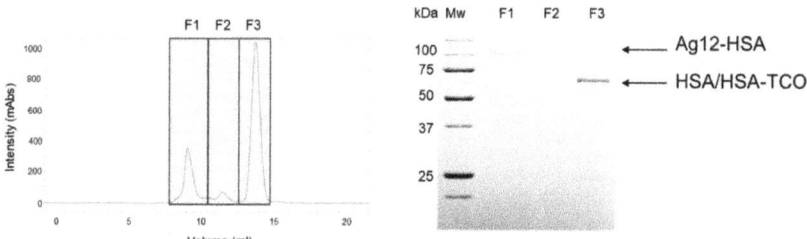

**Figure 6.** Purification of HSA-conjugated Ag12 variant (Ag12-HSA). Size-exclusion chromatography of Ag12-HSA conjugate mixture (**right**) and SDS-PAGE analysis of the eluted fractions (F1–F3) of Ag12-HSA (**left**). The protein gel was stained by Coomassie blue for the visualization of protein bands. Lanes: MW, molecular weight marker.

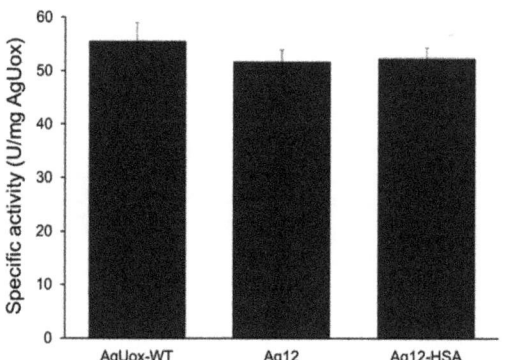

**Figure 7.** Specific activity of AgUox-WT, Ag12, and Ag12-HSA. Experiments were performed in quadruplicate, and error bars indicate the standard deviation.

### 3.6. Pharmacokinetic Study of AgUox-WT and Ag12-HSA

We measured the serum half-lives of AgUox-WT and Ag12-HSA after intravenous administration to mice. Moreover, the enzymatic activity of AgUox species in the serum samples was monitored. The serum half-life of AgUox-WT was about 1.7 h (Figure 8), which was longer than that of AfUox-WT (1.3 h) [30]. We also observed that the serum half-life of the Ag12-HSA conjugate was 29 h, which was approximately 17-times higher than that of AgUox-WT (Figure 8), indicating that HSA conjugation effectively prolonged the serum half-life of AgUox. Noteworthily, the serum half-life of Ag12-HSA conjugate was longer than that of AfUox-HSA (21 h) [30]. Considering that both Ag12-HSA and AfUox-HSA have four HSA molecules conjugated to each Uox molecule with the same linker, we believe that the difference observed in their serum half-life results from thermostability differences. In the case of AfUox-HSA, the serum half-life of Ag12-HSA was assessed by measuring the enzyme activity of the AgUox variant remaining in the serum. Taken together, these results highlight the thermostability of AgUox and how it retains its enzymatic activity in vivo. Furthermore, these data indicate that the conjugation of HSA to AgUox, which has high thermostability, results in a significantly longer serum half-life in vivo.

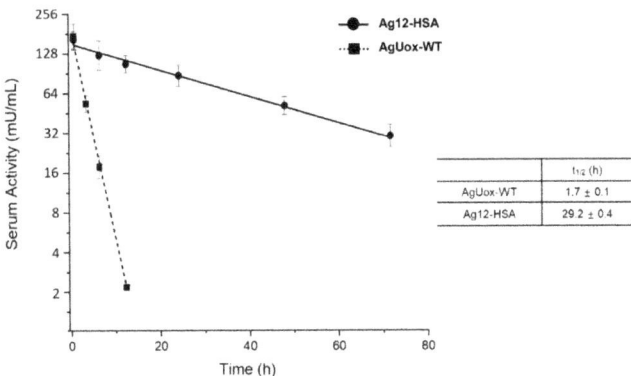

**Figure 8.** Pharmacokinetic studies of AgUox-WT and Ag12-HSA in mice. Enzymatic activity of residual AgUox-WT and Ag12-HSA conjugate samples was measured at 15 min; at 3, 6, and 12 h for AgUox-WT; and 15 min and 12, 24, 48, and 72 h for Ag12-HSA. The samples for pharmacokinetic studies were intravenously injected into BALB/c female mice ($n$ = 4). Error bars indicate the standard deviation.

## 4. Conclusions

AgUox is a promising therapeutic candidate for gout treatment because of its high thermostability and low immunogenicity. To further develop AgUox as a therapeutic agent, we achieved site-specific HSA conjugation to AgUox, resulting in the significantly prolonged circulation time in vivo compared with AgUox-WT and AfUox-HSA, likely due to the high thermostability of AgUox and the FcRn-mediated recycling of HSA. We demonstrated that the computational stability prediction of AgUox variants containing frTet successfully led to identification of 14 stable AgUox-frTet variants. As expected, approximately half of these variants retained enzymatic activity and relatively high thermostability. In particular, AgUox-196frTet (Ag12) showed enzyme activity and thermostability comparable to those of AgUox-WT. Pharmacokinetic studies further showed that the serum half-life of Ag12-HSA was extended to 29 h, which was approximately 17 times longer than that of AgUox-WT. Hence, we believe that the HSA-conjugated AgUox would be a good therapeutic candidate for severe gout treatment. Since the Uox-based therapeutics are very expensive compared to other small molecule-based urate lowering drugs, their use would be limited to patients with severe and refractory gout.

**Supplementary Materials:** The following are available online at https://www.mdpi.com/article/10.3390/pharmaceutics13081298/s1, Figure S1. Time-course enzymatic activity of AfUox-WT and AgUox-WT; Figure S2. Alignment of the amino acid sequences of AgUox and AfUox; Figure S3. The crystal structures of (**a**) AgUox, (**b**) AfUox, and (**c**) The overlapped structures of AgUox and AfUox; Figure S4. Matrix-assisted laser desorption/ionization-time of flight mass spectra (MALDI-TOF MS) of trypsin-digested (**a**) Ag1, (**b**) Ag6, (**c**) Ag8, (**d**) Ag10, and (**e**) Ag12; Figure S5. MALDI-TOF mass spectra of AgUox-WT (**a**) and the conjugate mixture generating Ag12-HSA (**b**); Table S1. Primers used for the site-directed mutagenesis of AgUox; Table S2. Rosetta scores of AgUox after point mutation into tryptophan or tyrosine; Table S3. List of masses of trypsin-digested AgUox-frTet variants.

**Author Contributions:** Conceptualization, B.Y. and I.K.; formal analysis, B.Y. and I.K.; investigation, B.Y.; methodology, B.Y.; resources, I.K.; supervision, I.K.; writing—original draft preparation, B.Y. and I.K.; writing—review and editing, B.Y. and I.K. Both authors have read and agreed to the published version of the manuscript.

**Funding:** This research was funded by the National Research Foundation of Korea (NRF), funded by the Ministry of Science and ICT (Grant No. 2019R1A2C1084910 and 2021R1A5A1028138).

**Institutional Review Board Statement:** All animal studies were conducted according to the Guidelines for Care and Use of Laboratory Animals proposed by GIST and approved by the Animal Ethics Committee of GIST (Approval number: GIST-2020-037 [6 April 2020]).

**Informed Consent Statement:** Not applicable.

**Data Availability Statement:** The supporting data presented in this study are available in Supplementary Materials.

**Acknowledgments:** The authors are grateful to George Church at Harvard Medical School for a generous gift of 321.ΔA.exp (Addgene plasmid #49018).

**Conflicts of Interest:** The authors declare no conflict of interest.

# References

1. Mccarty, D.J.; Hollander, J.L. Identification of urate crystals in gouty synovial fluid. *Ann. Intern. Med.* **1961**, *54*, 452–460. [CrossRef]
2. Harris, M.D.; Siegel, L.B.; Alloway, J.A. Gout and Hyperuricemia. *Am. Fam. Physician* **1999**, *59*, 925. [PubMed]
3. Burns, C.M.; Wortmann, R.L. Gout therapeutics: New drugs for an old disease. *Lancet* **2011**, *377*, 165–177. [CrossRef]
4. Nyborg, A.C.; Ward, C.; Zacco, A.; Chacko, B.; Grinberg, L.; Geoghegan, J.C.; Bean, R.; Wendeler, M.; Bartnik, F.; O'Connor, E.; et al. A therapeutic uricase with reduced immunogenicity risk and improved development properties. *PLoS ONE* **2016**, *11*, e0167935. [CrossRef] [PubMed]
5. Ramazzina, I.; Folli, C.; Secchi, A.; Berni, R.; Percudani, R. Completing the uric acid degradation pathway through phylogenetic comparison of whole genomes. *Nat. Chem. Biol.* **2006**, *2*, 144–148. [CrossRef] [PubMed]
6. Kahn, K.; Serfozo, P.; Tipton, P.A. Identification of the true product of the urate oxidase reaction. *J. Am. Chem. Soc.* **1997**, *119*, 5435–5442. [CrossRef]
7. Iwata, H.; Nishio, S.; Yokoyama, M.; Matsumoto, A.; Takeuchi, M. Solubility of uric acid and supersaturation of monosodium urate: Why is uric acid so highly soluble in urine? *J. Urol.* **1989**, *142*, 1095–1098. [CrossRef]
8. Tetko, I.V.; Tanchuk, V.Y.; Kasheva, T.N.; Villa, A.E. Estimation of aqueous solubility of chemical compounds using E-state indices. *J. Chem. Inf. Comput. Sci.* **2001**, *41*, 1488–1493. [CrossRef]
9. Vogt, B. Urate oxidase (rasburicase) for treatment of severe tophaceous gout. *Nephrol. Dial. Transplant.* **2005**, *20*, 431–433. [CrossRef]
10. Coiffier, B.; Mounier, N.; Bologna, S.; Fermé, C.; Tilly, H.; Sonet, A.; Christian, B.; Casasnovas, O.; Jourdan, E.; Belhadj, K.; et al. Efficacy and safety of rasburicase (recombinant urate oxidase) for the prevention and treatment of hyperuricemia during induction chemotherapy of aggressive non-Hodgkin's lymphoma: Results of the GRAAL1 (Grouped'Etude des Lymphomes de l'Adulte Trial on Rasburicase Activity in Adult Lymphoma) study. *J. Clin. Oncol.* **2003**, *21*, 4402–4406. [CrossRef]
11. Ryu, J.K.; Kim, H.S.; Nam, D.H. Current status and perspectives of biopharmaceutical drugs. *Biotechnol. Bioprocess Eng.* **2012**, *17*, 900–911. [CrossRef]
12. Schlesinger, N.; Yasothan, U.; Kirkpatrick, P. Pegloticase. *Nat. Rev. Drug Discov.* **2011**, *10*, 17–18. [CrossRef] [PubMed]
13. Sundy, J.S.; Baraf, H.S.B.; Yood, R.A.; Edwards, N.L.; Gutierrez-Urena, S.R.; Treadwell, E.L.; Vázquez-Mellado, J.; White, W.B.; Lipsky, P.E.; Horowitz, Z.; et al. Efficacy and tolerability of pegloticase for the treatment of chronic gout in patients refractory to conventional treatment: Two randomized controlled trials. *J. Am. Med. Assoc.* **2011**, *306*, 711–720. [CrossRef]
14. Sundy, J.S.; Becker, M.A.; Baraf, H.S.B.; Barkhuizen, A.; Moreland, L.W.; Huang, W.; Waltrip, R.W.; Maroli, A.N.; Horowitz, Z. Reduction of plasma urate levels following treatment with multiple doses of pegloticase (polyethylene glycol-conjugated uricase) in patients with treatment-failure gout: Results of a phase II randomized study. *Arthritis Rheum.* **2008**, *58*, 2882–2891. [CrossRef] [PubMed]
15. Tao, L.; Li, D.; Li, Y.; Shi, X.; Wang, J.; Rao, C.; Zhang, Y. Designing a mutant Candida uricase with improved polymerization state and enzymatic activity. *Protein Eng. Des. Sel.* **2017**, *30*, 753–759. [CrossRef]
16. Kratz, F. Albumin as a drug carrier: Design of prodrugs, drug conjugates and nanoparticles. *J. Control. Release* **2008**, *132*, 171–183. [CrossRef]
17. Sleep, D. Albumin and its application in drug delivery. *Expert Opin. Drug Deliv.* **2015**, *12*, 793–812. [CrossRef]
18. Bern, M.; Sand, K.M.K.; Nilsen, J.; Sandlie, I.; Andersen, J.T. The role of albumin receptors in regulation of albumin homeostasis: Implications for drug delivery. *J. Control. Release* **2015**, *211*, 144–162. [CrossRef]
19. Curry, S.; Mandelkow, H.; Brick, P.; Franks, N. Crystal structure of human serum albumin complexed with fatty acid reveals an asymmetric distribution of binding sites. *Nat. Struct. Biol.* **1998**, *5*, 827–835. [CrossRef] [PubMed]
20. Elsadek, B.; Kratz, F. Impact of albumin on drug delivery—New applications on the horizon. *J. Control. Release* **2012**, *157*, 4–28. [CrossRef]
21. Lim, S.I.; Hahn, Y.S.; Kwon, I. Site-specific albumination of a therapeutic protein with multi-subunit to prolong activity in vivo. *J. Control. Release* **2015**, *207*, 93–100. [CrossRef]
22. Cho, J.; Park, J.; Kim, S.; Kim, J.C.; Tae, G.; Jin, M.S.; Kwon, I. Intramolecular distance in the conjugate of urate oxidase and fatty acid governs FcRn binding and serum half-life in vivo. *J. Control. Release* **2020**, *321*, 49–58. [CrossRef]

23. Deehan, M.; Garcês, S.; Kramer, D.; Baker, M.P.; Rat, D.; Roettger, Y.; Kromminga, A. Managing unwanted immunogenicity of biologicals. *Autoimmun. Rev.* **2015**, *14*, 569–574. [CrossRef]
24. Suzuki, K.; Sakasegawa, S.I.; Misaki, H.; Sugiyama, M. Molecular cloning and expression of uricase gene from *Arthrobacter globiformis* in *Escherichia coli* and characterization of the gene product. *J. Biosci. Bioeng.* **2004**, *98*, 153–158. [CrossRef]
25. Andersen, J.T.; Dalhus, B.; Viuff, D.; Ravn, B.T.; Gunnarsen, K.S.; Plumridge, A.; Bunting, K.; Antunes, F.; Williamson, R.; Athwal, S.; et al. Extending Serum Half-life of Albumin by Engineering Neonatal Fc Receptor (FcRn) Binding. *J. Biol. Chem.* **2014**, *289*, 13492. [CrossRef] [PubMed]
26. Duttaroy, A.; Kanakaraj, P.; Osborn, B.L.; Schneider, H.; Pickeral, O.K.; Chen, C.; Zhang, G.; Kaithamana, S.; Singh, M.; Schulingkamp, R.; et al. Development of a Long-Acting Insulin Analog Using Albumin Fusion Technology. *Diabetes* **2005**, *54*, 251–258. [CrossRef] [PubMed]
27. Chen, H.; Wang, G.; Lang, L.; Jacobson, O.; Kiesewetter, D.O.; Liu, Y.; Ma, Y.; Zhang, X.; Wu, H.; Zhu, L.; et al. Chemical conjugation of evans blue derivative: A strategy to develop long-acting therapeutics through albumin binding. *Theranostics* **2016**, *6*, 243–253. [CrossRef] [PubMed]
28. Chaudhury, S.; Lyskov, S.; Gray, J.J. PyRosetta: A script-based interface for implementing molecular modeling algorithms using Rosetta. *Bioinformatics* **2010**, *26*, 689–691. [CrossRef]
29. Alford, R.F.; Leaver-Fay, A.; Jeliazkov, J.R.; O'Meara, M.J.; DiMaio, F.P.; Park, H.; Shapovalov, M.V.; Renfrew, P.D.; Mulligan, V.K.; Kappel, K.; et al. The Rosetta All-Atom Energy Function for Macromolecular Modeling and Design. *J. Chem. Theory Comput.* **2017**, *13*, 3031–3048. [CrossRef]
30. Yang, B.; Kwon, I. Multivalent albumin-FcRn interactions mediate a prominent extension of the serum half-life of a therapeutic protein. *Mol. Pharm.* **2021**, *18*, 2397–2405. [CrossRef]
31. Yang, B.; Lim, S.I.; Kim, J.C.; Tae, G.; Kwon, I. Site-Specific Albumination as an Alternative to PEGylation for the Enhanced Serum Half-Life in Vivo. *Biomacromolecules* **2016**, *17*, 1811–1817. [CrossRef] [PubMed]
32. O'Meara, M.J.; Leaver-Fay, A.; Tyka, M.D.; Stein, A.; Houlihan, K.; Dimaio, F.; Bradley, P.; Kortemme, T.; Baker, D.; Snoeyink, J.; et al. Combined covalent-electrostatic model of hydrogen bonding improves structure prediction with Rosetta. *J. Chem. Theory Comput.* **2015**, *11*, 609–622. [CrossRef] [PubMed]
33. Park, H.; Bradley, P.; Greisen, P.; Liu, Y.; Mulligan, V.K.; Kim, D.E.; Baker, D.; Dimaio, F. Simultaneous Optimization of Biomolecular Energy Functions on Features from Small Molecules and Macromolecules. *J. Chem. Theory Comput.* **2016**, *12*, 6201–6212. [CrossRef] [PubMed]
34. Lajoie, M.J.; Rovner, A.J.; Goodman, D.B.; Aerni, H.-R.; Haimovich, A.D.; Kuznetsov, G.; Mercer, J.A.; Wang, H.H.; Carr, P.A.; Mosberg, J.A.; et al. Genomically recoded organisms expand biological functions. *Science* **2013**, *342*, 357–360. [CrossRef] [PubMed]
35. Yang, B.; Kwon, K.; Jana, S.; Kim, S.; Avila-Crump, S.; Tae, G.; Mehl, R.A.; Kwon, I. Temporal control of efficient in vivo bioconjugation using a genetically encoded tetrazine-mediated inverse-electron-demand Diels-Alder reaction. *Bioconjug. Chem.* **2020**, *31*, 2456–2464. [CrossRef] [PubMed]
36. Juan, E.C.M.; Hoque, M.M.; Shimizu, S.; Hossain, M.T.; Yamamoto, T.; Imamura, S.; Suzuki, K.; Tsunoda, M.; Amano, H.; Sekiguchi, T.; et al. Structures of Arthrobacterglobiformis urate oxidase-ligand complexes. *Acta Crystallogr. Sect. D Biol. Crystallogr.* **2008**, *64*, 815–822. [CrossRef]
37. Schmidt, M.M.; Townson, S.A.; Andreucci, A.J.; King, B.M.; Schirmer, E.B.; Murillo, A.J.; Dombrowski, C.; Tisdale, A.W.; Lowden, P.A.; Masci, A.L.; et al. Crystal structure of an HSA/FcRn complex reveals recycling by competitive mimicry of HSA ligands at a pH-dependent hydrophobic interface. *Structure* **2013**, *21*, 1966–1978. [CrossRef]
38. Anderson, B.J.; Holford, N.H.G. Mechanistic basis of using body size and maturation to predict clearance in humans. *Drug Metab. Pharmacokinet.* **2009**, *24*, 25–36. [CrossRef]
39. Andersen, J.T.; Dalhus, B.; Cameron, J.; Daba, M.B.; Plumridge, A.; Evans, L.; Brennan, S.O.; Gunnarsen, K.S.; Bjørås, M.; Sleep, D.; et al. Structure-based mutagenesis reveals the albumin-binding site of the neonatal Fc receptor. *Nat. Commun.* **2012**, *3*, 610. [CrossRef] [PubMed]
40. Rahimizadeh, P.; Yang, S.; Lim, S.I. Albumin: An emerging opportunity in drug delivery. *Biotechnol. Bioprocess Eng.* **2020**, *25*, 985–995. [CrossRef]

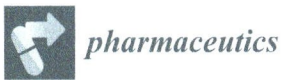

Article

# A Recombinant Fusion Construct between Human Serum Albumin and NTPDase CD39 Allows Anti-Inflammatory and Anti-Thrombotic Coating of Medical Devices

Meike-Kristin Abraham [1,2,3,†], Elena Jost [1,2,3,†], Jan David Hohmann [2,†], Amy Kate Searle [2,3,4], Viktoria Bongcaron [2,3], Yuyang Song [3,5], Hans Peter Wendel [1], Karlheinz Peter [2,4,5,6,*,‡], Stefanie Krajewski [1,‡] and Xiaowei Wang [3,4,5,6,*,‡]

1. Clinical Research Laboratory, Department of Thoracic, Cardiac and Vascular Surgery, University Hospital Tübingen, 72076 Tübingen, Germany; meike-kristin.abraham@hotmail.de (M.-K.A.); elenabarb.jost@gmail.com (E.J.); hans-peter.wendel@med.uni-tuebingen.de (H.P.W.); stefanie.krajewski@med.uni-tuebingen.de (S.K.)
2. Atherothrombosis and Vascular Biology, Baker Heart & Diabetes Institute, Melbourne, VIC 3004, Australia; jan_david_hohmann@outlook.com (J.D.H.); asearle@student.unimelb.edu.au (A.K.S.); viktoria.bongcaron@baker.edu.au (V.B.)
3. Molecular Imaging and Theranostics Laboratory, Baker Heart & Diabetes Institute, Melbourne, VIC 3004, Australia; yuyang.song@baker.edu.au
4. Department of Medicine, Monash University, Melbourne, VIC 3800, Australia
5. Department of Cardiometabolic Health, University of Melbourne, Melbourne, VIC 3010, Australia
6. La Trobe Institute for Molecular Science, La Trobe University, Melbourne, VIC 3086, Australia
\* Correspondence: karlheinz.peter@baker.edu.au (K.P.); xiaowei.wang@baker.edu.au (X.W.)
† Equally contributing first authors.
‡ Equally contributing senior authors.

**Abstract:** Medical devices directly exposed to blood are commonly used to treat cardiovascular diseases. However, these devices are associated with inflammatory reactions leading to delayed healing, rejection of foreign material or device-associated thrombus formation. We developed a novel recombinant fusion protein as a new biocompatible coating strategy for medical devices with direct blood contact. We genetically fused human serum albumin (HSA) with ectonucleoside triphosphate diphosphohydrolase-1 (CD39), a promising anti-thrombotic and anti-inflammatory drug candidate. The HSA-CD39 fusion protein is highly functional in degrading ATP and ADP, major pro-inflammatory reagents and platelet agonists. Their enzymatic properties result in the generation of AMP, which is further degraded by CD73 to adenosine, an anti-inflammatory and anti-platelet reagent. HSA-CD39 is functional after lyophilisation, coating and storage of coated materials for up to 8 weeks. HSA-CD39 coating shows promising and stable functionality even after sterilisation and does not hinder endothelialisation of primary human endothelial cells. It shows a high level of haemocompatibility and diminished blood cell adhesion when coated on nitinol stents or polyvinylchloride tubes. In conclusion, we developed a new recombinant fusion protein combining HSA and CD39, and demonstrated that it has potential to reduce thrombotic and inflammatory complications often associated with medical devices directly exposed to blood.

**Keywords:** albumin; anti-thrombotic; CD39; coating of medical devices; stent coating; therapeutic fusion protein

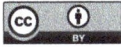

## 1. Introduction

Cardiovascular diseases such as ischemic heart disease and stroke are the world's leading causes of death. The World Health Organization states that 16% of total deaths can be traced back to these diseases [1]. Treatment of patients with cardiovascular problems often includes the invasive application of medical devices. Often these medical devices will be directly exposed to blood, e.g., vascular grafts, stents, permanently implantable biosensors such as pacemakers and defibrillators. The biomaterials used for blood-contacting devices represent foreign surfaces to human blood and therefore have the potential to induce specific inflammatory and pro-thrombotic reactions that can lead to clinical complications. The underlying pathological mechanisms of these complications are surface-induced reactions of plasma proteins, platelets and leukocytes. Uncoated medical devices often adsorb blood plasma proteins, such as fibrinogen, on their surfaces, thereby inducing an inflammatory process, platelet adhesion and activation of the coagulation [2–6]. Adsorbed proteins further mediate platelet aggregation and, in combination with fibrin, can form a platelet-fibrin thrombus [7]. The activation of platelet aggregation and the coagulation cascade may lead to severe and life-threatening thrombosis on the surfaces of biomaterials [3,7].

Both long-term medical devices (often used for a patient's lifetime) and short-term blood-contacting systems (mainly used for short-term treatment of critically ill patients) need to be examined for their haemocompatibility and thrombogenicity. During extracorporeal membrane oxygenation, the patient's blood comes into contact with foreign material such as silicone, polyvinylchloride (PVC) or polypropylene. In a heart–lung machine, the contact of blood with the surfaces of PVC (used for tubing) and polypropylene (used in oxygenators) are the main reasons for postoperative thrombotic and bleeding complications [8,9].

Therefore, major efforts have been undertaken by material scientists and engineers with the aim of designing medical device surfaces that can resist adsorption of blood proteins and adhesion of cells, and thus be less thrombogenic and pro-inflammatory [3]. Different materials and surface coatings have been developed to enhance biocompatibility and reduce device-associated complications [2,3]. Surface modification strategies are classified in two groups: (1) surface passivation; and (2) bioactive surface coatings or treatments [2,10]. With the passivation strategy, physical and chemical modifications are made to the materials and surfaces to reduce their inherent thrombogenicity. Bioactive surface coatings are achieved by permanent immobilization via an active agent or drug to directly inhibit the coagulation cascade and prevent neointimal hyperplasia [11–13]. In addition to these, administration of anti-platelet or anti-coagulation therapeutics is used as a treatment to prevent device-induced thrombosis [13–16].

Other considerations in relation to long-term blood-exposed devices include mechanical adaption to stress. Aortic valve prostheses need to resist constantly changing pressures and high shear stress [17,18]. Permanent implantation of stents for treatment of cardiovascular diseases have shown that drug-eluting stents (DES), with a surface coating of drugs, polymers, growth factors or proteins, promise a superior healing function compared to bare-metal stents [14,17,19,20]. DES have been shown to improve the outcome of revascularization therapy by preventing neointimal hyperplasia and in-stent restenosis (ISR) [21–23]. Although the incidence of ISR can be lessened using DES, there is an increased risk of in-stent thrombosis, which requires the application of dual anti-platelet therapy. Overall, this current stent therapy has been associated with adverse bleeding events, hypersensitivity reactions and delayed endothelialisation after implantation [24,25]. Therefore, there is a clinical need for the development of safe and biocompatible surface coatings that eliminate device-induced thrombosis and inflammation.

Human serum albumin (HSA) is widely used in the medical industry for coating of stents and tubings [26,27]. Being a highly abundant protein in the blood, HSA has been shown to have anti-thrombotic properties and corrosion resistance based on its electrostatic and hydrophilic properties [18,26,28]. Additionally, HSA adsorbs easily on surfaces, prevents endothelial apoptosis, provides antioxidant protection and also inhibits platelet activation and aggregation [27,29,30]. Therefore, albumin has played a central role in many drug delivery systems [31]. HSA coating has also been applied to various biomaterials, including titanium (Ti), stainless steel and nanoparticles [26,28,32,33]. For example, dopamine-modified albumin coating showed an attenuated immune and inflammatory response on xenogeneic grafts [34]. Additionally, Oriňaková et al. demonstrated that bovine serum albumin coating changed the corrosion resistance of sintered iron biomaterials [35].

The ectonucleoside triphosphate diphosphohydrolase-1, an NTPDase (CD39), is a promising anti-thrombotic and anti-inflammatory agent [36–40]. Normally expressed on the surface of endothelial cells (ECs), CD39 prevents platelet activation and attachment through hydrolysis of the phosphate residue of ATP and ADP [38,41–43]. ATP triggers pro-inflammatory pathways, so the degradation of ATP to ADP by CD39 reduces the pro-inflammatory effect of ATP. ADP is a major player in the platelet-activation cascade [39,44]. Through further hydrolysis of ADP to AMP by CD73, CD39 is responsible for a shift from a pro-inflammatory to an anti-inflammatory environment [39,40,45]. Several studies have confirmed that CD39 activity is substantively reduced in injured or rejected grafts, and that administration of soluble CD39 may be a useful substitute post implantation [41,46].

Here, we have designed, generated and analysed a novel anti-thrombotic and anti-inflammatory recombinant fusion protein consisting of HSA and CD39 as a highly promising bioactive coating for medical devices and PVC tubes to guarantee an active, safe and natural interface between blood and medical devices.

## 2. Materials and Methods

A more detailed description of the methods is provided in the Supplementary Material.

### 2.1. Generation of Recombinant Fusion Construct, Production, Expression of Protein and Purification

Details of HSA-CD39 origin, polymerase chain reaction (PCR)-based fusion, mammalian production (HEK293 cells) and purification are provided as Supplementary Methods. The quantity of the purified protein was measured using a Pierce Protein Assay Kit (ThermoFisher Scientific, Waltham, MA, USA). The samples from purification steps were loaded onto a 12% sodium dodecyl sulfate–polyacrylamide gel for electrophoresis under denaturing conditions and visualized via Coomassie staining. The same samples were also stained on a Western blot (BioRad, Hercules, CA, USA) using an anti-Penta-His antibody (Roche, Basel, Switzerland) coupled with horseradish peroxidase.

### 2.2. Blood Sampling from Healthy Human Volunteers

All blood sampling procedures were approved by the Research and Ethics Unit of the University of Tübingen, Germany (project number 270/2010BO1) and the Ethics Committee of the Alfred Hospital, Melbourne, Australia. Unless otherwise specified, blood was collected by venepuncture from healthy volunteers who provided informed consent and was anticoagulated with citrate. All subjects were free of platelet-affecting drugs for $\geq 14$ days.

### 2.3. Preparation of Platelet-Rich Plasma

Citrated blood from volunteers was centrifuged at $180\times g$ for 10 min. Platelet-rich plasma (PRP) was collected and stored at 37 °C. Before usage it was diluted 1:10 with phosphate-buffered saline plus (PBS+; 100 mg/L calcium chloride, 100 mg/L magnesium chloride; ThermoFisher Scientific, Waltham, MA, USA). Blood and PRP were used within the first 6 h after venepuncture.

### 2.4. Flow Cytometry

The efficiency and functionality of the HSA-CD39 protein were determined using flow cytometry. The protein was incubated with 20 µM ADP (MoeLab, Langenfeld, Germany) or 5 µL PBS for 20 min. The active protein will hydrolyse ADP to AMP. Diluted PRP was added and incubated for 5 min. Platelet activation status was measured by a fluorescein isothiocyanate (FITC)-labelled monoclonal antibody PAC-1 (BD Bioscience, Franklin Lakes, NJ, USA), a R-phycoerythrin (PE)-labelled monoclonal antibody directed against CD62P (P-Selectin) (BD Bioscience, Franklin Lakes, NJ, USA) or their respective isotype antibody controls (ThermoFisher Scientific, Waltham, MA, USA). Samples were fixed using Cellfix (BD Bioscience, Franklin Lakes, NJ, USA) and analysed via fluorescence-activated cell sorting (FACS) Calibur (BD Bioscience, Franklin Lakes, NJ, USA). A total of 10,000 events were acquired in each sample.

### 2.5. ADP Bioluminescence Assay

HSA-CD39's function to directly hydrolyse ADP was measured using an ATP bioluminescence assay according to the manufacturer's description (Kit CLS II, Roche, Basel, Switzerland) [39,41]. HSA-CD39 was incubated with 20 µM ADP for 20 min. The remaining ADP was converted to ATP by the pyruvate kinase reaction, and measured using the ATP bioluminescence assay via a microplate luminometer (Mithras LB 940, Berthold Technologies, Bad Wildbad, Germany). Different concentrations of ADP, PBS and HSA (Alburex Human albumin 5%, CSL Behring, Hattersheim am Main, Germany) were also used as controls.

### 2.6. Lyophilisation of Protein

To analyse the possibility of lyophilising the HSA-CD39 protein, different concentrations were lyophilised using the CoolSafe ScanVac (LaboGene ApS, Lynge, Denmark) according to the manufacturer's description. The lyophilised samples were stored for 14 days at room temperature (RT) before rehydration and analysis of platelet activation using flow cytometry.

### 2.7. Coating of Stent Material for In Vitro Analysis

HSA-CD39 and HSA (CSL Behring, Hattersheim am Main, Germany) proteins were passively adsorbed by the different materials. The samples were diluted in PBS, added, incubated and dried on the materials with HSA-CD39 and HSA (CSL Behring, Hattersheim am Main, Germany). Materials were then stored for 24 h before flow cytometric analysis of CD39 activity. Polystyrene (BD Bioscience, Franklin Lakes, NJ, USA), 316L stainless-steel plates, Ti plates (Acandis, Pforzheim, Germany), polyurethane-coated stents (Acandis, Pforzheim, Germany) and nitinol BlueOxide stents (Acandis, Pforzheim, Germany) were coated with different protein concentrations (0.05 µg, 0.1 µg, 0.25 µg and 0.5 µg) and PBS as the control. Coated 316L stainless-steel plates were washed 3× with PBS and dried again prior to functional testing. Coated Ti plates were sterilized with ethylene oxide (EO) according to the sterilization protocol for medical devices of the University Hospital of Tübingen, Germany. Long-term-coated material was stored at RT. DERIVO nitinol BlueOxide stents (3.3 × 15 mm, Acandis, Pforzheim, Germany) were coated by dip-coating of stents with 100 µg/mL HSA-CD39 in PBS 10× and dried with argon gas between dipping steps. Coated stents were also sterilized by EO according to the sterilization protocol.

### 2.8. Endothelialisation Analysis of Protein-Coated Nitinol BlueOxide Plates

The endothelialisation efficiency of HSA-CD39-coated plates was analysed using nitinol BlueOxide plates coated with 4.0 µg/cm$^2$ HSA-CD39. Coated plates were dried at RT followed by sterilisation under UV light for 30 min. Human ECs (hECs) were isolated from saphenous vein biopsies of patients who had undergone coronary artery bypass graft surgery as previously described by Avci-Adali et al. [47]. hECs were cultivated in cell-culture flasks pre-coated with 0.1% gelatine in Vasculife® EnGS EC culture medium (CellSystems, Troisdorf, Germany) containing VascuLife EnGS LifeFactors Kit, 50 mg/mL gentamicin and 0.05 mg/mL amphotericin B (GE Healthcare, Boston, MA, USA). Cells were kept at 37 °C/5% CO$_2$ and passaged using trypsin/ethylenediaminetetraacetic acid (EDTA) (0.04%/0.03%, PromoCell, Heidelberg, Germany). For endothelialisation analysis, 150,000 cells/well were seeded on coated nitinol BlueOxide plates and incubated for 48 h. Cells were fixed and stained with 4′,6-diamidino-2-phenylindole (DAPI) (Sigma-Aldrich, Sankt Gallen, Switzerland) and analysed via epifluorescence microscopy (Blue UV2A Nikon Optiphot 2, Tokyo, Japan).

*2.9. In Vitro Haemocompatibility Testing Using Roller Pump and Modified Chandler Loop Model*

To investigate the influence of HSA-CD39-coated nitinol BlueOxide stents (nitinol BlueOxide DERIVO embolisation device, Acandis, Pforzheim, Germany) in vitro, coated plates were loaded into heparin-coated Tygon tubes (Saint Gobain Performance Plastics, Wertheim, Germany). PVC tubes (inner diameter 3.2 mm, length 75 cm) were coated with heparin by Ension (Pittsburgh, PA, USA). Through this model, the haemocompatibility of the coated stents, i.e., activation of the coagulation cascade, the complement system and inflammation, were analysed after perfusion of blood, as described in detail by Krajewski et al. [48]. Human whole blood was anticoagulated with heparin (1.5 IE/mL, Ratiopharm GmbH, Ulm, Germany). Then, each tube was filled with 6 mL freshly heparinised human blood, connected by a silicon connection tubing and circulated by a roller pump (BVP Ismatec, Wertheim, Germany) in a water bath at 37 °C for 60 min at 150 mL/min. For each of the 5 donors, 6 mL heparinised blood was used for baseline measurements before circulation. Before and after circulation, blood was taken, measured with a haematolyser (ABX Micros 60, Axon Lab AG, Baden, Switzerland) for blood cell count and further used for enzyme-linked immunosorbent assays (ELISA) (Echelon Biosciences, Salt Lake City, UT, USA) [45,46]. For measuring thrombin–antithrombin III complex (TAT complex; Enzygnost TAT Micro, Siemens Healthcare, Erlangen, Germany) via ELISA, blood was directly filled in citrate S-Monovettes® (Sarstedt AG & Co, Nümbrecht, Germany) and centrifuged at $1800 \times g$ at 22 °C for 18 min. Resulting plasma was deep-frozen in liquid nitrogen and stored at −20 °C until performance of ELISA, according to the manufacturer's description. Stents were prepared for scanning electron microscopy (SEM).

In a second experimental setup, the previously established modified chandler loop was used to test the haemocompatibility of coated ECC tubes [10,48]. PCV tubes (lengths of 50 cm; Raumedic® ECC BloodLine 1/4 × 1/16, Raumedic AG, Helmbrechts, Germany) were coated via rotating incubation with 12 mL of 20 µg/mL (240 µg) HSA or 20 µg/mL (240 µg) HSA-CD39 at RT for 3 h followed by storage at 4 °C overnight. The pH of the protein solutions were adjusted to 4.6 prior to incubation. After incubation, tubes were rinsed with PBS prior to being filled with blood. An untreated tube without blood contact, an untreated tube and a commercially available heparin-coated tube (Carmeda BioActive Surface®, Medtronic, Dublin, Ireland) were used as controls. Coated tubes were filled with fresh, pooled and heparinised blood (1 IE/mL) and closed into a ring. Blood was circulated in a water bath at 37 °C for 90 min (30 rotations/min). Afterwards, tubes were washed with PBS and fixed with 2% glutaraldehyde (GA), then PVC pieces were prepared for SEM.

*2.10. Statistical Analysis*

Unless otherwise specified, data are represented as mean ± standard deviation (SD). All analyses containing more than two groups were analysed with one-way analysis of variance (ANOVA), comparing all groups with one another, corrected by post hoc Bonferroni analysis or Dunnett's/Sidak's test, and the corrected *p*-values are given. Multiple comparisons were analysed with two-way ANOVA and Dunnett's multiple comparison. All analyses for two groups were performed using Student's t-tests. The statistical analyses were performed with the statistical software package GraphPad Prism (version 6.0, GraphPad Software, San Diego, CA, USA). Statistical significance was defined as $p < 0.05$.

## 3. Results

*3.1. Generation, Production and Enzymatic Activity of Recombinant Fusion Protein HSA-CD39*

For the generation of our recombinant fusion protein consisting of HSA and CD39, the DNA sequence of HSA was inserted into a previously described pSectag2A vector containing the CD39 sequence [39]. The resulting HSA-CD39 was further digested, purified and inserted into a gWiz vector to yield a higher production rate (Figure 1A). Following double digestion of both constructs, the HSA-CD39 insert was visualised via agarose gel at 3235 bp (Figure 1A). Confirmation of successful molecular biology was made by colony screening of clones via PCR sequencing, where positive clones resulted in a 2149 bp

DNA strain (Figure 1C). After DNA sequencing confirmation, the DNA was produced by HEK293F cells and purified afterwards. The protein purity of the HSA-CD39 fusion protein was analysed on SDS–PAGE and a band was observed between the 100 kDa and 150 kDa marks (Figure 1D). Specificity of the HSA-CD39 construct was shown by Western blotting via the use of an anti-Penta-His antibody, which was coupled with horseradish peroxidase (141 kDa, Figure 1E).

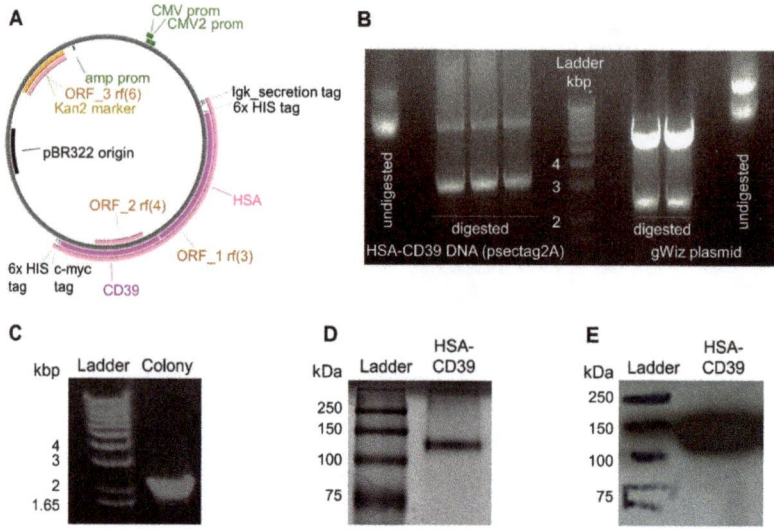

**Figure 1.** Vector map, generation, purification and characterisation of the HSA-CD39 construct. (**A**) Gene map of the HSA-CD39 construct (8585 bp) within the gWiz vector. The restriction enzymes for inserting the construct are EcoR1-HF and PsPOMI. (**B**) HSA-CD39 cut from pSectag2A (3235 bp) and ligated into gWiz by 1% agarose electrophoresis gel, double digested using EcoR1-HF and PsPOMI. (**C**) Control PCR on 1% agarose electrophoresis gel using gWiz forward primer and Not-1 reverse primer to detect HSA in gWiz (2149 bp). (**D**) Visualized via Coomassie staining, 12% sodium dodecyl sulfate-polyacrylamide gel electrophoresis of the HSA-CD39 construct. (**E**) Western blot analysis using a horseradish-peroxidase-coupled anti-6x-his to detect the 6x-his-tag of the HSA-CD39 construct (141 kDa).

The enzymatic activity of the HSA-CD39 fusion protein in hydrolysing ADP to AMP was determined using flow cytometry. While ADP is a platelet agonist, the resulting AMP is unable to activate platelets in vitro. Flow cytometry demonstrated that PAC-1 FITC and anti-CD62P PE bound to 20 µM ADP-activated platelets, but not to non-activated platelets incubated with PBS as control (Figures 2A and S1). By pre-incubating 0.05 µg of the HSA-CD39 protein with 20 µM ADP, we observed a strong reduction in PAC-1 binding as compared to using no protein control (0 µg), indicating successful hydrolysis of ADP to AMP (39.70 ± 7.25 vs. 66.56 ± 5.27, respectively; % activated platelets ± SD, $p < 0.0001$). Higher concentrations of HSA-CD39 (0.1 µg, 0.25 µg and 0.5 µg) resulted in complete dephosphorylation of ADP and therefore showed no PAC-1 binding (0.44 ± 0.28; 0.30 ± 0.16; 0.30 ± 0.20, respectively; % activated platelets ± SD, $p < 0.0001$) (Figure 2A,B).

*3.2. In Vitro Analysis of Environmental Stability of HSA-CD39 Fusion Protein and Coating*

HSA-CD39 was dried or lyophilised and stored to determine the ease of storage and handling. Flow cytometry analysis confirmed that our HSA-CD39 protein had active enzymatic properties after being dried in polystyrene tubes (Figure 3A,B). Twenty-four hours after air-drying and storage at RT, rehydration of the HSA-CD39 protein hydrolysed ADP at 0.05 µg, 0.1 µg, 0.25 µg and 0.5 µg, thereby preventing the binding of PAC-1, as compared to samples without HSA-CD39 (40.40 ± 15.28; 0.40 ± 0.26; 0.35 ± 0.30;

0.33 ± 0.15 vs. 67.93 ± 4.96, respectively; % activated platelets ± SD, $p < 0.0001$). Similarly, storage at 4 °C resulted in successful hydrolysis of ADP; therefore, HSA-CD39 at 0.05 µg, 0.1 µg, 0.25 µg and 0.5 µg prevented PAC-1 binding shown by flow cytometry, compared to samples without HSA-CD39 (37.38 ± 6.70; 0.70 ± 0.26; 0.50 ± 0.17; 0.50 ± 0.00 vs. 65.03 ± 6.81, respectively; % activated platelets ± SD, $p < 0.0001$).

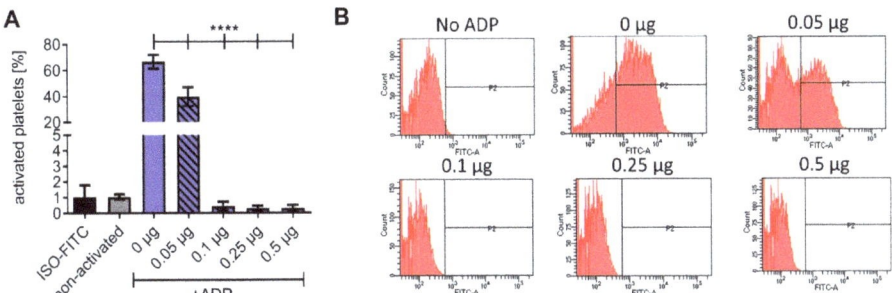

**Figure 2.** Functionality analysis of different concentrations of the HSA-CD39 construct. (**A**) Functionality analysis using flow cytometry detecting activated platelets through binding of the PAC-1 antibody, showing hydrolysing effects of CD39. (**B**) Representative fluorescence histograms of functionality analysis using flow cytometry. The different groups were compared using repeated-measures ANOVA and Bonferroni post hoc test. Values of 5 independent experiments are shown (% activated platelets ± SD, **** $p < 0.0001$).

The functionality of HSA-CD39 was investigated every week for two months (dried in polystyrene tubes and stored at RT) via flow cytometry (Figures 3C and S2). HSA-CD39 hydrolysed ADP and stopped platelet activation at ≥0.25 µg protein after rehydration, compared to samples without HAS-CD39 after week 1 (0.40 ± 0.17 vs. 59.33 ± 30.28; $p < 0.001$) and week 8 (3.80 ± 2.33 vs. 43.23 ± 6.73; % activated platelets ± SD, $p < 0.001$). The enzymatic properties of HAS-CD39 were similarly active through the 8 weeks of storage.

Direct analysis of ADP dephosphorylation by HSA-CD39 was conducted using an ATP bioluminescence assay. Increasing concentrations of HSA-CD39 resulted in linear and significant reductions in ADP concentration in comparison to the HSA control (Figure 4A). Similar effects were observed using lyophilised HSA-CD39, which demonstrates its long-term stability (Figure 4B).

### 3.3. HSA-CD39 Fusion Protein as an Anti-Thrombotic Coating for Different Medical Materials

HSA-CD39 was coated onto surface materials of medical devices such as stainless steel, polyurethane, nitinol BlueOxide and Ti. Stainless-steel plates were coated at 0.05 µg/mm$^2$ (0.25 µg of HSA-CD39 on about 0.5 mm$^2$) and resulted in a significant reduction in platelet activation. Direct HSA-CD39 coating on the plates resulted in successful ADP dephosphorylation as compared to non-coated plates (Figure 5A; 0.17 ± 0.06 vs. 70.70 ± 22.55; % activated platelets ± SD, $p < 0.0001$) and similar results were observed when the plates were washed thrice prior to exposure of ADP (Figure 5B; 0.93 ± 0.80 vs. 69.43 ± 21.99; $p < 0.0001$). Likewise, HSA-CD39 coating demonstrated good enzymatic activity for hydrolysing ADP on polyurethane, compared to HSA-coated stents (Figure 5C; 1.88 ± 1.25 vs. 65.23 ± 17.71; $p < 0.001$) and nitinol BlueOxide stents (Figure 5D; 0.30 ± 0.20 vs. 34.53 ± 5.13; $p < 0.001$). Furthermore, we investigated the stability of HSA-CD39 after coating on Ti plates and sterilisation with EO (Figure 5E). HSA-CD39 coating at 0.1 µg/mm$^2$ (0.5 µg of HSA-CD39 on about 0.5 mm$^2$ of plate) resulted in successful ADP dephosphorylation as compared to the control HSA coating, both before (0.57 ± 0.29 vs. 36.73 ± 8.88; $p < 0.001$) and after EO sterilisation (0.22 ± 0.17 vs. 37.44 ± 8.17; $p < 0.001$). No difference was noted in the function of HSA-CD39 after sterilisation with EO (0.57 ± 0.29 vs. 0.22 ± 0.17; ns).

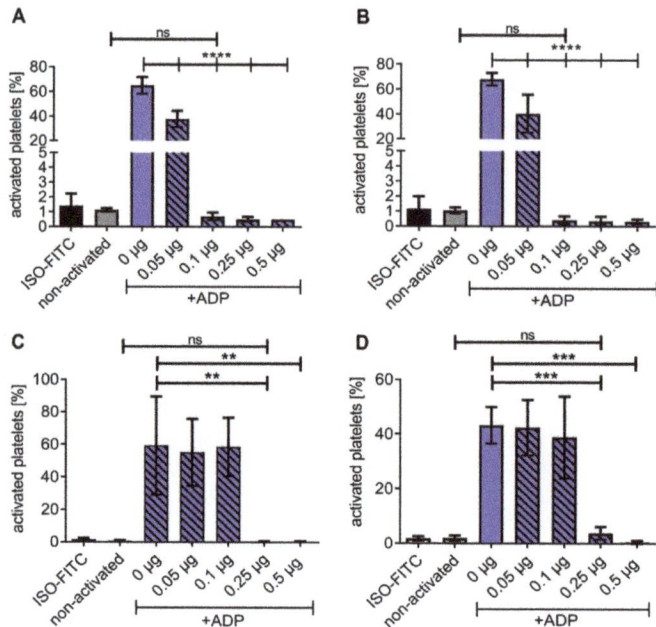

**Figure 3.** Flow cytometry demonstrating HSA-CD39 functionality when dried in polystyrene tubes and stored at RT for at least 8 weeks. Functionality of HSA-CD39 in hydrolysing ADP is still seen after drying in polystyrene tubes and storage at (**A**) 4 °C for 24 h or (**B**) at RT for 24 h. Flow cytometry was performed to determine the % of activated platelets. (**C**) HSA-CD39 is still functional after 7 days of storage at RT. (**D**) HSA-CD39 is still functional after 8 weeks of storage at RT. The different groups were compared using repeated-measures ANOVA and Bonferroni post hoc tests. ns = non-significant. Values of at least 3 independent experiments are depicted (% activated platelets ± SD, ** $p < 0.01$, *** $p < 0.001$, **** $p < 0.0001$).

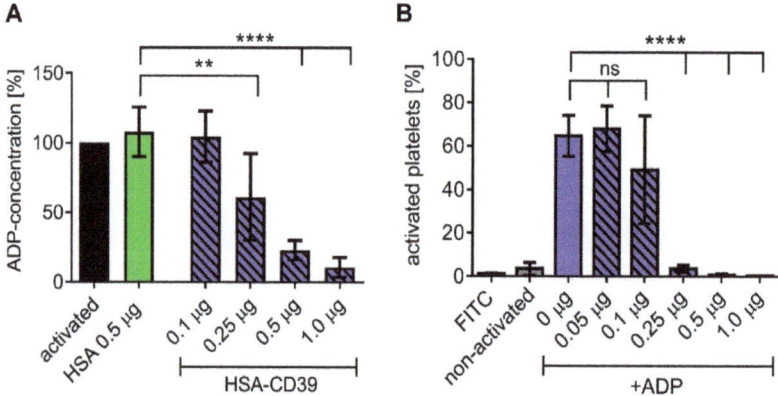

**Figure 4.** HSA-CD39 shows efficient ADP hydrolysis and can be lyophilised at higher concentrations without reduction in functionality. (**A**) Bioluminescence assay showing a reduced ADP concentration (%) for increased HSA-CD39 concentrations compared to the HSA control (** $p < 0.01$; **** $p < 0.0001$ compared to 0.5 µg HSA control, $n = 4$). Different groups were compared using repeated-measures ANOVA and Sidak's test. (**B**) Functionality of lyophilised HSA-CD39 shows that high amounts of the fusion protein (>1.0 µg) are still active after lyophilisation ($n = 4$, **** $p < 0.0001$ compared to PBS control). Values of at least 3 independent experiments are depicted.

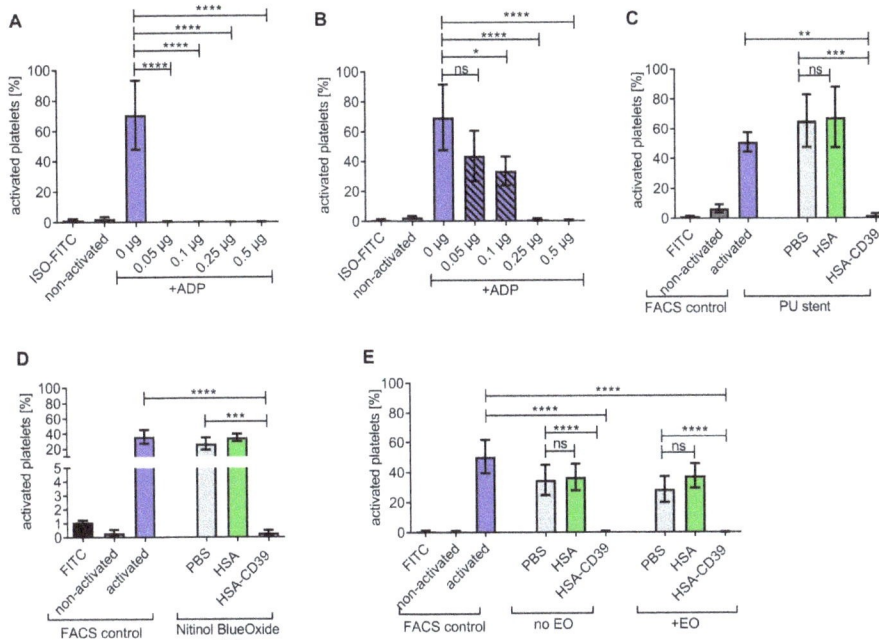

**Figure 5.** HSA-CD39 can be coated onto stainless steel, polyurethane stents and nitinol BlueOxide stents even after sterilisation with EO without reducing its functionality. (**A**) Significant reductions in platelet activation can be seen with different concentrations of HSA-CD39-coated stainless-steel plates without washing. (**B**) HSA-CD39 coated onto stainless-steel plates displays a reduced but still significant reduction in platelet activation after washing with PBS before analysis in flow cytometry. Bar graphs depict % of activated platelets. (**C**) Dried and coated HSA-CD39 on polyurethane stents as well as nitinol BlueOxide stents. (**D**) Shows effective prevention of platelet activation as analysed via flow cytometry. (**E**) HSA-CD39 and HSA for comparison, coated on Ti plates, shown to be still functional in hydrolysing ADP after EO sterilisation. The different groups were compared using repeated-measures ANOVA and Bonferroni post hoc tests. ns = non-significant. Values of at least 3 independent experiments are depicted (% activated platelets ± SD, * $p < 0.05$, ** $p < 0.01$, *** $p < 0.001$ **** $p < 0.0001$).

### 3.4. HSA-CD39 Fusion Protein Coating Allows for Endothelialisation

Fluorescence microscopy images of the HSA-CD39-coated nitinol BlueOxide plates displayed good endothelialisation performance. Sterilised plates were coated with HSA-CD39 or just PBS. hECs were seeded onto the coated plates, followed by incubation for 48 h. No differences between the DAPI-stained hECs regarding cell morphology, cell growth and cell count could be detected compared to the non-coated bare nitinol BlueOxide plates (Figure 6A,B). Additional quantitative analysis of the microscope pictures using ImageJ confirmed this result (Figure 6C).

### 3.5. Haemocompatibility and In Vitro Proof of Function of HSA-CD39-Coated Nitinol Blue Oxide Stents and PVC Tubes

HSA-CD39-coated nitinol BlueOxide stents and uncoated stents were loaded into PCV tubes and incubated with fresh human blood to determine their haemocompatibility and thrombogenicity [22,38]. PVC tubes without stents were used as an additional control. A baseline reading was analysed before the blood was placed into circulation through the stents or tubes. At the endpoint, the blood was collected for comparison analysis. No significant changes were measured in white blood cells, red blood cells, haemoglobin or haematocrit compared to the baseline, the control tube without stent and the uncoated stent (Figure 7A–D). Significant reductions in the number of platelets were found when blood was circulated in the PVC control tube and the uncoated groups, compared to the baseline (221,000.6 ± 23,000.84 and 133,000.2 ± 24,000.3 vs. 259,000 ± 36,000, respectively; number of platelets/µL ± SD, $p < 0.05$). However, no difference was observed in the HSA-CD39-coated nitinol BlueOxide stents as compared to the baseline reading (229,000.0 ± 27,000.74 vs. 259,000 ± 36,000; ns) (Figure 7E). These results indicate that the platelets in the PVC tube control and the uncoated groups aggregated, whereas no aggregation occurred in the HSA-CD39-coated nitinol BlueOxide stents. Activation of the coagulation cascade was determined by measuring the formation of the TAT complex before and after perfusion (Figure 7F). An increased readout of the TAT complex for the uncoated stent group was shown compared to the baseline, the control and also the HSA-CD39-coated stent group (446.4 ± 225.5 vs. 2.37 ± 0.45; 24.02 ± 11.45; 42.72 ± 11.26, respectively; µg/L TAT complex formation ± SD, $p < 0.01$).

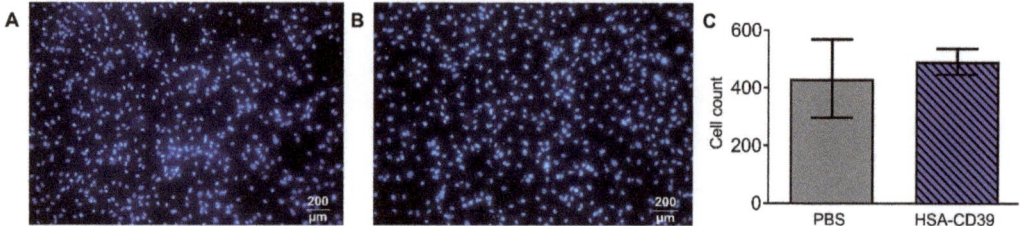

**Figure 6.** HSA-CD39 coated onto nitinol BlueOxide plates has no negative impact on endothelialisation. Incubation of HSA-CD39-coated nitinol BlueOxide stents with hECs. Analysis performed after 48 h with DAPI staining under epifluorescence microscopy. (**A**) Blank plate incubated with hECs. (**B**) HSA-CD39-coated plate incubated with hECs. (**C**) Quantitative analysis of coated (HSA-CD39) and uncoated (PBS control) plates. Original magnification: 10×. Values of at least 3 independent experiments are depicted.

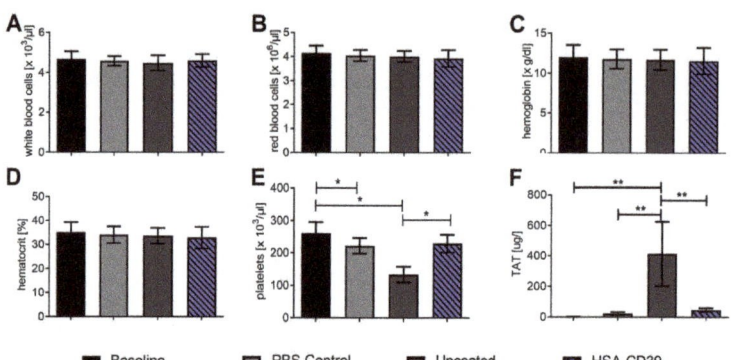

**Figure 7.** HSA-CD39 coated onto nitinol BlueOxide stents shows no effect on blood haematology or haemocompatibility using a dynamic in vitro thrombogenicity model. Haematology analysis of coated stents before and after circulation for 60 min at 150 mL/min (thrombogenicity model). (**A**) White blood cells. (**B**) Red blood cells. (**C**) Haemoglobin. (**D**) Haematocrit. (**E**) Platelets. (**F**) TAT complex using ELISA measurements. Baseline: directly after venepuncture. Control: tube only. Uncoated: bare nitinol BlueOxide stent. The different groups were compared using repeated-measures ANOVA and Bonferroni post hoc tests (% activated platelets ± SD, * $p < 0.05$, ** $p < 0.01$). Values of at least 4 independent experiments are depicted.

After circulation, uncoated and HSA-CD39-coated stents were also analysed via SEM. Representative SEM images of each stent from the same blood donor, displayed at different magnifications, showed distinct differences in the blood cell adhesion (Figure 8). The uncoated stent showed homogenous adhesion of several blood cells, especially platelets, and an increased fibrin network for all blood donors, such that only a few platelets could be detected on the surface of the HSA-CD39-coated stent (Figure 8). SEM imaging of HSA-CD39 coating on the PVC tubes showed a reduction in cell adhesion on the inner surface of the HSA-CD39-coated tube after circulation as compared to the other control groups (Figure 9). In particular, the non-treated and HSA-coated tubes showed more cell adhesion compared to the HSA-CD39-coated tube.

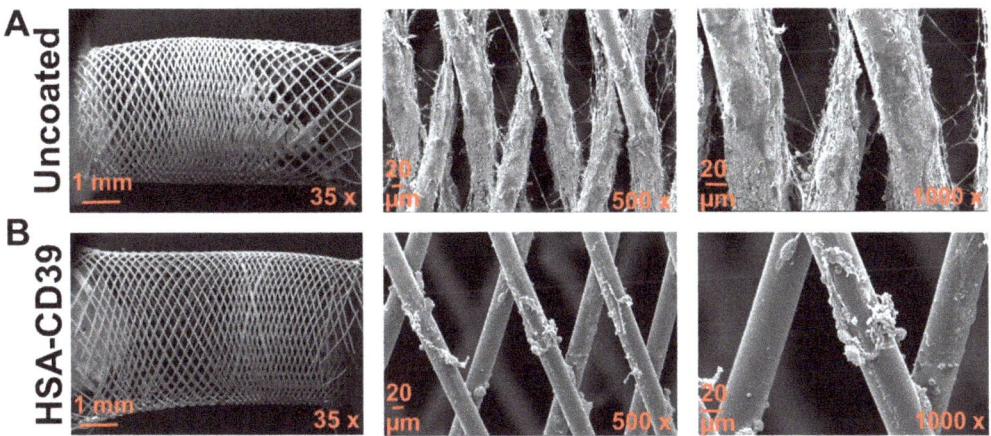

**Figure 8.** HSA-CD39 coated onto nitinol BlueOxide stents reduces blood cell adhesion during incubation in a dynamic in vitro model. SEM analysis of coated nitinol BlueOxide stents after circulation with human whole blood for 60 min at 150 mL/min (thrombogenicity model). Uncoated: bare nitinol BlueOxide stent. Different magnifications (35×, 500× and 1000×) show the amount of blood cell adhesion.

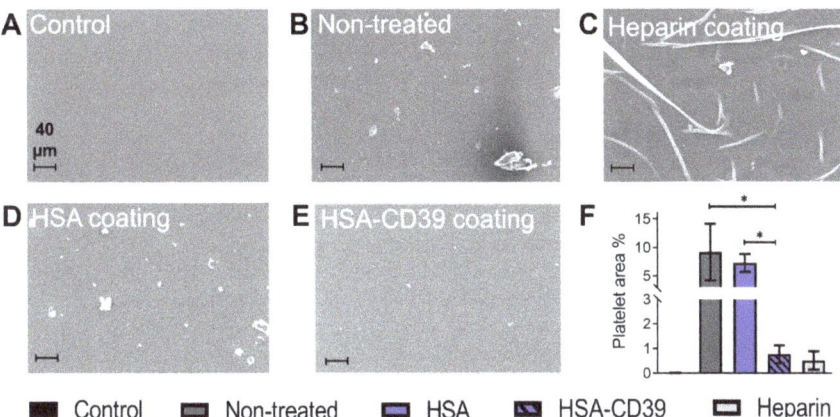

**Figure 9.** HSA-CD39 coated onto PCV tubes reduces blood cell adhesion as analysed in a modified chandler loop model. SEM analysis of PVC tubes to visualise the adhesion of platelets after circulation with human whole blood. (**A**) PVC tube without blood contact. (**B**) Non-treated PVC tube incubated with blood. (**C**) Commercially available heparin coating (Carmeda BioActive Surface®, Medtronic, Ireland). (**D**) HSA-coated PVC tube. (**E**) HSA-CD39-coated PVC tube (magnification: 250×). Less adhesion of platelets was measured in HSA-CD39-coated tubes as compared to HSA or non-treated controls. (**F**) Quantitative analysis of the percentage of area covered by platelets was performed using ImageJ (% activated platelets ± SD, * $p < 0.05$). Values of at least 3 independent experiments are depicted.

## 4. Discussion

Medical devices that are directly exposed to blood are often associated with inflammation and thrombus formation [2,3]. The lack of biocompatibility of foreign materials triggers inflammatory processes and activation of the coagulation cascade, as well as activation and aggregation of platelets in the blood [49–51]. The use of drug-eluting materials and extensive anti-platelet therapy after surgery have shown improvements in safety and efficiency. However, adverse drug interactions, pro-thrombotic events, poor endothelialisation, hypersensitivity and bleeding complications still occur frequently [24]. Therefore, research on a natural, non-allergic, bio- and haemo-compatible medical coating is required. In this study, we genetically designed the fusion of HSA to CD39 in order to engineer a recombinant multifunctional fusion protein which provides an ideal coating strategy for blood-contacting material. The HSA component allows adherence of our fusion protein to be passively adsorbed onto the materials, whilst the attached CD39 component prevents thrombotic actions from occurring. The data indicate that our HSA-CD39 fusion protein is stable in storage and is still highly functional in reducing platelet activation and adhesion for up to 8 weeks (Figures 3 and 4B). HSA-CD39 also protects platelet activation and inflammation processes, which are commonly evoked by foreign materials such as stainless steel, Ti, nitinol (an alloy of nickel and Ti), polyurethane stents and PVC (Figure 5).

CD39 is a membrane-bound enzyme constitutively expressed on intact ECs. This NTPDase hydrolyses the nucleotides ATP and ADP [39,42,45]. CD39 has attracted major attention as a pharmacological agent [39,42,52,53]. Several studies have shown that the administration of CD39 decreases the risk of thrombosis and protects against myocardial infarction and stroke [54,55]. A hallmark study conducted in transgenic mice expressing CD39 demonstrated increased resistance to thrombosis when challenged by an acute ferric-chloride-induced injury to their carotid artery [56]. Furthermore, overexpression of CD39 in rat aortas diminishes the proliferation of smooth vascular cells and prevents neointimal formation after angioplasty [46]. However, direct injection of CD39 is associated with concentration-dependent bleeding complications [39,54]. To overcome this obstacle, our laboratory genetically fused CD39 to a single-chain antibody that was specific to activated platelets, resulting in a successful and bleeding-free targeted therapy in vivo [38–40]. We further investigated this construct in a murine model of myocardial ischemia/reperfusion injury, where we demonstrated that the activated-platelet-targeted CD39 provides significant myocardial protection and preserves heart function [40]. Furthermore, using CD39 mRNA, we showed the CD39 protein has active enzymatic properties and can hydrolyse ADP to AMP, thereby preventing platelet activation and proving the therapeutic potential of CD39 [42]. In this current study, we harness the enzymatic properties of CD39 and further utilise HSA for coating on several medically used materials. To demonstrate the anti-thrombotic effects of this fusion protein, we used two markers of platelet activation, the monoclonal antibody PAC-1 (specific for activated GPIIb/IIIa) and an antibody against P-selectin (anti-CD62P) (Figure S1). Upon platelet activation, GPIIb/IIIa changes from a low-affinity state to a high-binding-affinity state for fibrinogen/fibrin, thereby mediating platelet aggregation [57–59]. Being the most abundant platelet receptor, with the high density of 60,000 to 80,000 receptors per platelet, the activation of GPIIb/IIIa and its resulting aggregation is a main contributor to thrombosis [58,60]. P-selectin's role in platelet aggregation is not as dominant, but it is seen as a sensitive marker of platelet activation [41]. Since most blood-contact medical device failures are due to thrombosis, our study has chosen to focus on platelet activation as a readout. Overall, our studies indicated HSA-CD39 fusion protein is highly functional in hydrolysing ADP, a major player in the platelet activation cascade, and at preventing platelet activation, adhesion and aggregation.

HSA has been widely used for the coating of medical products, possibly owing to its inferred safety and stability given its abundance in human serum [61–64]. Serum hypoalbuminemia has been observed during inflammatory processes and in cardiovascular events [29]. HSA is physiochemically stable and has been studied extensively in relation to clinical use for the maintenance of blood homeostasis in medical conditions [61,63].

Blood contact with foreign materials leads to the adherence of pro-thrombotic plasma proteins (e.g., fibrinogen) on the materials' surfaces, but studies have shown that adsorbed albumin is able to passivate various materials, thereby providing an anti-thrombotic effect by minimising platelet adhesion [26,64,65]. Furthermore, HSA is known to provide an antioxidant effect, reducing complement cascade activation [62,65,66]. Clinically, HSA is used in combination therapy with various drugs and bioactive proteins, or as an encapsulation agent [64].

HSA coated on an arterial polyester prosthesis (Dacron®) displayed reduction in platelet adhesion, less activation of the coagulation cascade and decreased formation of fibrinopeptide A, as an index for decreased thrombin action, highlighting the importance of structural design and surface chemistry [67,68]. Additionally, a HSA/polyethylenimine multilayer coating on plasma-treated PVC was shown to resist platelet adhesion effectively [69].

Ti is a material frequently used for orthopaedic implants and cardiovascular devices. Adsorption of HSA into Ti has been shown to prevent adhesion of other blood proteins and reduce bacterial adherence [70,71]. We harnessed these advantages of HSA, especially its passive binding capacity, as part of our fusion protein to improve the biocompatibility of medical devices. Our HSA-CD39 fusion protein provides protection against device-induced platelet activation and inflammation processes, and thus minimises bleeding risk and promotes adaptation of the surrounding tissue to the foreign material in situ. We demonstrate the maintained functionality of our generated fusion protein HSA-CD39 on Ti even after sterilisation with EO (Figure 5E). After radiation, sterilisation via EO is the most commonly used process in the medical device industry and is performed after standard protocols [72,73]. Therefore, we demonstrate a highly stable device coating already suited to clinical translation.

The application of therapeutic recombinant proteins for a safe, biocompatible interface on medical devices has attracted major interest in the biopharmaceutical industry. This includes the pursuit of a perfectly haemocompatible, biopassive surface and the progress in the application of active therapeutic compounds [74,75]. In the development of stents, nitinol combines the properties of elasticity, biocompatibility and the shape-memory effect, which makes it suitable for self-expanding stents. The native oxide layer formed on the surface prevents nickel ions from binding to Ti, resulting in a nickel-free environment and substantially reducing allergic reactions and toxicity [74,75]. To analyse our HSA-CD39 fusion protein in vitro, we used a flow diverter nitinol BlueOxide DERIVO embolisation device, which has been evaluated for the treatment of intracranial aneurysms in clinical trials (Figures 7 and 8) [76].

In the area of coating strategies, antibodies against CD34 and CD133 coated onto stents have been evaluated in a rabbit model, showing reduced intimal proliferation and re-stenosis as compared to bare metal stents and gelatine-coated stents [62,63,75,76]. Using these antibodies to attract vascular-circulating endothelial progenitor cells (EPCs) leads to adhesion of a functional endothelial layer of EPCs on the stent surface after vascular injury. Murine monoclonal CD34-coated stents (GenousTM, OrbusNeich) were proven to be safe and enhance endothelialisation in various clinical trials [77,78]. Our study demonstrates good endothelialisation rates and a reduction in platelet activation (Figure 6).

Haemocompatibility analysis of our HSA-CD39 protein showed no influence on whole human blood. Using uncoated bare metal nitinol BlueOxide stents, we noted a significant reduction in platelet count, which also implies increased platelet aggregation. Our HSA-CD39-coated stents, on the other hand, showed no significant decrease in platelet count and additionally showed a reduced TAT complex, indicating minimal platelet aggregation and minimal coagulation cascade activation, respectively (Figure 7) [28].

Addressing the issue of the handling and storage of sensitive medical products, our data demonstrate preserved enzymatic activity of HSA-CD39 after drying, lyophilisation, coating, washing, sterilisation and 8 weeks of storage. We have shown that HSA-CD39 can be used as a new coating strategy across various devices and blood-contacting materials.

Our HSA-CD39 protein approach reduces platelet adhesion, activation and further inflammatory processes, therefore providing a great clinical advancement in the realm of bioprostheses by minimising the need for anti-thrombotic therapy, which is inherently linked to potential bleeding complications. There are some limitations to our study. We have shown that HSA-CD39 coating on our materials was present after washing steps were conducted and remained highly functional in its activity to hydrolyse ADP. However, we have not directly measured the amount of protein lost. Different materials may require other coating methods, which may expose our fusion protein to heat or other storage conditions. Although we have demonstrated that our fusion protein is more effective in reducing platelet activation, adhesion and aggregation, we have not systematically defined which of the individual components, HSA or CD39, are the cause of the described benefits. Further characterisations of HSA-CD39 should include the contributions of the individual fusion protein components. We have conducted ex vivo blood circulation and demonstrated that HSA-CD39 coating resulted in less platelet aggregation; however, future in vivo experiments will be conducted to determine the anti-thrombotic and anti-inflammatory properties of the materials post implantation. Additionally, the contribution of reduced ADP levels, in comparison to the generation of adenosine via the use of P2Y receptor inhibitors or A2A adenosine receptor blockers in vivo, will allow us to define the effects of HSA-CD39 more thoroughly. In addition, future investigations into the coating strategies, temperature changes and storage conditions, as well as a diverse range of biomaterials, will be explored.

## 5. Conclusions

In this study, we have generated a recombinant fusion protein combining the anti-thrombotic and anti-inflammatory properties of CD39 with HSA as a suitable coating for medical devices in order to reduce foreign-material-associated complications. Our newly designed HSA-CD39 fusion protein is highly functional in preventing platelet activation, adhesion and aggregation. It is also stable after EO sterilisation and can be coated onto several materials typically used in medical devices. HSA-CD39 coating can mitigate the healing process, improve the incorporation of foreign material into the surrounding tissue and reduce interactions with blood components such as coagulation proteins, platelets and leukocytes. Overall, our HSA-CD39 fusion protein is a natural bioactive interface which is highly potent in the prevention of platelet activation and inflammation; therefore, its use for medical device coating provides potential benefits for patients.

**Supplementary Materials:** The following are available online at https://www.mdpi.com/article/10.3390/pharmaceutics13091504/s1, Figure S1: Representative images of fluorescence histograms via flow cytometry demonstrating HSA-CD39 prevents platelet activation using two markers of platelet activation; Figure S2: Flow cytometry demonstrating HSA-CD39 can be dried in polystyrene tubes and stored at RT for up to 7 weeks.

**Author Contributions:** Conceptualisation, K.P. and X.W.; Methodology, M.-K.A., E.J., J.D.H., A.K.S., V.B., Y.S. and X.W.; Validation, M.-K.A., E.J., J.D.H., A.K.S., V.B., Y.S., H.P.W., K.P., S.K. and X.W.; Investigation, M.-K.A., E.J., J.D.H., A.K.S., V.B. and Y.S.; Resources, H.P.W., K.P., S.K. and X.W.; Writing—Original Draft Preparation, M.-K.A. and E.J.; Writing—Review and Editing, J.D.H., A.K.S., H.P.W., K.P., S.K. and X.W.; Supervision, H.P.W., K.P., S.K. and X.W.; Project Administration, S.K. and X.W.; Funding Acquisition, K.P., S.K. and X.W. All authors have read and agreed to the published version of the manuscript.

**Funding:** This work was funded by the Australian National Health and Medical Research Council (NHMRC) and in part by the Victorian Government Operational Infrastructure Support Program. M.-K.A. was supported by the German Research Association (Deutsche Forschungsgemeinschaft); E.J. was supported by the Promotionskolleg des interdisziplinären Zentrums für Klinische Forschung (IZKF); A.S.K. was supported by the National Heart Foundation (NHF) Australian Indigenous Scholarship; K.P. was supported by a National Health and Medical Research Council Investigator Fellowship; S.K. was supported by the Margarete von Wrangell-Habilitationsstipendium des Ministeriums für Wissenschaft, Forschung und Kunst Baden-Württemberg; and X.W. was supported by an NHF Future Leader Fellowship with the Paul Korner Innovation Award and a Baker Fellowship.

**Institutional Review Board Statement:** The study was conducted according to the guidelines of the Declaration of Helsinki, and approved by the Ethics Committee of the Alfred Hospital, Melbourne, Australia. (project number 627/17, approved 12 December 2017).

**Informed Consent Statement:** Informed consent was obtained from all healthy volunteers involved in the study.

**Data Availability Statement:** Data is contained within the article or Supplementary Material.

**Acknowledgments:** We would like to thank Giorgio Cattaneo and Acandis GmbH, Pforzheim, Germany, for providing the nitinol BlueOxide stents and plates.

**Conflicts of Interest:** The authors declare no conflict of interest.

## References

1. WHO. The Top 10 Causes of Death. Available online: http://www.who.int/mediacentre/factsheets/fs310/en/ (accessed on 21 August 2020).
2. Biran, R.; Pond, D. Heparin coatings for improving blood compatibility of medical devices. *Adv. Drug Deliv. Rev.* **2017**, *112*, 12–23. [CrossRef]
3. Jaffer, I.H.; Fredenburgh, J.C.; Hirsh, J.; Weitz, J.I. Medical device-induced thrombosis: What causes it and how can we prevent it? *J. Thromb. Haemost. JTH* **2015**, *13* (Suppl. S1), S72–S81. [CrossRef]
4. Hickman, D.A.; Pawlowski, C.L.; Sekhon, U.D.S.; Marks, J.; Gupta, A.S. Biomaterials and Advanced Technologies for Hemostatic Management of Bleeding. *Adv. Mater.* **2018**, *30*, 1700859. [CrossRef]
5. Asada, Y.; Yamashita, A.; Sato, Y.; Hatakeyama, K. Thrombus Formation and Propagation in the Onset of Cardiovascular Events. *J. Atheroscler. Thromb.* **2018**, *25*, 653–664. [CrossRef]
6. Dutra, G.V.S.; Neto, W.S.; Dutra, J.P.S.; Machado, F. Implantable Medical Devices and Tissue Engineering: An Overview of Manufacturing Processes and the Use of Polymeric Matrices for Manufacturing and Coating their Surfaces. *Curr. Med. Chem.* **2020**, *27*, 1580–1599. [CrossRef] [PubMed]
7. Lavery, K.S.; Rhodes, C.; Mcgraw, A.; Eppihimer, M.J. Anti-thrombotic technologies for medical devices. *Adv. Drug Deliv. Rev.* **2017**, *112*, 2–11. [CrossRef] [PubMed]
8. Thomas, J.; Kostousov, V.; Teruya, J. Bleeding and Thrombotic Complications in the Use of Extracorporeal Membrane Oxygenation. *Semin. Thromb. Hemost.* **2018**, *44*, 20–29. [CrossRef]
9. Sun, W.; Wang, S.; Chen, Z.; Zhang, J.; Li, T.; Arias, K.; Griffith, B.P.; Wu, Z.J. Impact of high mechanical shear stress and oxygenator membrane surface on blood damage relevant to thrombosis and bleeding in a pediatric ECMO circuit. *Artif. Organs* **2020**, *44*, 717–726. [CrossRef]
10. Wendel, H.P.; Hauser, N.; Briquet, F.; Ziemer, G. Hemocompatibility of medical connectors with biopassive or bioactive surface coatings. *J. Biomater. Appl.* **2002**, *17*, 5–17. [CrossRef] [PubMed]
11. Bertrand, O.F.; Sipehia, R.; Mongrain, R.; Rodés, J.; Tardif, J.C.; Bilodeau, L.; Côté, G.; Bourassa, M.G. Biocompatibility aspects of new stent technology. *J. Am. Coll. Cardiol.* **1998**, *32*, 562–571. [CrossRef]
12. Hoffman, J.I.E.; Kaplan, S. The incidence of congenital heart disease. *J. Am. Coll. Cardiol.* **2002**, *39*, 1890–1900. [CrossRef]
13. Lukovic, D.; Nyolczas, N.; Hemetsberger, R.; Pavo, I.J.; Pósa, A.; Behnisch, B.; Horak, G.; Zlabinger, K.; Gyöngyösi, M. Human recombinant activated protein C-coated stent for the prevention of restenosis in porcine coronary arteries. *J. Mater. Sci. Mater. Med.* **2015**, *26*, 241. [CrossRef]
14. Buccheri, D.; Piraino, D.; Andolina, G.; Cortese, B. Understanding and managing in-stent restenosis: A review of clinical data, from pathogenesis to treatment. *J. Thorac. Dis.* **2016**, *8*, E1150–E1162. [CrossRef]
15. Khan, S.U.; Singh, M.; Valavoor, S.; Khan, M.U.; Lone, A.N.; Khan, M.Z.; Khan, M.S.; Mani, P.; Kapadia, S.R.; Michos, E.D.; et al. Dual Antiplatelet Therapy After Percutaneous Coronary Intervention and Drug-Eluting Stents: A Systematic Review and Network Meta-Analysis. *Circulation* **2020**, *142*, 1425–1436. [CrossRef]
16. Nicolais, C.; Lakhter, V.; Virk, H.U.H.; Sardar, P.; Bavishi, C.; O'Murchu, B.; Chatterjee, S. Therapeutic Options for In-Stent Restenosis. *Curr. Cardiol. Rep.* **2018**, *20*, 7. [CrossRef]
17. Li, Q.; Hegner, F.; Bruecker, C.H. Comparative Study of Wall-Shear Stress at the Ascending Aorta for Different Mechanical Heart Valve Prostheses. *J. Biomech. Eng.* **2020**, *142*, 011006. [CrossRef]
18. Labarrere, C.A.; Dabiri, A.E.; Kassab, G.S. Thrombogenic and Inflammatory Reactions to Biomaterials in Medical Devices. *Front. Bioeng. Biotechnol.* **2020**, *8*, 123. [CrossRef] [PubMed]
19. McGinty, S. A decade of modelling drug release from arterial stents. *Math. Biosci.* **2014**, *257*, 80–90. [CrossRef] [PubMed]
20. Rykowska, I.; Nowak, I.; Nowak, R. Drug-Eluting Stents and Balloons-Materials, Structure Designs, and Coating Techniques: A Review. *Molecules* **2020**, *25*, 4624. [CrossRef] [PubMed]

21. Lekshmi, K.M.; Che, H.-L.; Cho, C.-S.; Park, I.-K. Drug- and Gene-eluting Stents for Preventing Coronary Restenosis. *Chonnam Med. J.* **2017**, *53*, 14–27. [CrossRef] [PubMed]
22. Busch, R.; Strohbach, A.; Rethfeldt, S.; Walz, S.; Busch, M.; Petersen, S.; Felix, S.; Sternberg, K. New stent surface materials: The impact of polymer-dependent interactions of human endothelial cells, smooth muscle cells, and platelets. *Acta Biomater.* **2014**, *10*, 688–700. [CrossRef] [PubMed]
23. Torii, S.; Jinnouchi, H.; Sakamoto, A.; Mori, H.; Park, J.; Amoa, F.C.; Sawan, M.; Sato, Y.; Cornelissen, A.; Kuntz, S.H.; et al. Vascular responses to coronary calcification following implantation of newer-generation drug-eluting stents in humans: Impact on healing. *Eur. Heart J.* **2020**, *41*, 786–796. [CrossRef] [PubMed]
24. Essandoh, M.; Dalia, A.A.; Albaghdadi, M.; George, B.; Stoicea, N.; Shabsigh, M.; Rao, S.V. Perioperative Management of Dual-Antiplatelet Therapy in Patients With New-Generation Drug-Eluting Metallic Stents and Bioresorbable Vascular Scaffolds Undergoing Elective Noncardiac Surgery. *J. Cardiothorac. Vasc. Anesth.* **2017**, *31*, 1857–1864. [CrossRef] [PubMed]
25. Shlofmitz, E.; Iantorno, M.; Waksman, R. Restenosis of Drug-Eluting Stents: A New Classification System Based on Disease Mechanism to Guide Treatment and State-of-the-Art Review. *Circ. Cardiovasc. Interv.* **2019**, *12*, e007023. [CrossRef]
26. Freitas, S.C.; Maia, S.; Figueiredo, A.C.; Gomes, P.; Pereira, P.J.B.; Barbosa, M.A.; Martins, M.C.L. Selective albumin-binding surfaces modified with a thrombin-inhibiting peptide. *Acta Biomater.* **2014**, *10*, 1227–1237. [CrossRef]
27. Zoellner, H.; Höfler, M.; Beckmann, R.; Hufnagl, P.; Vanyek, E.; Bielek, E.; Wojta, J.; Fabry, A.; Lockie, S.; Binder, B.R. Serum albumin is a specific inhibitor of apoptosis in human endothelial cells. *J. Cell Sci.* **1996**, *109*, 2571–2580. [CrossRef]
28. Krajewski, S.; Neumann, B.; Kurz, J.; Perle, N.; Avci-Adali, M.; Cattaneo, G.; Wendel, H.P. Preclinical Evaluation of the Thrombogenicity and Endothelialization of Bare Metal and Surface-Coated Neurovascular Stents. *Am. J. Neuroradiol.* **2015**, *36*, 133–139. [CrossRef]
29. Celik, I.E.; Yarlioglues, M.; Kurtul, A.; Duran, M.; Koseoglu, C.; Oksuz, F.; Aksoy, O.; Murat, S.N. Preprocedural Albumin Levels and Risk of In-Stent Restenosis After Coronary Stenting With Bare-Metal Stent. *Angiology* **2016**, *67*, 478–483. [CrossRef]
30. Mulvihill, J.N.; Faradji, A.; Oberling, F.; Cazenave, J.P. Surface passivation by human albumin of plasmapheresis circuits reduces platelet accumulation and thrombus formation. Experimental and clinical studies. *J. Biomed. Mater. Res.* **1990**, *24*, 155–163. [CrossRef] [PubMed]
31. Hyun, H.; Park, J.; Willis, K.; Park, J.E.; Lyle, L.T.; Lee, W.; Yeo, Y. Surface modification of polymer nanoparticles with native albumin for enhancing drug delivery to solid tumors. *Biomaterials* **2018**, *180*, 206–224. [CrossRef] [PubMed]
32. Klinger, A.; Steinberg, D.; Kohavi, D.; Sela, M.N. Mechanism of adsorption of human albumin to titanium in vitro. *J. Biomed. Mater. Res.* **1997**, *36*, 387–392. [CrossRef]
33. D'Elia, N.L.; Gravina, N.; Ruso, J.M.; Marco-Brown, J.L.; Sieben, J.M.; Messina, P.V. Albumin-mediated deposition of bone-like apatite onto nano-sized surfaces: Effect of surface reactivity and interfacial hydration. *J. Colloid Interface Sci.* **2017**, *494*, 345–354. [CrossRef]
34. Tao, C.; Zhu, W.; Iqbal, J.; Xu, C.; Wang, D.-A. Stabilized albumin coatings on engineered xenografts for attenuation of acute immune and inflammatory responses. *J. Mater. Chem. B* **2020**, *8*, 6080–6091. [CrossRef] [PubMed]
35. Oriňaková, R.; Gorejová, R.; Králová, Z.O.; Oriňak, A.; Shepa, I.; Hovancová, J.; Kovalčíková, A.; Bujňáková, Z.L.; Király, N.; Kaňuchová, M.; et al. Influence of albumin interaction on corrosion resistance of sintered iron biomaterials with polyethyleneimine coating. *Appl. Surf. Sci.* **2020**, *509*, 145379. [CrossRef]
36. Kaczmarek, E.; Koziak, K.; Sévigny, J.; Siegel, J.B.; Anrather, J.; Beaudoin, A.R.; Bach, F.H.; Robson, S.C. Identification and characterization of CD39/vascular ATP diphosphohydrolase. *J. Biol. Chem.* **1996**, *271*, 33116–33122. [CrossRef]
37. Fung, C.Y.E.; Marcus, A.J.; Broekman, M.J.; Mahaut-Smith, M.P. P2x1 receptor inhibition and soluble CD39 administration as novel approaches to widen the cardiovascular therapeutic window. *Trends Cardiovasc. Med.* **2009**, *19*, 1–5. [CrossRef] [PubMed]
38. Granja, T.; Körner, A.; Glück, C.; Hohmann, J.D.; Wang, X.; Köhler, D.; Streißenberger, A.; Nandurkar, H.H.; Mirakaj, V.; Rosenberger, P.; et al. Targeting CD39 Toward Activated Platelets Reduces Systemic Inflammation and Improves Survival in Sepsis: A Preclinical Pilot Study. *Crit. Care Med.* **2019**, *47*, e420–e427. [CrossRef]
39. Hohmann, J.D.; Wang, X.; Krajewski, S.; Selan, C.; Haller, C.A.; Straub, A.; Chaikof, E.L.; Nandurkar, H.H.; Hagemeyer, C.E.; Peter, K. Delayed targeting of CD39 to activated platelet GPIIb/IIIa via a single-chain antibody: Breaking the link between antithrombotic potency and bleeding? *Blood* **2013**, *121*, 3067–3075. [CrossRef]
40. Ziegler, M.; Hohmann, J.D.; Searle, A.K.; Abraham, M.-K.; Nandurkar, H.H.; Wang, X.; Peter, K. A single-chain antibody-CD39 fusion protein targeting activated platelets protects from cardiac ischaemia/reperfusion injury. *Eur. Heart J.* **2018**, *39*, 111–116. [CrossRef] [PubMed]
41. Straub, A.; Krajewski, S.; Hohmann, J.D.; Westein, E.; Jia, F.; Bassler, N.; Selan, C.; Kurz, J.; Wendel, H.P.; Dezfouli, S.; et al. Evidence of platelet activation at medically used hypothermia and mechanistic data indicating ADP as a key mediator and therapeutic target. *Arterioscler. Thromb. Vasc. Biol.* **2011**, *31*, 1607–1616. [CrossRef]
42. Abraham, M.-K.; Nolte, A.; Reus, R.; Behring, A.; Zengerle, D.; Avci-Adali, M.; Hohmann, J.D.; Peter, K.; Schlensak, C.; Wendel, H.P.; et al. In vitro Study of a Novel Stent Coating Using Modified CD39 Messenger RNA to Potentially Reduce Stent Angioplasty-Associated Complications. *PLoS ONE* **2015**, *10*, e0138375. [CrossRef] [PubMed]
43. Abraham, M.-K.; Peter, K.; Michel, T.; Wendel, H.P.; Krajewski, S.; Wang, X. Nanoliposomes for Safe and Efficient Therapeutic mRNA Delivery: A Step Toward Nanotheranostics in Inflammatory and Cardiovascular Diseases as well as Cancer. *Nanotheranostics* **2017**, *1*, 154–165. [CrossRef] [PubMed]

44. Covarrubias, R.; Chepurko, E.; Reynolds, A.; Huttinger, Z.M.; Huttinger, R.; Stanfill, K.; Wheeler, D.G.; Novitskaya, T.; Robson, S.C.; Dwyer, K.M.; et al. Role of the CD39/CD73 Purinergic Pathway in Modulating Arterial Thrombosis in Mice. *Arterioscler. Thromb. Vasc. Biol.* **2016**, *36*, 1809–1820. [CrossRef] [PubMed]
45. Allard, B.; Longhi, M.S.; Robson, S.C.; Stagg, J. The ectonucleotidases CD39 and CD73: Novel checkpoint inhibitor targets. *Immunol. Rev.* **2017**, *276*, 121–144. [CrossRef]
46. Robson, S.C.; Wu, Y.; Sun, X.; Knosalla, C.; Dwyer, K.; Enjyoji, K. Ectonucleotidases of CD39 family modulate vascular inflammation and thrombosis in transplantation. *Semin. Thromb. Hemost.* **2005**, *31*, 217–233. [CrossRef] [PubMed]
47. Avci-Adali, M.; Kobba, J.; Neumann, B.; Lescan, M.; Perle, N.; Wilhelm, N.; Wiedmaier, H.; Schlensak, C.; Wendel, H.P. Application of a rotating bioreactor consisting of low-cost and ready-to-use medical disposables for in vitro evaluation of the endothelialization efficiency of small-caliber vascular prostheses: Rotating Bioreactor for Investigation of Endothelialization. *J. Biomed. Mater. Res. B Appl. Biomater.* **2013**, *101B*, 1061–1068. [CrossRef] [PubMed]
48. Krajewski, S.; Prucek, R.; Panacek, A.; Avci-Adali, M.; Nolte, A.; Straub, A.; Zboril, R.; Wendel, H.P.; Kvitek, L. Hemocompatibility evaluation of different silver nanoparticle concentrations employing a modified Chandler-loop in vitro assay on human blood. *Acta Biomater.* **2013**, *9*, 7460–7468. [CrossRef]
49. Wendel, H.P.; Ziemer, G. Coating-techniques to improve the hemocompatibility of artificial devices used for extracorporeal circulation. *Eur. J. Cardio-Thorac. Surg.* **1999**, *16*, 342–350. [CrossRef]
50. Farhatnia, Y.; Tan, A.; Motiwala, A.; Cousins, B.G.; Seifalian, A.M. Evolution of covered stents in the contemporary era: Clinical application, materials and manufacturing strategies using nanotechnology. *Biotechnol. Adv.* **2013**, *31*, 524–542. [CrossRef]
51. Joung, Y.-H. Development of implantable medical devices: From an engineering perspective. *Int. Neurourol. J.* **2013**, *17*, 98–106. [CrossRef]
52. Marcus, A.J.; Broekman, M.J.; Drosopoulos, J.H.; Islam, N.; Alyonycheva, T.N.; Safier, L.B.; Hajjar, K.A.; Posnett, D.N.; Schoenborn, M.A.; Schooley, K.A.; et al. The endothelial cell ecto-ADPase responsible for inhibition of platelet function is CD39. *J. Clin. Investig.* **1997**, *99*, 1351–1360. [CrossRef]
53. Marcus, A.J.; Broekman, M.J.; Drosopoulos, J.H.; Pinsky, D.J.; Islam, N.; Maliszewsk, C.R. Inhibition of platelet recruitment by endothelial cell CD39/ecto-ADPase: Significance for occlusive vascular diseases. *Ital. Heart J.* **2001**, *2*, 824–830. [PubMed]
54. Cai, M.; Huttinger, Z.M.; He, H.; Zhang, W.; Li, F.; Goodman, L.A.; Wheeler, D.G.; Druhan, L.J.; Zweier, J.L.; Dwyer, K.M.; et al. Transgenic over expression of ectonucleotide triphosphate diphosphohydrolase-1 protects against murine myocardial ischemic injury. *J. Mol. Cell. Cardiol.* **2011**, *51*, 927–935. [CrossRef]
55. Marcus, A.J.; Broekman, M.J.; Drosopoulos, J.H.F.; Olson, K.E.; Islam, N.; Pinsky, D.J.; Levi, R. Role of CD39 (NTPDase-1) in thromboregulation, cerebroprotection, and cardioprotection. *Semin. Thromb. Hemost.* **2005**, *31*, 234–246. [CrossRef]
56. Huttinger, Z.M.; Milks, M.W.; Nickoli, M.S.; Aurand, W.L.; Long, L.C.; Wheeler, D.G.; Dwyer, K.M.; d'Apice, A.J.F.; Robson, S.C.; Cowan, P.J.; et al. Ectonucleotide Triphosphate Diphosphohydrolase-1 (CD39) Mediates Resistance to Occlusive Arterial Thrombus Formation after Vascular Injury in Mice. *Am. J. Pathol.* **2012**, *181*, 322–333. [CrossRef] [PubMed]
57. Wang, X.; Peter, K. Molecular Imaging of Atherothrombotic Diseases: Seeing Is Believing. *Arterioscler. Thromb. Vasc. Biol.* **2017**, *37*, 1029–1040. [CrossRef] [PubMed]
58. Wang, X.; Hagemeyer, C.E.; Hohmann, J.D.; Leitner, E.; Armstrong, P.C.; Jia, F.; Olschewski, M.; Needles, A.; Peter, K.; Ahrens, I. Novel Single-Chain Antibody-Targeted Microbubbles for Molecular Ultrasound Imaging of Thrombosis: Validation of a Unique Noninvasive Method for Rapid and Sensitive Detection of Thrombi and Monitoring of Success or Failure of Thrombolysis in Mice. *Circulation* **2012**, *125*, 3117–3126. [CrossRef]
59. Hanjaya-Putra, D.; Haller, C.; Wang, X.; Dai, E.; Lim, B.; Liu, L.; Jaminet, P.; Yao, J.; Searle, A.; Bonnard, T.; et al. Platelet-targeted dual pathway antithrombotic inhibits thrombosis with preserved hemostasis. *JCI Insight* **2018**, *3*, e99329. [CrossRef]
60. Wang, X.; Gkanatsas, Y.; Palasubramaniam, J.; Hohmann, J.D.; Chen, Y.C.; Lim, B.; Hagemeyer, C.; Peter, K. Thrombus-Targeted Theranostic Microbubbles: A New Technology towards Concurrent Rapid Ultrasound Diagnosis and Bleeding-free Fibrinolytic Treatment of Thrombosis. *Theranostics* **2016**, *6*, 726–738. [CrossRef]
61. Tao, C.; Chuah, Y.J.; Xu, C.; Wang, D.-A. Albumin conjugates and assemblies as versatile bio-functional additives and carriers for biomedical applications. *J. Mater. Chem. B* **2019**, *7*, 357–367. [CrossRef]
62. Merlot, A.M.; Kalinowski, D.S.; Richardson, D.R. Unraveling the mysteries of serum albumin-more than just a serum protein. *Front. Physiol.* **2014**, *5*, 299. [CrossRef]
63. Kratz, F. Albumin as a drug carrier: Design of prodrugs, drug conjugates and nanoparticles. *J. Control. Release* **2008**, *132*, 171–183. [CrossRef] [PubMed]
64. Höhn, S.; Braem, A.; Neirinck, B.; Virtanen, S. Albumin coatings by alternating current electrophoretic deposition for improving corrosion resistance and bioactivity of titanium implants. *Mater. Sci. Eng. C* **2017**, *73*, 798–807. [CrossRef] [PubMed]
65. Goodman, S.L.; Cooper, S.L.; Albrecht, R.M. The effects of substrate-adsorbed albumin on platelet spreading. *J. Biomater. Sci. Polym. Ed.* **1991**, *2*, 147–159. [CrossRef]
66. Mason, R.G.; Shermer, R.W.; Zucker, W.H. Effects of certain purified plasma proteins on the compatibility of glass with blood. *Am. J. Pathol.* **1973**, *73*, 183–200.
67. Kottke-Marchant, K.; Anderson, J.M.; Umemura, Y.; Marchant, R.E. Effect of albumin coating on the in vitro blood compatibility of Dacron® arterial prostheses. *Biomaterials* **1989**, *10*, 147–155. [CrossRef]

68. Guidoin, R.; Snyder, R.; Martin, L.; Botzko, K.; Marois, M.; Awad, J.; King, M.; Domurado, D.; Bedros, M.; Gosselin, C. Albumin coating of a knitted polyester arterial prosthesis: An alternative to preclotting. *Ann. Thorac. Surg.* **1984**, *37*, 457–465. [CrossRef]
69. Ji, J.; Tan, Q.; Fan, D.-Z.; Sun, F.-Y.; Barbosa, M.A.; Shen, J. Fabrication of alternating polycation and albumin multilayer coating onto stainless steel by electrostatic layer-by-layer adsorption. *Colloids Surf. B Biointerfaces* **2004**, *34*, 185–190. [CrossRef] [PubMed]
70. Kinnari, T.J.; Peltonen, L.I.; Kuusela, P.; Kivilahti, J.; Könönen, M.; Jero, J. Bacterial adherence to titanium surface coated with human serum albumin. *Otol. Neurotol.* **2005**, *26*, 380–384. [CrossRef]
71. Van De Keere, I.; Willaert, R.; Tourwé, E.; Hubin, A.; Vereecken, J. The interaction of human serum albumin with titanium studied by means of atomic force microscopy. *Surf. Interface Anal.* **2008**, *40*, 157–161. [CrossRef]
72. Lambert, B.J.; Mendelson, T.A.; Craven, M.D. Radiation and Ethylene Oxide Terminal Sterilization Experiences with Drug Eluting Stent Products. *AAPS PharmSciTech* **2011**, *12*, 1116–1126. [CrossRef]
73. Shintani, H. Ethylene Oxide Gas Sterilization of Medical Devices. *Biocontrol Sci.* **2017**, *22*, 1–16. [CrossRef]
74. Barras, C.D.; Myers, K.A. Nitinol—its use in vascular surgery and other applications. *Eur. J. Vasc. Endovasc. Surg.* **2000**, *19*, 564–569. [CrossRef] [PubMed]
75. Nathan, A.; Kobayashi, T.; Giri, J. Nitinol Self-Expanding Stents for the Superficial Femoral Artery. *Interv. Cardiol. Clin.* **2017**, *6*, 227–233. [CrossRef] [PubMed]
76. Akgul, E.; Onan, H.B.; Akpinar, S.; Balli, H.T.; Aksungur, E.H. The DERIVO Embolization Device in the Treatment of Intracranial Aneurysms: Short- and Midterm Results. *World Neurosurg.* **2016**, *95*, 229–240. [CrossRef] [PubMed]
77. Wu, X.; Yin, T.; Tian, J.; Tang, C.; Huang, J.; Zhao, Y.; Zhang, X.; Deng, X.; Fan, Y.; Yu, D.; et al. Distinctive effects of CD34- and CD133-specific antibody-coated stents on re-endothelialization and in-stent restenosis at the early phase of vascular injury. *Regen. Biomater.* **2015**, *2*, 87–96. [CrossRef]
78. Aoki, J.; Serruys, P.W.; van Beusekom, H.; Ong, A.T.L.; McFadden, E.P.; Sianos, G.; van der Giessen, W.J.; Regar, E.; de Feyter, P.J.; Davis, H.R.; et al. Endothelial Progenitor Cell Capture by Stents Coated With Antibody Against CD34: The HEALING-FIM (Healthy Endothelial Accelerated Lining Inhibits Neointimal Growth-First In Man) Registry. *J. Am. Coll. Cardiol.* **2005**, *45*, 1574–1579. [CrossRef] [PubMed]

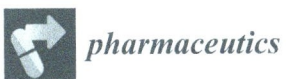

Article

# Albumin-EDTA-Vanadium Is a Powerful Anti-Proliferative Agent, Following Entrance into Glioma Cells via Caveolae-Mediated Endocytosis

Itzik Cooper [1,2,3,*], Orly Ravid [1], Daniel Rand [1], Dana Atrakchi [1], Chen Shemesh [1], Yael Bresler [1,4], Gili Ben-Nissan [5], Michal Sharon [5], Mati Fridkin [6] and Yoram Shechter [5]

1. The Joseph Sagol Neuroscience Center, Sheba Medical Center, Ramat-Gan 52620, Israel; Orly.ravid@sheba.health.gov.il (O.R.); Daniel.Rand@sheba.health.gov.il (D.R.); Dana.Atrakchi@sheba.health.gov.il (D.A.); Chen.Shemesh@sheba.health.gov.il (C.S.); Yael.Bresler@sheba.health.gov.il (Y.B.)
2. School of Psychology, The Reichman University, Herzliya 4610101, Israel
3. The Nehemia Rubin Excellence in Biomedical Research, The TELEM Program, Sheba Medical Center, Tel-Hashomer, Ramat Gan 52620, Israel
4. Sackler Faculty of Medicine, Tel-Aviv University, Tel-Aviv 69978, Israel
5. Department of Biomolecular Sciences, The Weizmann Institute of Science, Rehovot 76100, Israel; Gili.Ben-nissan@weizmann.ac.il (G.B.-N.); michal.sharon@weizmann.ac.il (M.S.); yoram.shechter@weizmann.ac.il (Y.S.)
6. Department of Organic Chemistry, The Weizmann Institute of Science, Rehovot 76100, Israel; mati.fridkin@weizmann.ac.il
* Correspondence: Itzik.Cooper@sheba.helath.gov.il; Tel.: +972-3-5303693; Fax: +972-3-5304752

**Abstract:** Human serum albumin (HSA) is efficiently taken up by cancer cells as a source of carbon and energy. In this study, we prepared a monomodified derivative of HSA covalently linked to an EDTA derivative and investigated its efficacy to shuttle weakly anti-proliferative EDTA associating ligands such as vanadium, into a cancer cell line. HSA-S-MAL-$(CH_2)_2$-NH-CO-EDTA was found to associate both with the vanadium anion (+5) and the vanadium cation (+4) with more than thrice the associating affinity of those ligands toward EDTA. Both conjugates internalized into glioma tumor cell line via caveolae-mediated endocytosis pathway and showed potent anti-proliferative capacities. $IC_{50}$ values were in the range of 0.2 to 0.3 µM, potentiating the anti-proliferative efficacies of vanadium (+4) and vanadium (+5) twenty to thirty fold, respectively. HSA-EDTA-VO$^{++}$ in particular is a cancer permeable prodrug conjugate. The associated vanadium (+4) is not released, nor is it active anti-proliferatively prior to its engagement with the cancerous cells. The bound vanadium (+4) dissociates from the conjugate under acidic conditions with half maximal value at pH 5.8. In conclusion, the anti-proliferative activity feature of vanadium can be amplified and directed toward a cancer cell line. This is accomplished using a specially designed HSA-EDTA-shuttling vehicle, enabling vanadium to be anti-proliferatively active at the low micromolar range of concentration.

**Keywords:** albumin; conjugates; vanadium; cancer; prodrug

## 1. Introduction

Intensive studies have been carried out on the insulin-like effects of vanadium salts. Vanadium mimics the action of insulin in insulin responsive tissues and in diabetic rodents via insulin-independent pathways [1–3], which is reviewed in [4,5]. Vanadium belongs to a family of metals, which interferes with cellular redox homeostasis [6], and as such was investigated also for its anti-cancer efficacy. Vanadium is an element with a wide range of effects on the mammalian organism. In recent years, many studies were published regarding its various organic complexes in view of their application in medicine and the fact that the bioactive complexes/compounds of this metal can be therapeutically active at low concentrations [7]. With its physiological duality, vanadium is essential in trace amounts and toxic at concentrations above 10 µM. Its biological activities include anti-viral, antibacterial, anti-parasitic, anti-fungal, anti-cancer, anti-diabetic, anti-hypercholesterolemic, cardio-protective, and neuroprotective activity [8]. Moreover, in vivo studies reported chemo-preventive effects of vanadium complexes, whereas observations regarding therapeutic activities were limited [9–14]. Indeed vanadium can act in two opposing directions: as a metabolic factor, it might promote proliferation, and on the other hand due to its ability to generate ROS and/or to inhibit a large variety of phosphatases and hydrolases, it can act as an anticancer agent [6]. Consequently, the question arose whether these two opposing effects can be dissociated to permit conversion of vanadium exclusively into an anticancer agent.

In this study, we initially turned vanadium into a prodrug, capable of uptake preferentially by cancerous cells. A derivative of EDTA was covalently linked to HSA in a monomodified fashion. Albumin is largely taken by malignant tissues as a source of carbon and energy [15]. Albumin is also a natural transport protein with long circulatory half-life, which promotes it as an attractive candidate for half-life extension and targeted intracellular delivery of drugs attached by covalent conjugation or association [16].

Both vanadium (+4) and vanadium (+5) associate with EDTA at physiological pH [17]. We assumed that the resultant HSA- EDTA-vanadium conjugates will be inactive extracellularly, but will release bound vanadium both in the cytosol and even more efficiently at the acidic pH of the lysosome, following internalization.

Here, we wished to determine whether vanadium (+4) or vanadium (+5) generate intracellular cytotoxicity, if shuttled into a cancerous cell line with this HSA-EDTA carrier. Likewise, we attempted to identify conditions that eliminate the proliferative effects of vanadium and preserve solely its anti-proliferative efficacy. Our efforts in those directions are presented here in detail.

## 2. Materials and Methods

### 2.1. Materials

Dulbecco's Modified Earl's medium (DMEM) was purchased from Gibco (Life Technologies, Carlsbad, CA, USA). Gentamicin, glutamine, fetal calf serum (FCS), and penicillin/streptomycin were obtained from Biological Industries (Kibbutz Beit Haemek, Galilee, Israel). Human serum albumin (HSA), diethylenetriamine pentaacetic dianhydride (EDTA-dianhyride), $N$(2-aminethyl) malemide, 4.4' dithiodipyridine (4.4DTDP), dithiothreitol (DTT), phosphatase acid from potato (#P-3762), pNitrophenyl phosphate (pNPP), phenylarsine oxide (PAO), indomethacin (IND), nystatin, methyl β cyclodextrin (MCD), and bafilomycin A1 (BAF) were purchased from Sigma Aldrich (Jerusalem, Israel). Sodium metavanadate ($NaVO_3$) and Vanadyl chloride ($VOCl_2$) were from BDH Chemicals Ltd. Poole England. Ethylenediaminetetraacetic acid (EDTA) from Baker Analyzed A.C.S Reagents, and $PEG_{30}$-SH (M-SH-30K) were purchased from Jenkem Technology (Plano, TX, USA). All other materials used in this study were of analytical grade.

### 2.2. Preparation of Mercaptoalbumin

About one third of cysteine-34 of HSA is disulfide-bonded to glutathione or cysteine and this can be reversed by mild reduction with dithioerithritol [18]. This allows us to obtain conjugates containing 0.56 mole EDTA per mole of human serum albumin (Supplementary Table S1). HSA (1.4 g, 20 µmol) dissolved in 0.1 M Hepes buffer (pH 7.3) followed by the addition of one equivalent of dithiothreitol (20 µmol). The reaction was carried out for 1 h at 0 °C and dialyzed over a period of two days with several changes of $H_2O$ and lyophilized. This procedure removes mixed disulfide bonded glutathione or cystine from the cysteinyl moiety of HSA [19]. Mercapto-HSA prepared by this procedure contains 0.7 + 0.05 mole-SH per mole human serum albumin, as determined with 4.4 dithiodipyridine (4.4' DTDP) using $\varepsilon_{324} = 19,800$ [20].

## 2.3. Preparation of EDTA-NH-(CH$_2$)$_2$-Maleimide (EDTA-Maleimide)

EDTA-Dianhydride (38 mg, 100 µmol) suspended in 1.0 mL DMSO and transferred to a tube containing 110 µmol (27 mg) MAL-(CH$_2$)$_2$-NH$_2$. DIPEA (N,N-Disopropylethylamine) was then added in aliquots to achieve neutral pH value, upon 100 times dilution of aliquots in H$_2$O. Following one hour, the product EDTA-maleimide was obtained by centrifugation, washed twice with DMSO and stored at −70 °C until used.

## 2.4. Preparation of HSA-S-MAL-EDTA

N-(2 aminoethyl) maleimide (2.5 mg, 10 µmol) was dissolved in 1.0 mL of 1 M Hepes buffer (pH 7.3) and transferred immediately to a glass tube containing 38 mg (100 µmol) of EDTA-dianhydride. The reaction mixture was stirred for 30 min and combined with a solution of Mercapto-HSA (210 mg/3.0 mL H$_2$O, 3 µmol). Following 1 h, the product (HSA-S-MAL-(CH$_2$)$_2$-NH-CO-EDTA) was dialyzed against H$_2$O over a period of three days with several changes of H$_2$O and lyophilized.

## 2.5. Characterization of HSA-S-MAL-(CH$_2$)$_2$-NHCO-EDTA by Reversed Phase Liquid Chromatography, Coupled to Mass Spectrometry (LC-MS) Analysis

The different protein samples were diluted to 0.17 µM in 100 mM ammonium acetate, pH 6.8. A total of 5 µL from each sample were loaded onto a monolithic reversed phase column [21] and eluted over a gradient of 10–60% acetonitrile, during 15 min, at column temperature of 60 °C. The HSA proteins eluted at 43% acetonitrile and were directly sprayed into a modified Q Exactive Plus EMR Orbitrap mass spectrometer [21], for intact mass measurements. The instrument was operated using the HESI source, at a flow rate of 15 µL/min, using sheath gas 10 and auxiliary gas 3. The inlet capillary was set to 320 °C, capillary voltage 4.3 kV, fore vacuum pressure 1.54 mbar, and trapping gas pressure 0.8, corresponding to HV pressure of $3.0 \times 10^{-5}$ mbar and UHV pressure of $2.2 \times 10^{-10}$ mbar. The source was operated at a constant energy of 2 V in the flatapole bias and interflatapole lens. Bent flatapole DC bias and gradient were set to 1.7 and 10 V, respectively, and the HCD cell was operated at 15 V. Measurements were performed at inject time of 250 and resolution of 10,000. Masses were calculated by the computational suite UniDec v. 4.1.1 [22] (2019, University of Arizona, Tucson, AZ, USA).

## 2.6. Evaluating the Affinities of HSA-EDTA to Vanadium: Reversal of Vanadium-Evoked Inhibition of Acid Phosphatase

This assay was carried out essentially according to reference [4] with slight modifications. It evaluates the efficacy of vanadium chelators toward vanadium, by determining their potency to reverse vanadium-evoked inhibition of acid phosphatase at pH 7.3. Each tube contains 0.5 mL of 0.05 M Hepes buffer pH 7.3, 1.0 M KCl, p-nitophenylphosphate, (0.2 mM) either NaVO$_3$ or VOCl$_2$ (5 µM), increasing concentration of the studied chelator and acid phosphatase (50 µg/tube). Following 40 min at 25 °C, NaOH (20 µL from 4 M NaOH) was added and the absorbance corresponding to the formed p-nitrophenolate was determined at 410 nm. IC$_{50}$ is defined here as the concentration of the vanadium chelator that reversed half maximally vanadium (+4) or vanadium (+5) evoked inhibition of acid phosphatase. It should be noticed that since this is an in-direct method, direct measurements of released vanadium using procedures such as ICP-MS, should be conducted in future studies.

## 2.7. Preparation of HSA-EDTA-Vanadium

HSA-EDTA (25 mg, 0.37 µmol) dissolved in 0.2 mL H$_2$O and VOCl$_2$, or NaVO$_3$, 4 molar excess was then added. The reaction mixture was loaded on a Sephadex G-50 column (12 × 1.7 cm) pre-equilibrated and run with 0.01 M NaHCO$_3$ (pH 8.22). The peak corresponding to the protein fraction was pooled and lyophilized.

## 2.8. Preparation of Rhodamine-Labeled HSA-EDTA

Rhodamine-labeled HSA and HSA-EDTA were prepared by dissolving 17 mg of each (~0.25 μmol) in 0.2 mL of 0.1 M $Na_2CO_3$ (pH 10.3). Rhodamine B isothiocyanate 0.9 mg (2.5 molar excess over HSA) was then added and the reaction was carried out for 1 h at 25 °C. The reaction mixture was loaded on a Sephadex G-50 column (1.7 × 14 cm) equilibrated and run in the same buffer. The tubes containing rhodamine-labeled HSA were pooled, dialyzed against water, and lyophilized. Rhodamine-HSA and rhodamine-HSA-EDTA prepared by this procedure contain 0.95 ± 0.1 mole of rhodamine/mole of HSA as determined by its absorbance at 550 nm using $\varepsilon_{550}$ = 11,400.

## 2.9. Growth Inhibitory Effects of EDTA and Vanadium Containing Conjugates

The glioma cell line CNS-1 (obtained from Mariano S. Viapiano [23]) was grown in 96 well plates in DMEM containing 10% fetal calf serum; 2 mM L-glutamine, penicillin (100 units/mL), and streptomycin (0.1 mg/mL) under humidified atmosphere containing 5% $CO_2$. Cells were seeded at 1000 cells/well. Twenty-four hours later, the EDTA and vanadium containing conjugates were added to each plate to give concentrations as indicated in the text. Control experiments using non-cancer cells were conducted with primary bovine brain pericytes and CD34+ human endothelial cells (both obtained and characterized at the Artois University, France [24–26]) treated with the HSA-EDTA-$VO^{++}$ conjugate. These cells were seeded at 15,000 cells/well in ECM medium (Sciencell, Carlsbad, CA, USA), which was composed as follows: 5% fetal calf serum (Gibco, Gaithersburg, MD, USA), ECGS supplements, and 50 mg/mL gentamicin (Biological industries, Beit-Haemek, Israel). Cells were treated the day after. Cell viability was measured after 72 h using a standard MTT (3-(4,5-dimethylthiazol-2-yl)-2,5-diphenyltetrazolium bromide) assay as described before [27]. Experiments were repeated at least 3 times in quadruplicate. $IC_{50}$ values were calculated from the dose response curves using a median-effect plot.

## 2.10. Immunocytochemistry

CNS-1 cells (60,000/well) were seeded on cover slips in 24 well-plates. After 24 h, growth medium (10% FCS, penicillin (100 U/mL) streptomycin (0.1 mg/mL) and L-glutamine (2 mmol/L) dissolved in DMEM was replaced with fresh medium containing 5 μM rhodamine-labeled HSA or HSA-EDTA-$VO^{++}$. After 5 min, 1 h, or 24 h, the cells were washed with cold PBS and fixed with 4% paraformaldehyde for 15 min. The cells were then stained with Alexa fluor 488-phalloidin (Thermo Fisher Scientific, Waltham, MA, USA) for 20 min and 2 min with Hoechst (Sigma, Burlington, MA, USA). Cells were rinsed with PBS and coverslips were mounted and observed with Olympus IX43 fluorescence microscope.

## 2.11. Uptake of Rhodamine-HSA and Rhodamine-HSA-EDTA-$VO^{++}$

CNS-1 cells (50,000/well) were seeded in 24 well plates. After 48 h, cells were washed with 37 °C phosphate buffer saline (PBS) and pre-incubated in the absence or presence of different blockers in serum-free medium. Pre-incubation conditions of the different blockers were as follows: PAO (clathrin-mediated endocytosis inhibitor, 3 μM) and BAF (metabolic inhibitor, 100 nM) were added only during the pre-incubation period for 30 min. The caveolae-mediated endocytosis inhibitors MCD (5 mM), nystatin (54 μM), and IND (100 μM) were added for 10 min at the pre-incubation period and also during the uptake. After pre-incubation, the cells were incubated with rhodamine-labeled HSA or HSA-EDTA-$VO^{++}$ (0.25 μM) with or without the blockers for 1 h at 37 °C. Cells were then rinsed twice with ice-cold PBS and solubilized with 0.5 M NaOH/0.05% SDS (500 μL/well). A total of 200 μL from each well were transferred to black 96 well plate and the fluorescence was measured using TECAN infinite 200 Pro plate reader at excitation/emission wavelengths of 544/576 nm. A total of 50 μL from each well were evaluated for protein content using a standard BCA assay (Thermo Scientific, Waltham, MA, USA). The effect of the different blockers was calculated after reduction of blanks (the fluorescence of supernatants without rhodamine labeled compounds) and normalization for protein content. Data are presented as the percentage of uptake relative to cells without blockers.

*2.12. Statistical Analysis*

Statistical analyses were performed using the Prism 6 software. Data are presented as the means ± standard error of the mean (SEM). Differences between two groups were assessed by an unpaired *t*-test and among three or more groups by a one-way analysis of variance followed by Tukey's Multiple Comparison Test. A *p*-value of less than 0.05 was considered to be statistically significant.

## 3. Results

*3.1. Preparation of Monomodified HSA-EDTA Derivative*

HSA contains a single cysteinyl moiety at position 34, and its derivatization has little or no effect on the three-dimensional configuration of this carrier protein [15]. Our initial intention was therefore to obtain a monomodified derivative of HSA, containing a single moiety of EDTA. Since EDTA-dianhydride is insoluble in organic solvents the synthesis was carried out under aqueous conditions in 1.0 M Hepes buffer (pH 7.3) for a period of 30 min. During this period, unreacted EDTA-dianhydride is fully hydrolyzed, avoiding the risk of reacting with the amino side chains of HSA (preliminary observation). MAL-containing compounds lose a significant amount of their alkylating capacity under these conditions [28]; however, a sufficient level of MAL-$(CH_2)_2$-NH-CO-EDTA remained for alkylating the single cysteinyl moiety of HSA. All non-covalently linked low molecular-weight molecules were then removed by extensive dialysis, prior to lyophilization (Experimental part). Figure 1 shows a schematic presentation of EDTA and the monomodified HSA-EDTA derivative (HSA-S-MAL-$(CH_2)_2$-NH-CO-EDTA) prepared.

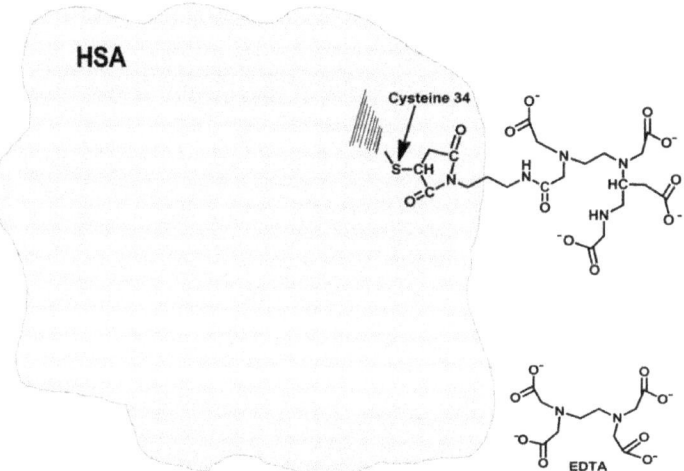

**Figure 1.** Schematic representation of EDTA and the monomodified HSA-EDTA derivative (HSA-S-MAL-$(CH_2)_2$-NH-CO-EDTA).

*3.2. Characterization of HSA-S-MAL-$(CH_2)_2$-NHCO-EDTA by LC-MS*

This procedure was found particularly suitable for HSA-derivatives, since the first stage (denaturation under acidic conditions at 60 °C) eliminates non-covalent interactions (like binding of long-chain free fatty acids) from the protein. Supplementary Materials Table S1 summarizes the MW of mercapto-HSA and two batches of HSA-S-MAL-$(CH_2)_2$-NHCO-EDTA prepared by us. Interestingly enough, the two batches showed additional masses in the vicinity of 150 Da, rather than 530 Da, which was expected for the covalently linked MAL-(CH$_2$)$_2$-NHCO-EDTA to HSA. We therefore postulated that the peptide bond connecting HSA to EDTA, namely HSA-MAL-(CH$_2$)$_2$-NH–CO-EDTA is cleaved during the first stage of the procedure, via a mechanism resembling the hydrolysis of maleyllysine, described by Butler et al. [29]. The MW of the "tail" linked to HSA was calculated to be 156 Da, and additions of 159 and 147 Da were obtained for the two different batches of HSA-S-MAL-(CH$_2$)$_2$-NHCO-EDTA prepared by us (summarized in Supplementary Table S1). Supplementary Figure S1 shows the deconvoluted mass distribution of mercapto-HSA and of HSA-S-MAL-(CH$_2$)$_2$-NHCO-EDTA. This analyses suggested that about 56% of the molecules were modified. Cysteine 34 of albumin is known to "resist" derivatization of somewhat larger –SH reagent, due to its orientation in the three dimensional structure of albumin. These analyses also suggested that these conjugates are mono-modified, in spite of the fact that associating affinity towards vanadium was elevated 3–4 times (Figure 2).

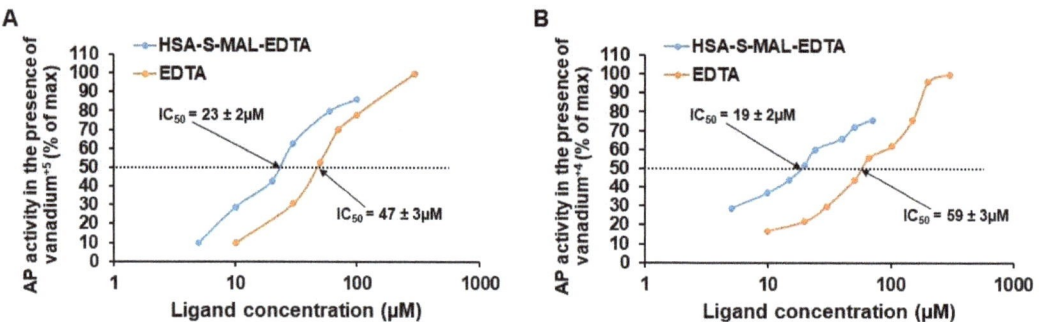

**Figure 2.** Reversal of inhibition of acid phosphatase (AP) by EDTA and HSA-EDTA at pH 7.3. (**A**) Reversal of NaVO$_3$ (+5) evoked inhibition of acid phosphatase and; (**B**) reversal of VOCl$_2$ (+4) evoked inhibition of acid phosphatase. Vanadium concentration was 5 µM. AP, acid phosphatase.

*3.3. Association of Vanadium with HSA-EDTA: Comparison to EDTA and EDTA-Maleimide*

Figure 2A shows the reversal of NaVO$_3$ (+5) evoked inhibition of acid phosphatase by EDTA, EDTA-maleimide and HSA-EDTA at pH 7.3. Half-maximal values were 47, 56 and 23 µM for EDTA, EDTA-maleimide and HSA-EDTA respectively. Figure 2B demonstrates the reversal of VOCl$_2$ (+4) evoked inhibition of acid phosphatase by those ligands. In this case, half maximal values amounted to 59, 71 and 19 µM for EDTA, EDTA-maleimide and HSA-EDTA respectively. Thus the associating affinity toward both forms of this metalooxide increased 3–4 folds (Figure 2) when this chelator is linked to cysteine-34 of this carrier protein.

*3.4. Preparation of HSA-EDTA Vanadium Conjugates*

HSA-S-MAL-EDTA was treated with four-fold molar excess of NaVO$_3$ or VOCl$_2$ and the resultant conjugates were purified on a Sephadex G-50 column (Experimental procedures). This purification step removed unbound vanadium as well as vanadium molecules adsorbed to HSA in an EDTA-independent fashion (in control experiments we added to native HSA 4-fold molar excess of vanadium, transferred them on the Sephadex G-50 column, pooled and lyophilized the void volume, and examined it for the presence of vanadium by the acid phosphatase assay. No vanadium could be detected). Following gel-filtration, both conjugates contain 0.56 ± 0.005 mole vanadium per mole HSA-EDTA. This was quantitated by determining their dose-dependent inhibitory potencies toward acid-phosphatase at pH 5.0 (Figure 3A,B). At this pH (or lower), vanadium dissociates fully from the conjugates, regaining the efficacy of the free metalooxide to inhibit this enzymatic activity (subsequent paragraph). IC$_{50}$ values were 0.40 ± 0.03 µM for vanadium (+5) and 0.45 ± 0.02 µM for HSA-EDTA-VO$_3^-$ (Figure 3A). Vanadium (+4) and HSA-EDTA-VO$^{++}$ inhibits this enzymatic activity at pH 5.0 with IC$_{50}$ values of 0.8 ± 0.04 and 0.7 ± 0.03 µM respectively (Figure 3B). For comparison, the efficacy of vanadium (+4) and HSA-EDTA-VO$^{++}$ to inhibit acid phosphatase at pH 7.3 is shown in Figure 3C. IC$_{50}$ values amounted to 0.7 ± 0.03 and 8.1 ± 0.3 for vanadium (+4) and HSA-EDTA-VO$^{++}$, respectively.

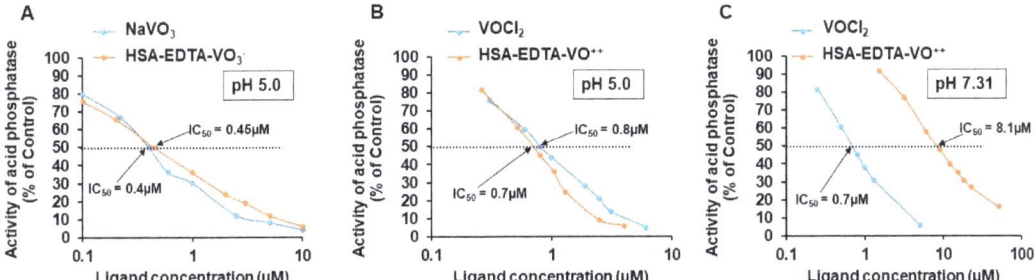

**Figure 3.** Dose-dependent inhibition of acid phosphatase at pH 5.0 and 7.31 by Sephadex-purified HSA-EDTA-vanadium and the free metalooxides. The incubation assay was run for 40–60 min at 25 °C in tubes (0.6 mL) containing 0.1 M KCl-1 mM HCl (pH 5.0, **A,B**) or 0.1 M KCl-100 mM Hepes buffer (pH 7.31, **C**). Each tube contained PNPP (0.2 mM), 5 µg acid phosphatase (**A,B**) or 25 µg (**C**) and the indicated concentrations of HSA-EDTA-vanadium or the free metalooxide. The assay was terminated with NaOH, upon reaching OD$_{410}$ = 0.9 ± 0.1 in tubes having no HSA-EDTA-vanadium or the free metalooxide. Results are expressed as the mean ± SEM of three independent experiments.

*3.5. Stability of HSA-EDTA-VO$^{++}$ as a Function of pH*

As shown in Figure 3B, the vanadium (+4) dissociates fully at pH 5.0 from the conjugate, regaining the efficacy of the free metalooxide to inhibit acid-phosphatase. Table 1 summarizes the IC$_{50}$ values for the inhibition of this enzymatic activity at varying pH values. The dissociated fraction of vanadium (+4) from the conjugate as a function of pH was calculated. IC$_{50}$ values varied between 1.0 ± 0.03 µM at pH 5.4 (corresponding to 70% dissociation) to 5 µM at pH 7.15 (corresponding to 14% dissociation). Extrapolation of these values revealed that half maximal dissociation of vanadium (+4) from the conjugate takes place at pH 5.8.

**Table 1.** IC$_{50}$ values for the inhibition of acid phosphatase at varying pH values [1].

| pH | IC$_{50}$ (µM) [2] | % Dissociated [3] | Comments |
|---|---|---|---|
| 5.0 | 0.7 [4] | 100 | Full dissociation |
| 5.4 | 1.0 | 70 | |
| 6.0 | 1.57 | 44 | |
| 7.0 | 3.7 | 19 | |
| 7.15 | 5.0 | 14 | |
| 7.31 | 8.1 [4] | 9 | Relatively stable |

[1] IC$_{50}$ values for free vanadium (+4) amounted to 0.7 ± 0.1 µM in all pH tested. [2] Assays were carried out for a period of 20 to 60 min with acid phosphatase concentrations of 5 µg/tube at pH 5 to 6 and 25 µg/tube at pH 7–7.31. Reaction was terminated by adding NaOH upon reaching OD$_{410}$ = 0.9 ± 0.1 in the absence of HSA-EDTA-VO$^{++}$. [3] Calculated by dividing IC$_{50}$ value of pH 5.0 with the IC$_{50}$ values obtained at each pH measured. [4] Valued obtained from Figure 3.

*3.6. HSA-EDTA-Vanadium Conjugates Are Powerful Anti-Proliferative Agents*

Figure 4A shows the dose-dependent anti-proliferative efficacy of HSA-EDTA-VO$_3^-$ in the CNS-1 cell line. This was compared to that of free vanadate (+5) and to a 1:1 complex of EDTA with VO$_3^-$. HSA-EDTA-VO$_3^-$ facilitates its anti-proliferative effect with IC$_{50}$ value of 0.27 + 0.03 µM, potentiating the effect of vanadium (+5) about 20 folds (IC$_{50}$ = 5.3 µM, Table 2). The complex of EDTA with vanadium (+5) also facilitates a significant anti-proliferative effect (Table 2), suggesting that this metalooxide can significantly dissociate from EDTA during the three-day period of incubation with the cells. Figure 4B shows the dose-dependent anti-proliferative efficacy of HSA-EDTA-VO$^{++}$ as compared to that of the vanadyl cation and to a 1:1 complex of EDTA with VO$^{++}$. This conjugate was found to be a powerful anti-proliferative agent as well (IC$_{50}$ = 0.34 ± 0.03 µM, Table 2). It potentiated the effect of vanadyl about 26 times. (IC$_{50}$ = 8.9 µM). Unlike EDTA-VO$_3^-$ (Figure 4A), the one to one complex EDTA-VO$^{++}$ had negligible anti-proliferative efficacy at concentrations above 5 µM (Figure 4B, Table 2). Thus, HSA-EDTA-VO$^{++}$ appears to be a 'silent' prodrug prior of engagement with the CNS-1 cells, where a powerful anti-proliferative effect is developed. Neither one of the three components comprising HSA-EDTA, showed anti-proliferative efficacy with IC$_{50}$ lower than 10 µM (Table 2). The anti-proliferative effect of the HSA-EDTA-VO$^{++}$ conjugate was examined also in non-cancer cells (primary bovine brain pericytes and CD34+ human endothelial cells) and the potency towards these cells was found to be much lower than towards the CNS-1 glioma cells (IC$_{50}$ > 10 µM, Supplementary Materials Figure S2).

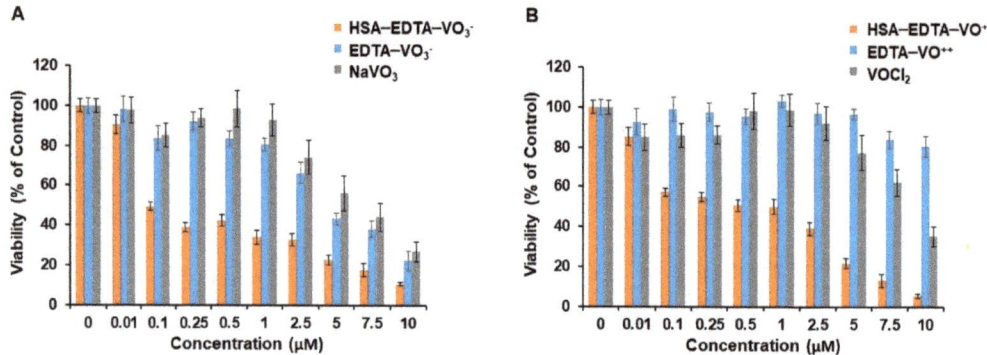

**Figure 4.** Anti-proliferative efficacies of free metalooxide, 1:1 complexes of EDTA and vanadium, and HSA-EDTA-vanadium conjugates in the CNS-1 glioma cell line. Dose-dependent toxicity experiments were conducted as described in the Section 2. HSA-EDTA-VO$_3^-$, NaVO$_3$, and EDTA-VO$_3^-$ (**A**) or HSA-EDTA-VO$^{++}$, VOCl$_2$, and EDTA-VO$^{++}$ (**B**) were added to the cell culture for 72 h before MTT toxicity assay was applied to determine their anti-proliferative efficacies. Experiments were repeated at least three times in quadruplicate. Data are presented as the mean percentage ±SEM. $n$ = 12 per treatment from at least 3 different experiments.

**Table 2.** Anti-proliferative efficacies of HSA-EDTA-vanadium conjugates, and of the building components of those conjugates, in the CNS-1 glioma cell line.

| Compound | IC$_{50}$ (µM) [1] | Potentiation Efficacy (Fold) |
|---|---|---|
| Vanadate (NaVO$_3$) | 5.3 | |
| Vanadyl (VOCl$_2$) | 8.9 | |
| HSA | >20 | |
| EDTA | >20 | |
| HSA-EDTA | >10 | |
| EDTA·VO$_3^-$ (1:1 complex) | 3.2 | |
| EDTA·VO$^{+2}$ (1:1 complex) | 16.0 | |
| HSA-EDTA-VO$_3^-$ | 0.27 | 19.6 |
| HSA-EDTA-VO$^{+2}$ | 0.34 | 26 |

[1] IC$_{50}$ values were calculated from dose response curves using a median-effect plot.

*3.7. HSA-EDTA-VO$^{++}$ Penetrates into CNS-1 Glioma Cell Line via Caveolae-Mediated Endocytosis*

In order to confirm that this conjugate acts intracellularly, we have prepared rhodamine-labeled HSA and rhodamine-labeled HSA-EDTA-VO$^{++}$ (Experimental part). These compounds were incubated with the cells for varying periods of time. Figure 5A,B show that both HSA and the conjugate were largely taken to the cell interior within 1 h of incubation, indicating that internalization at 37 °C is a rapid event. Uptake of these compounds was already shown after 5 min incubation and also after 24 h (not shown). We then tested a series of inhibitors targeting different endocytosis pathways. Figure 5C,D show that both the native HSA and the HSA-EDTA-VO$^{++}$ conjugate uptake into the CNS1 glioma cells were significantly blocked (58 and 61%, respectively) by MCD, which is a caveolae-mediated endocytosis inhibitor. Nystatin, another caveolae-mediated endocytosis inhibitor also blocked the uptake of HSA and HSA-EDTA-VO$^{++}$ by 20 and 34%, respectively. The clathrin-mediated endocytosis inhibitor PAO had no effect on the uptake of both compounds, nor did the metabolic inhibitor BAF or the caveolae-mediated endocytosis inhibitor IND, which blocks the internalization of caveolae and the return of plasmalemmal vesicles to the cell surface [30].

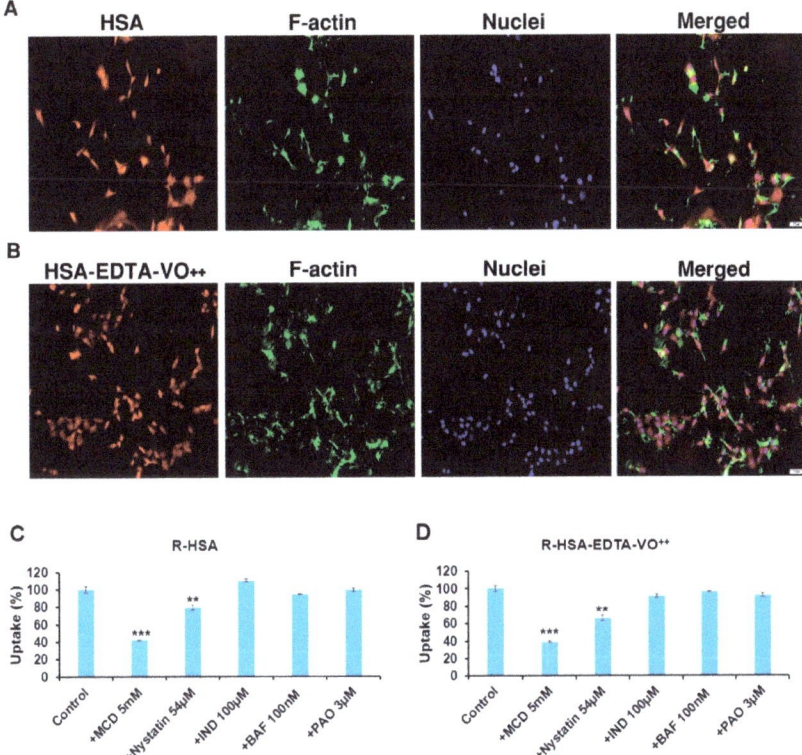

**Figure 5.** Uptake of HSA and HSA-EDTA-VO$^{++}$ into CNS-1 glioma cell line is a caveolae-mediated endocytosis process. Rhodamine-labeled HSA (**A**) and HSA-EDTA-VO$^{++}$ (**B**) (5 µM) were incubated with the cells for 1 h. The cells were washed, fixed, and mounted on cover slips. The uptake of the compounds was visualized with a fluorescence microscope. The cells were counter stained with phalloidin (green) and Hoechst (blue) for actin filaments and nuclei, respectively. Different blockers were used to determine the mechanism of entry of Rhodamine-labeled HSA (R-HSA) (**C**) and R-HSA-EDTA-VO$^{++}$ (**D**). Data presented as mean ± SEM, $n$ = 9 from three different experiments. ** $p$ < 0.01, *** $p$ < 0.001. Bar, 50 µm.

## 4. Discussion

Vanadium, an anabolic metalooxide in insulin responsive tissues, inhibits a wide variety of phosphohydrolases [31]. As such, it facilitates a variety of biological responses in different directions [32]. In cancer cells, both anti-proliferative and proliferative responses were observed [4]. The question arose whether the anti-proliferative effect of vanadium can be isolated, magnified, and specifically directed toward a tumor cell line.

In this study, we selected HSA as the protein carrier for obtaining selectivity toward cancer cell lines [15]. Albumin is taken up by malignant tissues as a source of carbon and energy [33,34]. The protein has a single cysteinyl moiety enabling preparation of a monomodified conjugate with MAL-containing compounds [27]. Cysteine-34 is located on the outer surface of HSA distant from the main interior drug binding sites, making it attractive for covalent conjugation of drugs [16]. Derivatization of this moiety with low molecular weight compounds has no or little effect on its native structure and was shown to be efficiently pinocytosed by cancer cells [33,34]. Initially, we treated HSA by one equivalent of DTT, to release disulfide bonded cysteine-34. This procedure yielded HSA having $0.85 \pm 0.05$ mole-SH/mole protein. Although cysteine-34 is located in a hydrophobic crevice of depth 10–12 Å [35], it reacted with the unbranched MAL-$(CH_2)_2$-NH-CO-EDTA to obtain the macromolecular chelator shown in Figure 1.

Interestingly enough, HSA-EDTA associated with both forms of vanadium at 3–4 fold higher affinity as compared to EDTA or to EDTA-maleimide (Figure 2). Cysteine-34 is positioned in a 10–12 Å deep hydrophobic crevice on the surface of HSA [36]. It therefore appears that the vicinity of this cysteine moiety contributes significantly in elevating the associating affinity of this chelator toward vanadium. PEG30-S-MAL-EDTA showed no higher affinity toward vanadium as compared to that of EDTA (unpublished observation). Both HSA-EDTA-vanadium conjugates studied here were purified on a Sephadex G-50 column prior to analyses for anti-proliferative efficacies. This procedure removed unbound vanadium and vanadium ions that associate with HSA in an EDTA-independent fashion. This purification step demonstrated that the conjugates are stable in the presence of 0.01 M NaHCO$_3$ (pH 8.2).

Although not in the frame work of this study, we noted that stable-Sephadex purified complexes of HSA-EDTA with $Zn^{+2}$, $Fe^{+2}$, $Mn^{+2}$, $Co^{+2}$, $MOO_4^{-2}$, and $WOO_4^{-2}$ could also be obtained (not shown) despite the fact that $Zn^{+2}$, $Fe^{+2}$, $Mn^{+2}$, and $Co^{+2}$ have considerably lower binding affinities than vanadium toward EDTA [37]. Finally, we demonstrated the superiority of both conjugates in facilitating the anti-proliferative effect in the CNS-1 cell line as opposed to free vanadium (Figure 4). Since the complex of vanadium (+4) with EDTA displays negligible effects on cells, our preference is given to HSA-EDTA-VO$^{++}$.

We refer to HSA-EDTA-VO$^{++}$ as the first example of a possible 'peripherally non-toxic chemotherapeutically active prodrug conjugate'. Vanadium (+4), a rather anabolic metalooxide, exhibited low peripheral toxicity in rodents and in human diabetic patients [2,38–42]. This is most likely valid for HSA-EDTA, which associates with vanadium (+4) with considerably higher affinity (Figure 2). Reactivation is exclusively an intracellular mediated event and as opposed to other previously studied albumin-drug conjugates [15], the release of the chemotherapeutically active component is a simple intracellular dissociation that takes place half maximally at pH $5.8 \pm 0.1$ (Table 1). The cytosolic pH of cancer cells is lower than 7.0 [43], suggesting that a sufficient amount of VO$^{++}$ can be released at the cytosol following internalization and more so at the acidic pH of the lysosome [44]. In this context, some tumor cell-related properties may hinder the efficiency of these albumin-vanadium conjugates and should be considered in preclinical and clinical settings. For example, extracellular pH of tumor cells (pHe) is usually mildly acidic [45]. pHe values greatly vary between different tumors and also spatiotemporally within a certain tumor [46]. Thus, certain part of vanadium ions may be released prior to its internalization into the cells depending on the tumor type and location inside the tumor microenvironment. Yet, since the half maximal dissociation value of vanadium (+4) is at pH 5.8 (Table 1), most of the conjugate should remain intact prior to cell uptake.

HSA-EDTA-VO$^{++}$, similarly to native HSA, internalizes into CNS-1 glioma cells mainly through caveolae/lipid rafts-mediated endocytosis (Figure 5). The uptake of both compounds into the cells was blocked in a similar fashion, exhibiting the importance of monomodification [47]. Two common caveolae-mediated inhibitors, i.e., MCD, and to a lesser extent also nystatin, were the only drugs that significantly blocked the uptake into the cells (Figure 5). MCD and nystatin interfere with the caveolae-mediated endocytosis by binding sterols within the cell membrane. The differences in the magnitude of inhibition between the two drugs might result from their different patterns and/or capacity of sterols binding [48]. It is well documented that native albumin has several pathways to be internalized into cells depending on the cell type and physiological conditions [49]. This includes receptor-mediated endocytosis—a process that is generally blocked by Bafilomycin A1 (BAF)—a specific inhibitor of the vacuolar H$^+$-ATPase. H$^+$-ATPase localized in the endosomal membrane is responsible for lowering pH inside the endosome, which is an essential process for the dissociation of the ligands and receptors after receptor-mediated endocytosis. Thus, inhibition of vacuolar H$^+$-ATPase results in decreased activity of the receptor-mediated endocytosis process. It is reasonable that the CNS-1 glioma cells that originate in the brain, an organ mostly deprived of albumin, do not express receptor/s for albumin, explaining the lack of uptake inhibition by BAF in these cells. Clathrin-mediated endocytosis is also a pathway with which albumin is being internalized into various cells. For example, alveolar epithelial cells internalize albumin via clathrin-mediated endocytosis, but not by the caveolae-mediated pathway [49], demonstrating that albumin internalizes into cells by different pathways depending on the type of the cells and tissue. We also used indomethacin (IND), which blocks caveolae-mediated endocytosis differently than MCD and nystatin by inhibiting the internalization of caveolae and the return of plasmalemmal vesicles to the cell surface [49]. This blocker had no inhibitory effect neither on HSA nor on the conjugate, strengthening the conclusion that caveolae-mediated endocytosis through inhibition of cholesterol-related processes at the cell membrane is the most dominant pathway of HSA and HSA-EDTA-VO$^{++}$ internalization in these cells.

In conclusion, we have engineered a HSA-EDTA shuttling vehicle that can introduce EDTA-associating ligands into a glioma cell line via caveolae-mediated endocytosis, and demonstrated its efficacy to convert vanadium into a powerful anti-proliferative agent.

**Supplementary Materials:** The following are available online at https://www.mdpi.com/article/10.3390/pharmaceutics13101557/s1, Figure S1: Mass spectrometry measurements, Figure S2: Anti-proliferative efficacies of HSA-EDTA-VO$^{++}$ in non-cancer cells, Table S1: Mass spectroscopy; MW calculations of HSA derivatives.

**Author Contributions:** Investigation including acquisition, analysis and interpretation of data, I.C., Y.B., O.R., C.S., D.A., D.R., G.B.-N., M.S. and Y.S.; Conceptualization, I.C., M.F. and Y.S.; Writing—original draft: I.C., M.F. and Y.S.; Writing—review & editing including revising it critically for important intellectual content: I.C., M.F., Y.S., G.B.-N. and M.S.; Supervision: I.C. and Y.S. All authors have read and agreed to the published version of the manuscript.

**Funding:** This work was supported in whole or part by a Kimmelman grant from the Weizmann Institute.

**Institutional Review Board Statement:** Not applicable.

**Informed Consent Statement:** Not applicable.

**Data Availability Statement:** Data from this study is available from authors upon reasonable request.

**Acknowledgments:** We thank Steven J. D. Karlish from the Weizmann Institute for his insightful comments during the revision process.

**Conflicts of Interest:** The authors declare no conflict of interest.

## Abbreviations

BAF: bafilomycin A1; EDTA-dianhydride, diethylentriaminepentaacetic dianhydride; DTT-dithiothreitol; 4.4′ DTDP, 4,4 dithiodipyridine; DIPEA, N,N-Disopropylethylamine; HSA, Human–serum albumin; HSA-S-MAL-EDTA, a one to one conjugate of HSA in which EDTA is linked to its cysteinyl moiety through MAL(CH$_2$)$_3$-NH$_2$; IND, indomethacin; MAL, maleimide; MAL-(CH$_2$)$_2$-NH$_2$, N(2-aminoethyl) maleimide; MCD, methyl β cyclodextrin; Mercapto-HSA, HSA- containing mole cysteine (cysteine-34) per mole HSA; PEG$_{30}$-S-MAL-EDTA, a one to one conjugate of PEG$_{30}$-SH linked to MAL-(CH$_2$)$_2$-NH-CO-EDTA; PAO, phenylarsine oxide; PNPP, p-nihophenyl phosphate.

## References

1. Elberg, G.; Li, J.; Shechter, Y. Vanadium activates or inhibits receptor and non-receptor protein tyrosine kinases in cell-free experiments, depending on its oxidation state. Possible role of endogenous vanadium in controlling cellular protein tyrosine kinase activity. *J. Biol. Chem.* **1994**, *269*, 9521–9527. [CrossRef]
2. Meyerovitch, J.; Farfel, Z.; Sack, J.; Shechter, Y. Oral administration of vanadate normalizes blood glucose levels in streptozotocin-treated rats. Characterization and mode of action. *J. Biol. Chem.* **1987**, *262*, 6658–6662. [CrossRef]
3. Shechter, Y.; Karlish, S.J. Insulin-like stimulation of glucose oxidation in rat adipocytes by vanadyl (IV) ions. *Nature* **1980**, *284*, 556–558. [CrossRef]
4. Goldwaser, I.; Gefel, D.; Gershonov, E.; Fridkin, M.; Shechter, Y. Insulin-like effects of vanadium: Basic and clinical implications. *J. Inorg. Biochem.* **2000**, *80*, 21–25. [CrossRef]
5. Sekar, N.; Li, J.; Shechter, Y. Vanadium salts as insulin substitutes: Mechanisms of action, a scientific and therapeutic tool in diabetes mellitus research. *Crit. Rev. Biochem. Mol. Biol.* **1996**, *31*, 339–359. [CrossRef]
6. Jungwirth, U.; Kowol, C.R.; Keppler, B.K.; Hartinger, C.G.; Berger, W.; Heffeter, P. Anticancer activity of metal complexes: Involvement of redox processes. *Antioxid. Redox Signal.* **2011**, *15*, 1085–1127. [CrossRef] [PubMed]
7. Tracey, A.S.; Willsky, G.R.; Takeuchi, E.S. *Vanadium: Chemistry, Biochemistry, Pharmacological, and Practical Applications*; CRC Press, Taylor and Francis Group: Boca Raton, FL, USA, 2007.
8. Ścibior, A.; Pietrzyk, Ł.; Plewa, Z.; Skiba, A. Vanadium: Risks and possible benefits in the light of a comprehensive overview of its pharmacotoxicological mechanisms and multi-applications with a summary of further research trends. *J. Trace Elem. Med. Biol.* **2020**, *61*, 126508. [CrossRef] [PubMed]
9. Bishayee, A.; Waghray, A.; Patel, M.A.; Chatterjee, M. Vanadium in the detection, prevention and treatment of cancer: The in vivo evidence. *Cancer Lett.* **2010**, *294*, 1–12. [CrossRef]
10. Chakraborty, A.; Ghosh, R.; Roy, K.; Ghosh, S.; Chowdhury, P.; Chatterjee, M. Vanadium: A modifier of drug-metabolizing enzyme patterns and its critical role in cellular proliferation in transplantable murine lymphoma. *Oncology* **1995**, *52*, 310–314. [CrossRef]
11. El-Naggar, M.M.; El-Waseef, A.M.; El-Halafawy, K.M.; El-Sayed, I.H. Antitumor activities of vanadium(IV), manganese(IV), iron(III), cobalt(II) and copper(II) complexes of 2-methylaminopyridine. *Cancer Lett.* **1998**, *133*, 71–76. [CrossRef]
12. Evangelou, A.M. Vanadium in cancer treatment. *Crit. Rev. Oncol. Hematol.* **2002**, *42*, 249–265. [CrossRef]
13. Kostova, I. Titanium and vanadium complexes as anticancer agents. *Anticancer Agents Med. Chem.* **2009**, *9*, 827–842. [CrossRef] [PubMed]
14. Leon, I.E.; Cadavid-Vargas, J.F.; Di Virgilio, A.L.; Etcheverry, S.B. Vanadium, Ruthenium and Copper Compounds: A New Class of Nonplatinum Metallodrugs with Anticancer Activity. *Curr. Med. Chem.* **2017**, *24*, 112–148. [CrossRef] [PubMed]
15. Neumann, E.; Frei, E.; Funk, D.; Becker, M.D.; Schrenk, H.-H.; Müller-Ladner, U.; Fiehn, C. Native albumin for targeted drug delivery. *Expert Opin. Drug Deliv.* **2010**, *7*, 915–925. [CrossRef]
16. Larsen, M.T.; Kuhlmann, M.; Hvam, M.L.; Howard, K.A. Albumin-based drug delivery: Harnessing nature to cure disease. *Mol. Cell. Ther.* **2016**, *4*, 3. [CrossRef]
17. Crans, D.C.; Bunch, R.L.; Theisen, L.A. Interaction of trace levels of vanadium(IV) and vanadium(V) in biological systems. *J. Am. Chem. Soc.* **1989**, *111*, 7597–7607. [CrossRef]
18. Sogami, M.; Nagoka, S.; Era, S.; Honda, M.; Noguchi, K. Resolution of human mercapt- and nonmercaptalbumin by high-performance liquid chromatography. *Int. J. Pept. Protein Res.* **1984**, *24*, 96–103. [CrossRef]
19. Hartley, R.W.; Peterson, E.A.; Sober, H.A. The relation of free sulfhydryl groups to chromatographic heterogeneity and polymerization of bovine plasma albumin. *Biochemistry* **1962**, *1*, 60–68. [CrossRef]
20. Grassetti, D.R.; Murray, J.F. Determination of sulfhydryl groups with 2,2'- or 4,4'-dithiodipyridine. *Arch. Biochem. Biophys.* **1967**, *119*, 41–49. [CrossRef]
21. Rozen, S.; Tieri, A.; Ridner, G.; Stark, A.-K.; Schmaler, T.; Ben-Nissan, G.; Dubiel, W.; Sharon, M. Exposing the subunit diversity within protein complexes: A mass spectrometry approach. *Methods* **2013**, *59*, 270–277. [CrossRef]
22. Marty, M.T.; Baldwin, A.J.; Marklund, E.G.; Hochberg, G.K.A.; Benesch, J.L.P.; Robinson, C.V. Bayesian deconvolution of mass and ion mobility spectra: From binary interactions to polydisperse ensembles. *Anal. Chem.* **2015**, *87*, 4370–4376. [CrossRef]
23. Kruse, C.A.; Molleston, M.C.; Parks, E.P.; Schiltz, P.M.; Kleinschmidt-DeMasters, B.K.; Hickey, W.F. A rat glioma model, CNS-1, with invasive characteristics similar to those of human gliomas: A comparison to 9L gliosarcoma. *J. Neurooncol.* **1994**, *22*, 191–200. [CrossRef]
24. Cecchelli, R.; Aday, S.; Sevin, E.; Almeida, C.; Culot, M.; Dehouck, L.; Coisne, C.; Engelhardt, B.; Dehouck, M.-P.; Ferreira, L. A stable and reproducible human blood-brain barrier model derived from hematopoietic stem cells. *PLoS ONE* **2014**, *9*, e99733.
25. Shelly, S.; Liraz Zaltsman, S.; Ben-Gal, O.; Dayan, A.; Ganmore, I.; Shemesh, C.; Atrakchi, D.; Garra, S.; Ravid, O.; Rand, D.; et al. Potential neurotoxicity of titanium implants: Prospective, in-vivo and in-vitro study. *Biomaterials* **2021**, *276*, 121039. [CrossRef]
26. Israelov, H.; Ravid, O.; Atrakchi, D.; Rand, D.; Elhaik, S.; Bresler, Y.; Twitto-Greenberg, R.; Omesi, L.; Liraz-Zaltsman, S.; Gosselet, F.; et al. Caspase-1 has a critical role in blood-brain barrier injury and its inhibition contributes to multifaceted repair. *J. Neuroinflamma* **2020**, *17*, 267. [CrossRef]

27. Cooper, I.; Fridkin, M.; Shechter, Y. Conjugation of Methotrexate-Amino Derivatives to Macromolecules through Carboxylate Moieties Is Superior Over Conventional Linkage to Amino Residues: Chemical, Cell-Free and In Vitro Characterizations. *PLoS ONE* **2016**, *11*, e0158352. [CrossRef]
28. Hazum, E.; Shisheva, A.; Shechter, Y. Preparation and application of radioiodinated sulfhydryl reagents for the covalent labeling of SH-proteins present in minute quantities. *J. Biochem. Biophys. Methods* **1992**, *24*, 95–106. [CrossRef]
29. Butler, P.J.; Harris, J.I.; Hartley, B.S.; Lebeman, R. The use of maleic anhydride for the reversible blocking of amino groups in polypeptide chains. *Biochem. J.* **1969**, *112*, 679–689. [CrossRef]
30. Visser, C.C.; Stevanović, S.; Heleen Voorwinden, L.; Gaillard, P.J.; Crommelin, D.J.A.; Danhof, M.; De Boer, A.G. Validation of the transferrin receptor for drug targeting to brain capillary endothelial cells in vitro. *J. Drug Target* **2004**, *12*, 145–150. [CrossRef]
31. Shechter, Y.; Eldberg, G.; Shisheva, A.; Gefel, D.; Sekar, N.; Qian, S.; Bruck, R.; Gershonov, E.; Crans, D.C.; Goldwasser, Y.; et al. Insulin-like Effects of Vanadium; Reviewing In Vivo and In Vitro Studies and Mechanisms of Action. In *Vanadium Compounds: Chemistry, Biochemistry, and Therapeutic Applications*; Tracey, A.S., Crans, D.C., Eds.; ACS Symposium Series; American Chemical Society: Washington, DC, USA, 1998; Volume 711, pp. 308–315.
32. Mukherjee, B.; Patra, B.; Mahapatra, S.; Banerjee, P.; Tiwari, A.; Chatterjee, M. Vanadium—An element of atypical biological significance. *Toxicol. Lett.* **2004**, *150*, 135–143. [CrossRef]
33. Jain, R.K. Delivery of molecular and cellular medicine to solid tumors. *J. Control. Release* **1998**, *53*, 49–67. [CrossRef]
34. Maeda, H.; Wu, J.; Sawa, T.; Matsumura, Y.; Hori, K. Tumor vascular permeability and the EPR effect in macromolecular therapeutics: A review. *J. Control. Release* **2000**, *65*, 271–284. [CrossRef]
35. Carter, D.C.; Ho, J.X. Structure of serum albumin. In *Lipoproteins, Apolipoproteins, and Lipases*; Advances in Protein Chemistry; Elsevier: Amsterdam, The Netherlands, 1994; Volume 45, pp. 153–203.
36. Kratz, F.; Warnecke, A.; Scheuermann, K.; Stockmar, C.; Schwab, J.; Lazar, P.; Drückes, P.; Esser, N.; Drevs, J.; Rognan, D.; et al. Probing the cysteine-34 position of endogenous serum albumin with thiol-binding doxorubicin derivatives. Improved efficacy of an acid-sensitive doxorubicin derivative with specific albumin-binding properties compared to that of the parent compound. *J. Med. Chem.* **2002**, *45*, 5523–5533. [CrossRef]
37. Smith, S.W. The role of chelation in the treatment of other metal poisonings. *J. Med. Toxicol.* **2013**, *9*, 355–369. [CrossRef]
38. Boden, G.; Chen, X.; Ruiz, J.; van Rossum, G.D.; Turco, S. Effects of vanadyl sulfate on carbohydrate and lipid metabolism in patients with non-insulin-dependent diabetes mellitus. *Metab. Clin. Exp.* **1996**, *45*, 1130–1135. [CrossRef]
39. Cohen, N.; Halberstam, M.; Shlimovich, P.; Chang, C.J.; Shamoon, H.; Rossetti, L. Oral vanadyl sulfate improves hepatic and peripheral insulin sensitivity in patients with non-insulin-dependent diabetes mellitus. *J. Clin. Investg.* **1995**, *95*, 2501–2509. [CrossRef]
40. Halberstam, M.; Cohen, N.; Shlimovich, P.; Rossetti, L.; Shamoon, H. Oral vanadyl sulfate improves insulin sensitivity in NIDDM but not in obese nondiabetic subjects. *Diabetes* **1996**, *45*, 659–666. [CrossRef]
41. Heyliger, C.E.; Tahiliani, A.G.; McNeill, J.H. Effect of vanadate on elevated blood glucose and depressed cardiac performance of diabetic rats. *Science* **1985**, *227*, 1474–1477. [CrossRef]
42. Meyerovitch, J.; Rothenberg, P.; Shechter, Y.; Bonner-Weir, S.; Kahn, C.R. Vanadate normalizes hyperglycemia in two mouse models of non-insulin-dependent diabetes mellitus. *J. Clin. Investg.* **1991**, *87*, 1286–1294. [CrossRef]
43. Anderson, M.; Moshnikova, A.; Engelman, D.M.; Reshetnyak, Y.K.; Andreev, O.A. Probe for the measurement of cell surface pH in vivo and ex vivo. *Proc. Natl. Acad. Sci. USA* **2016**, *113*, 8177–8181. [CrossRef]
44. Yu, F.; Chen, Z.; Wang, B.; Jin, Z.; Hou, Y.; Ma, S.; Liu, X. The role of lysosome in cell death regulation. *Tumour Biol.* **2016**, *37*, 1427–1436. [CrossRef] [PubMed]
45. Corbet, C.; Feron, O. Tumour acidosis: From the passenger to the driver's seat. *Nat. Rev. Cancer* **2017**, *17*, 577–593. [CrossRef] [PubMed]
46. Korenchan, D.E.; Flavell, R.R. Spatiotemporal ph heterogeneity as a promoter of cancer progression and therapeutic resistance. *Cancers* **2019**, *11*, 1026. [CrossRef] [PubMed]
47. Stehle, G.; Sinn, H.; Wunder, A.; Schrenk, H.H.; Schütt, S.; Maier-Borst, W.; Heene, D.L. The loading rate determines tumor targeting properties of methotrexate-albumin conjugates in rats. *Anticancer Drugs* **1997**, *8*, 677–685. [CrossRef] [PubMed]
48. Valitova, J.; Sulkarnayeva, A.; Kotlova, E.; Ponomareva, A.; Mukhitova, F.K.; Murtazina, L.; Ryzhkina, I.; Beckett, R.; Minibayeva, F. Sterol binding by methyl-β-cyclodextrin and nystatin–comparative analysis of biochemical and physiological consequences for plants. *FEBS J.* **2014**, *281*, 2051–2060. [CrossRef]
49. Ikehata, M.; Yumoto, R.; Nakamura, K.; Nagai, J.; Takano, M. Comparison of albumin uptake in rat alveolar type II and type I-like epithelial cells in primary culture. *Pharm. Res.* **2008**, *25*, 913–922. [CrossRef]

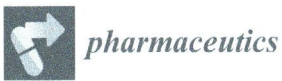

*Article*

# Molecular-Level Release of Coumarin-3-Carboxylic Acid and Warfarin-Derivatives from BSA-Based Hydrogels

Niuosha Sanaeifar [1], Karsten Mäder [2] and Dariush Hinderberger [1,*]

1. Institute of Chemistry, Martin Luther University Halle-Wittenberg, Von-Danckelmann-Platz 4, 06120 Halle (Saale), Germany; niuosha.sanaeifar@chemie.uni-halle.de
2. Institute of Pharmacy, Martin Luther University Halle-Wittenberg, Wolfgang-Langenbeck-Str. 4, 06120 Halle (Saale), Germany; karsten.maeder@pharmazie.uni-halle.de
* Correspondence: dariush.hinderberger@chemie.uni-halle.de

**Abstract:** This investigation aimed at developing BSA hydrogels as a controlled release system to study the release behavior of spin-labeled coumarin-3-carboxylic acid (SL-CCS) and warfarin (SL-WFR). The release profiles of these spin-labeled (SL-) pharmaceuticals from BSA hydrogels prepared with different procedures are compared in detail. The mechanical properties of the gels during formation and release were studied via rheology, while a nanoscopic view on the release behavior was achieved by analyzing SL-drugs–BSA interaction using continuous wave electron paramagnetic resonance (CW EPR) spectroscopy. The influence of type of drug, drug concentration, duration of gel formation, and gelation methods on release behavior were characterized by CW EPR spectroscopy, EPR imaging (EPRI), and dynamic light scattering (DLS), which provide information on the interaction of BSA with SL-drugs, the percentage of drug inside the hydrogel and the nature and size of the released structures, respectively. We found that the release rate of SL-CCS and SL-WFR from BSA hydrogels is tunable through drug ratios, hydrogel incubation time and gelation procedures. All of the results indicate that BSA hydrogels can be potentially exploited in controlled drug delivery applications.

**Keywords:** albumin; hydrogels; EPR/ESR spectroscopy; release behavior

**Citation:** Sanaeifar, N.; Mäder, K.; Hinderberger, D. Molecular-Level Release of Coumarin-3-Carboxylic Acid and Warfarin-Derivatives from BSA-Based Hydrogels. *Pharmaceutics* **2021**, *13*, 1661. https://doi.org/10.3390/pharmaceutics13101661

Academic Editor: Katona Gábor

Received: 1 September 2021
Accepted: 2 October 2021
Published: 11 October 2021

**Publisher's Note:** MDPI stays neutral with regard to jurisdictional claims in published maps and institutional affiliations.

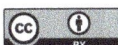

**Copyright:** © 2021 by the authors. Licensee MDPI, Basel, Switzerland. This article is an open access article distributed under the terms and conditions of the Creative Commons Attribution (CC BY) license (https://creativecommons.org/licenses/by/4.0/).

## 1. Introduction

Conventional drug administration leads to an elevated drug concentration in the blood followed by a drop until the next dosage is administered [1]. The administration of a single large dose causes the drug level to rise above the minimum toxic concentration (MTC), leading to harmful side effects, and then rapidly decreases below the minimum effective concentration (MEC). Frequent dosing may maintain the drug level within the therapeutic range, however, it can decrease patient compliance [2]. Controlled drug delivery systems in which the entire therapeutic dose is administered at once can avoid high fluctuations of the drug plasma level, minimize possible side effects, and release the drug in a well-defined behavior over extended periods of time [3]. Various systems have been developed as controlled drug delivery systems such as polylactic acid (PLA) and poly(lactic-*co*-glycolic acid) (PLGA) products [4,5], nanocarriers [6,7], smart polymers [8,9], hydroxyapatite (HA) [10], hydrogels [11–13], and others.

Hydrogels are entangled networks made from proteins, hydrophilic polymers, or small molecules with the capability to retain water and biological fluids in large amounts without dissolving, due to the presence of physical and chemical bonds between the polymeric chains [14–16]. Their swollen, soft, and rubbery nature resembles living tissues and minimizes negative immune reaction after implantation [14,17]. Since a drug can be incorporated in the water-swollen network and released gradually, hydrogels have emerged as excellent candidates for the controlled release of therapeutics [18].

In order to develop a novel drug delivery vehicle, we selected bovine serum albumin (see Figure 1A) as our drug carrier because of its high biocompatibility, availability, stability, and low cost [19,20]. Although albumins do show species-specific differences in solution structure and dynamics [21–23], from a general perspective, serum albumin is a heart-shaped molecule in the crystalline state, and the most abundant protein in the circulatory system of vertebrates [24]. In addition to maintaining osmotic pressure and blood pH, it transports a variety of ligands such as un-esterified fatty acids, hormones, proteins, and drug compounds to different tissues through physical or chemical bonding to the binding sites of this protein [17,25,26].

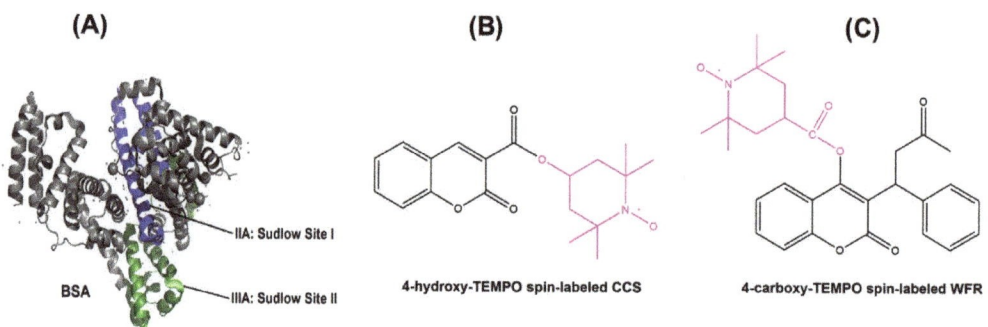

**Figure 1.** (**A**) Crystal structure of BSA and its drug-binding sites (PDB ID: 4f5s) and molecular structures of (**B**) SL-CCS and (**C**) SL-WFR.

The mechanism of hydrogel formation from albumin by heating and chemical crosslinking has been previously established [27]. Thermally induced gel formation requires conformational changes and unfolding of polypeptide segments induced by heating above denaturation temperature of the albumin, which results in the availability of functional groups present in intramolecular hydrogen bonding for intermolecular interactions, which are essential in the aggregation and build-up of the gel network [28]. Albumin hydrogels can be generated at 37 °C by lowering the pH to 3.5. In these pH-triggered gels, changes in the net charge of the protein from −16 mV at pH 7.4 to +100 mV at pH 3.5 cause the repulsion of protein domains and subsequent partial denaturation [29]. We recently elucidated the ability to form hydrogels from bovine and human serum albumin below their denaturation temperature and wide pH range [19]. Moreover, ethanol induced hydrogels can be formed at 37 °C by mixing different concentrations of BSA solution and chemical denaturant ethanol [27].

Several reports are available on the use of albumin for drug delivery purposes, but they have been largely based on nanocarrier systems. For instance, Pápay et al. studied the pulmonary delivery of apigenin, a natural polyphenol with antioxidant activity from BSA nanoparticles [30]. Gharbavi et al. developed a microemulsion system based on BSA nanoparticles to investigate the release behavior of paclitaxel and folate [31]. In another experiment by de Redín et al., human serum albumin nanoparticles were prepared to explore the ocular delivery of Bevacizumab [32].

Electron paramagnetic resonance (EPR) spectroscopy is a non-destructive and highly specific method used to monitor paramagnetic compounds containing unpaired electrons. The majority of materials, except for paramagnetic transition metal ions that possess intrinsic free radicals, are not detectable by EPR due to the absence of paramagnetic centers. Thus, by spin labeling or spin probing techniques, which are based on the covalent or non-covalent corporation of paramagnetic substances such as organic nitroxide radicals into the drug, the protein, or both, it is possible to study drug–protein interactions in drug delivery systems. Furthermore, through this method, information about the local environment, motional parameters, and ligand binding of the protein can be obtained, which allow for deep insights into the release properties [16,25,27,33]. Spectral information as well as spatial distribution of free radicals can be studied by EPR imaging. Thus, this method has been implemented as a useful technique to probe property changes in different parts of an object that releases drugs [34,35].

Coumarin (CCS) and warfarin (WFR) are widely prescribed as anticoagulant drugs for the treatment of thromboembolic disorders, which are among the most common and often fatal cardiovascular diseases. Moving toward a more controlled delivery of these types of drugs can avoid problems related to their oral administration including variability in dose response due to their narrow therapeutic window or considerable interaction with other medications [36–38]. Previously, our group synthesized various spin-labeled pharmaceuticals (SLP) including warfarin and coumarin-3-carboxylic acid (see Figure 1B,C) and analyzed drug binding to human serum albumin in solution with serum-like concentrations via the continuous-wave EPR spectroscopic approach [39]. Furthermore, the release of 16-doxyl stearic acid (16-DSA) as a model drug from BSA hydrogels and the nanoscopic properties of released components has been studied extensively [20]. In the present report, we aimed at developing and comparing controlled delivery systems based on BSA hydrogels and spin-labeled coumarin-3-carboxylic acid (SL-CCS) and warfarin (SL-WFR) as our candidate drugs to investigate the release behavior from the prepared gels. The parameters taken into consideration were the method of gel formation, the drug concentration, and the incubation time, which is the time required for gelation to process at specific temperature or pH. Our investigation is complemented by studying the influence of these parameters on the mechanical properties of the gels using rheology, the interaction and spatial distribution of SL-drugs with BSA gels by means of CW EPR spectroscopy and EPR imaging, and the size and nature of released components by DLS. From the combined data, we finally draw conclusions on the release mechanisms from the gels.

## 2. Experimental Section

### 2.1. Materials

Bovine serum albumin (fatty acid free, lyophilized powder, BSA > 96%) was purchased from Sigma-Aldrich (Taufkirchen, Germany) and used as received without any purification. 4-Hydroxy TEMPO-labeled coumarin-3-carboxylic acid (SL-CCS) and 4-carboxy-TEMPO-labeled warfarin (SL-WFR), synthesized previously [39], were used in this research. In our recent work [20], we introduced a concise notation, $BSA_i(\theta, p, t, r)$, to describe the gelation technique (i), which can be either thermally (T) or pH (P) induced methods, temperature ($\theta$) and pH (p) of hydrogel preparation, incubation time (t, in minutes), and time-release (r, in hours) indicating the release of drug over a specific time, respectively. For instance, $BSA_T$ (65, 7.4, 5, 48) refers to the thermally prepared gel at 65 °C for 5 min and pH 7.4, and the release behavior was studied 48 h after gelation.

### 2.2. Methods

The 3 mM precursor solution of BSA was prepared by dissolving BSA powder in deionized water. After 1 h of stirring at 100 rpm at room temperature, the final solution was sterilized by a 0.45 µm filter. SL-CCS and SL-WFR powders were dissolved separately in DMSO to obtain 26 mM stock solutions and added into the BSA precursor solution with three different drug:BSA molar ratios into glass vials. Hydrogels were prepared by adopting the procedures described in our paper [20]. Thermally induced gels were obtained by keeping the vials in a thermomixer at 65 °C and 59 °C, above and below the denaturation temperature of BSA, while some hydrogels were prepared at 37 °C by the addition of 2 M HCl and lowering the pH to 3.5 by the so-called pH induced method.

### 2.3. In Vitro Drug Release

Our release experiment was based on the addition of 1 mL 10× PBS on top of the hydrogels and incubating vials in a thermomixer at 37 °C. In order to maintain sink condition, after removal of 12 µL release medium at various time intervals for deeper analysis, this amount was replaced with fresh PBS.

### 2.4. Rheological Characterization

The mechanical properties and viscoelastic behavior during the formation of the hydrogels were investigated using rheological characterization. Evaluation of storage and loss moduli ($G'$ and $G''$, respectively) provides information on gelation point (i.e., the start-time for deviation of $G'$ from $G''$). According to the shape and magnitude of storage and loss moduli, it is possible to obtain an insight into the gel stability and define mechanically robust and weak hydrogels.

Rheological measurements of hydrogels were performed on a Physica MCR 301 rheometer (Anton Paar, Graz, Austria) using a CP50-2/TG plate as a measurement system. After placing the 2 mL of precursor solutions, namely BSA and different ratios of CCS/WFR:BSA, on the surface of the rheometer plate, the measurement gap was covered by silicon oil to avoid water evaporation. Time dependent curves of storage and loss moduli during gel formation were obtained using a 0.5% oscillatory strain and 1 rad s$^{-1}$ frequency.

### 2.5. Continuous Wave Electron Paramagnetic Resonance (CW EPR) Spectroscopy

CW EPR spectroscopy provides information on the release mechanisms by plotting the double integral of the released spin-labeled drugs in the EPR spectra versus release time intervals, which is a measure of the released molecules. Furthermore, a deeper understanding of the drug–protein interaction in the hydrogel and the release medium can be obtained by analyzing the rotational motion of the spin probe. For instance, immobilized radicals show slow rotational dynamics that are coupled to the much slower rotational motion of the protein, while freely tumbling spin probes show no or little attachment to proteins.

The CW EPR measurements were conducted on a Miniscope MS400 (Magnettech, Berlin, Germany) benchtop spectrometer with a microwave frequency of 9.4 GHz recorded with a frequency counter (Racal Dana 2101, Neu-Isenburg, Germany). The temperature of the samples was set to 37 °C using temperature controller H03 (Magnettech). All experiments were performed at a microwave power of 15 mW, a sweep width of 15 mT, and modulation amplitude of 0.2 or 0.03 mT (for analyzing release medium and hydrogels, respectively). Simulations of recorded EPR spectra were evaluated in MATLAB using the EasySpin program package. This program was based on applying the Schneider–Freed approach to solve the Schrödinger equation for slowly rotating nitroxides [40].

Sample preparation was as follows: about 12 µL of desired solution were filled into 50 µL glass capillary (Blaubrand, Wertheim, Germany) and capped with tube sealant (Leica Critoseal, Wetzlar, Germany).

### 2.6. Electron Paramagnetic Resonance Imaging

Spectral-spatial electron paramagnetic resonance imaging (EPRI) is a well-suited technique to reveal a spatial tomogram as well as an EPR spectrum. The former derives information on the macromolecular structure of the sample while the latter indicates the micromolecular structure arises from mobility of the paramagnetic center [41].

In this work, EPRI was used to monitor the release procedure by analyzing hydrogels, while the released substances in the medium were investigated by applying CW EPR.

The EPRI spectra were obtained using an L-band spectrometer (Magnettech, Berlin, Germany) equipped with a re-entrant resonator, operating at a microwave frequency of about 1.1–1.3 GHz.

The measurement parameters used for 2D spatial imaging were set as follows: center field 48.8 mT, scan width 8 mT, scan time 60 s, and modulation amplitude 0.02 mT.

The samples were prepared by placing 600 µL of precursor solution into cylindrical Teflon sample holders (9.3 mm diameters and 8.76 mm height) and keeping them in an oven (UE 400, Memmert, Büchenbach, Germany) with different incubation times. After gel formation, sample holders were placed into 100 mL flasks containing 65 mL 10× PBS and kept in an incubation shaker at 37 °C. For EPRI measurements, at different time intervals, the sample holders were taken out of the buffer, externally dried with a tissue and subsequently transferred into the spectrometer.

*2.7. Dynamic Light Scattering*

Dynamic light scattering (DLS) measures fluctuations of the scattering intensity arising from Brownian motion of particles in solution. By analyzing these fluctuations, information about the diffusion correlation and particle size can be obtained. DLS is one of the most popular techniques used as a non-destructive method to characterize complex liquids, proteins, and polymer structures [20,42,43].

A Litesizer 500 (Anton Paar GmbH, Graz, Austria) equipped with a 40 nm semiconductor laser with a wavelength of 658 nm was used for these experiments. The instrument measures with six runs and the duration of 30 s for each run and the temperature was set to 37 °C (with 4 min of equilibration time).

To obtain the hydrodynamic radius and intensity correlation function, the release medium was analyzed by transferring 100 µL of release sample into a Quartz cuvette (Hellma Analytics) with no further filtration. Thereafter, the samples were measured to gain insights into the nature of the released molecules and gel fragments.

## 3. Results and Discussion

*3.1. Rheological Measurement*

Mechanical and viscoelastic properties of hydrogels can be considered essential design parameters for pharmaceutical and biomedical applications. In the field of drug delivery, the integrity of the hydrogel plays a crucial role in protecting a therapeutic agent in the case of a non-biodegradable system until it is released out of the system, while the flow properties of some gels gain importance since they are used as injectable carriers for drug delivery purposes [44,45].

Physical protein gels are formed by non-covalent interchain associations involving hydrophobic, van der Waals, solvation, and electrostatic interactions determining the rheological behavior of proteins. The rigidity of the protein network arises from the strength and number as well as pattern of these interactions [19,46]. Figure 2A shows the time dependent storage (G′) and loss (G″) moduli of 3 mM BSA precursor solution at different temperatures.

For thermally induced hydrogels, the precursor solutions of BSA were heated and kept at 65 °C and 59 °C (slightly above and below the denaturation temperature of BSA, respectively). In both samples, the storage modulus dominated the loss modulus instantly, reflecting the gelation point. We defined a hydrogel to be mechanically tough when the G′ value exceeded 10,000 Pa after 1 h. The value of G′ for $BSA_T$(65, 7.4, 60) and $BSA_T$(59, 7.4, 60) increased up to 29,000 and 20,000 Pa after 60 min, respectively. Therefore, robust hydrogels can be formed by the heat induced technique even at 59 °C, which is slightly below the denaturation temperature of BSA. However, the G′ value of $BSA_T$(65, 7.4) was, as expected, considerably higher than that of the $BSA_T$(59, 7.4). In our previous work [20], we extensively studied changes in the secondary structure of BSA during gelation.

In Figure 2A, we also present gel formation (i.e., rheology at 37 °C) through the addition of 2 M HCl to a BSA precursor solution, which reduces the pH to 3.5. Gelation in this hydrogel sets in after 25 min, and is less rigid compared to hydrogels formed by heating. The gelation rate in pH-triggered hydrogels is relatively slow, so that in order to obtain mechanically tough hydrogels, much longer incubation times are required.

To probe the impact of CCS and WFR on albumin gelation kinetics, different ratios of these drugs were added to the precursor solutions of BSA and rheological measurements were repeated at different temperatures (see Figure S1 for CCS:BSA with different molar ratios at 59 °C). Due to the similarity in mechanical properties of WFR with CCS, the whole rheological characterization of WFR is explained in detail in the Supplementary Materials. Human serum albumin (HSA) has two main drug binding sites called Sudlow sites I and II, located in the hydrophobic cavities of subdomains IIA and IIIA, respectively. Sudlow site I can bind bulky heterocyclic compounds, while site II has a high binding affinity to aromatic compounds [47,48]. According to [39], HSA has only one high affinity binding site for SL-WFR, while SL-CCS occupied three binding sites of this protein, but with lower affinity. It is important to note that the binding characteristics of BSA show high resemblance to that of HSA [49].

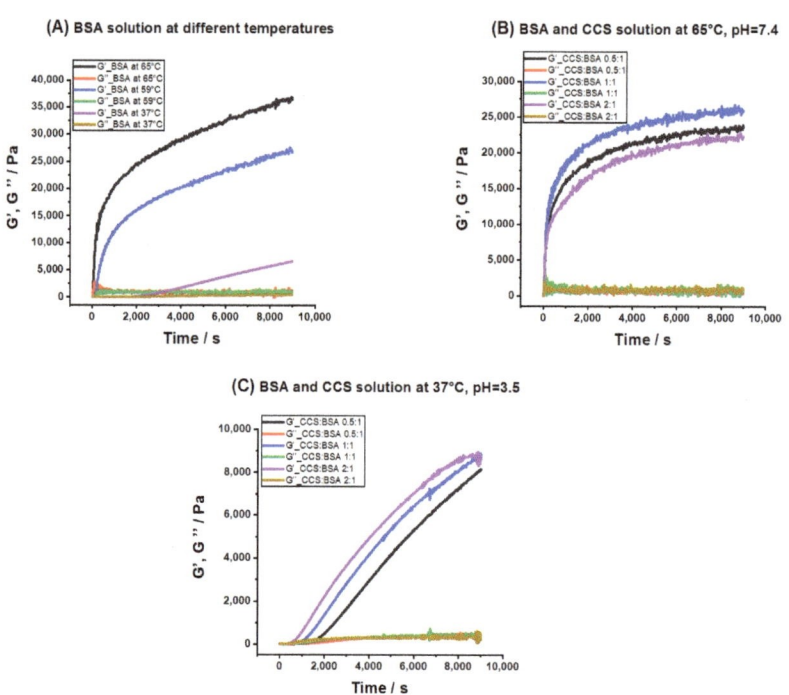

**Figure 2.** Storage (G′) and loss (G″) moduli as a function of time for (**A**) BSA$_T$(65, 7.4), BSA$_T$(59, 7.4), and BSA$_p$(37, 3.5); (**B**) different ratios of CCS:BSA at 65 °C, pH 7.4; and (**C**) different ratios of CCS:BSA at 37 °C, pH 3.5.

Time dependence of storage and loss moduli for the system including BSA and CCS with three different molar ratios at 65 °C are depicted in Figure 2B. It seems that the addition of CCS leads to a lower storage modulus (around 10,000 Pa) and weaker mechanical properties compared to the BSA hydrogel formed at the same temperature without CCS. This is due to the presence of CCS in the Sudlow binding sites in albumin (see Figure 1A), which stabilize BSA structure to some extent and thus impede the conformational changes. Similar effects are known for bound fatty acids [22,50]. Apparently, the concentration of CCS cannot deeply affect thermally-induced gelation, since the storage modulus values for three different ratios are similar. However, pH-triggered hydrogels demonstrate the opposite behavior (see Figure 2C). Gelation starts faster and the storage modulus increases slightly when CCS is added to the BSA precursor solution. As explained in the CW EPR section, the percentage of bound SL-CCR to BSA in pH-induced hydrogels is very low. It seems that CCS does not fully bind to Sudlow sites with this preparation method and instead may interact with the surface of the protein, which may facilitate denaturation and may then result in the observed earlier gelation starting point.

We have previously investigated the effect of fatty acids on gel formation by adding different concentrations of stearic acid (SA) to a BSA precursor solution (SA and 16-DSA are substitutable in their binding to BSA). Unlike CCS and WFR, fatty acids delay gelation onset time and considerably affect the mechanical properties. Generally, BSA consists of seven long chain fatty acid binding sites that obstruct protein denaturation and final gelation and increase the thermal stability of protein [20].

*3.2. Release Studies of SL-CCS and SL-WFR Loaded BSA Hydrogels and Gel Characterization*

Drug binding to HSA in solution has been well studied by a spin labeling and CW-EPR spectroscopy approach, which provides information on the maximum number of binding sites per protein as well as the dynamics of SL-pharmaceuticals [39].

CW EPR measurements have proven to be useful for quantitative characterization of drug and fatty acid binding processes to albumin-derived materials and the respective bound states [22,23,50,51]. For albumin hydrogels, results from a recent study on the interaction of 16-DSA with BSA and HSA hydrogels revealed that both proteins and their hydrogels have strong fatty acid binding capacities, however, the number and strength of their binding strongly depends on the gel preparation method [19]. Furthermore, the rotational reorientation as well as polarity around the nitroxide group can be gained from rigorous simulation of EPR spectra. The former, achieved from rotational correlation time $\tau_c$, which is calculated from diffusion tensor $D$ ($\tau_c = \frac{1}{6}(DxxDyyDzz)^{-\frac{1}{3}}$), is in the range of 10 ps for fast rotation components to a few microseconds for tightly immobilized molecules. The latter can be determined from the isotropic $^{14}N$-hyperfine coupling constant $\alpha_{iso}$. High polar environments result in larger $\alpha_{iso}$ values, while smaller hyperfine couplings are indicative of lower polarities [19,20,39]. In the following, we describe the influence of differences in chemical substitution of SL-CCS and SL-WFR on gel formation and their release behavior from BSA hydrogels.

Figure 3A shows the spectral features (simulated) of ligands that are freely tumbling ligands, intermediately, or strongly immobilized in the EPR spectra separately, while in Figure 3B, the features of different spectroscopic species of nitroxide spin probe are displayed in the measured spectrum that essentially is a superposition of these three spectral components of Figure 3A with varying amplitudes (weights). Figure 3C,D shows $BSA_T$(65, 7.4, 10) and $BSA_P$(37, 3.5, 30) at 2:1 SL-CCS:BSA ratios, respectively. Due to the delayed gel formation of samples prepared by the pH-induced method, much longer incubation times were required. Results from spectral simulation revealed that in a hydrogel prepared by the thermally induced method at 65 °C, almost 26% of SL-CCS showed freely tumbling rotation, 29% were strongly bound to BSA, and 44% had intermediate rotational motion. However, with the addition of acid, the percentage of freely rotating and intermediately immobilized SL-CCS increased to 33% and 51% while that of the strongly bound ligand to BSA decreased to 14%. In general, the strongly immobilized state in BSA could stem from ligand binding sites, which are located at the interfaces of α-helices. The intermediately immobilized ligand with faster rotation is typically situated in water swollen regions of BSA with a β-sheet structure [19]. Acidic conditions affect the helical content in BSA differently to temperature denaturation. In other words, more α-helix content is preserved in pH-induced hydrogels since intermolecular β-sheets formed at the cost of both α-helix and random coils [19]. Figure 3E,F shows the spectra of SL-WFR loaded hydrogels at a 2:1 SL-WFR:BSA molar ratio prepared by heat and pH-change, respectively. Remarkably, the percentage of tightly immobilized and intermediately bound SL-WFR was higher in these hydrogels than in SL-CCS loaded BSA and only less than 10% of SL-WFR rotated freely. The reason for this may be explained by considering the difference in the chemical substitution of both pharmaceuticals (see Figure 1B,C). The free 3-oxo-1-phenyl-butyl group can increase the average binding affinity by providing flexibility to its coumarin backbone in a way that the 3-oxo group can facilitate hydrogen bonding in protein. Compared with SL-WFR, SL-CCS without the additional group has less flexibility and only the carbonyl group at position 2 may have a hydrogen-bond acceptor function. The parameters obtained from simulation of the EPR spectra in Figure 3 are illustrated in Table 1. The results of Figure 3 are comparable to the rheological characterization, as thermally induced hydrogels containing CCS and WFR show more mechanical robustness than the same gels prepared through reducing pH. Moreover, as will be explained later, there were high percentages of freely tumbling SL-pharmaceuticals in the release medium of samples prepared by the thermally induced method, and there was no sign of strongly bound components. Therefore, we can conclude that the SL-pharmaceuticals are also bound more strongly to these types of hydrogels. The hydrogel characterization for both SL-pharmaceuticals at other ratios and temperatures is described in more detail in the Supplementary Materials.

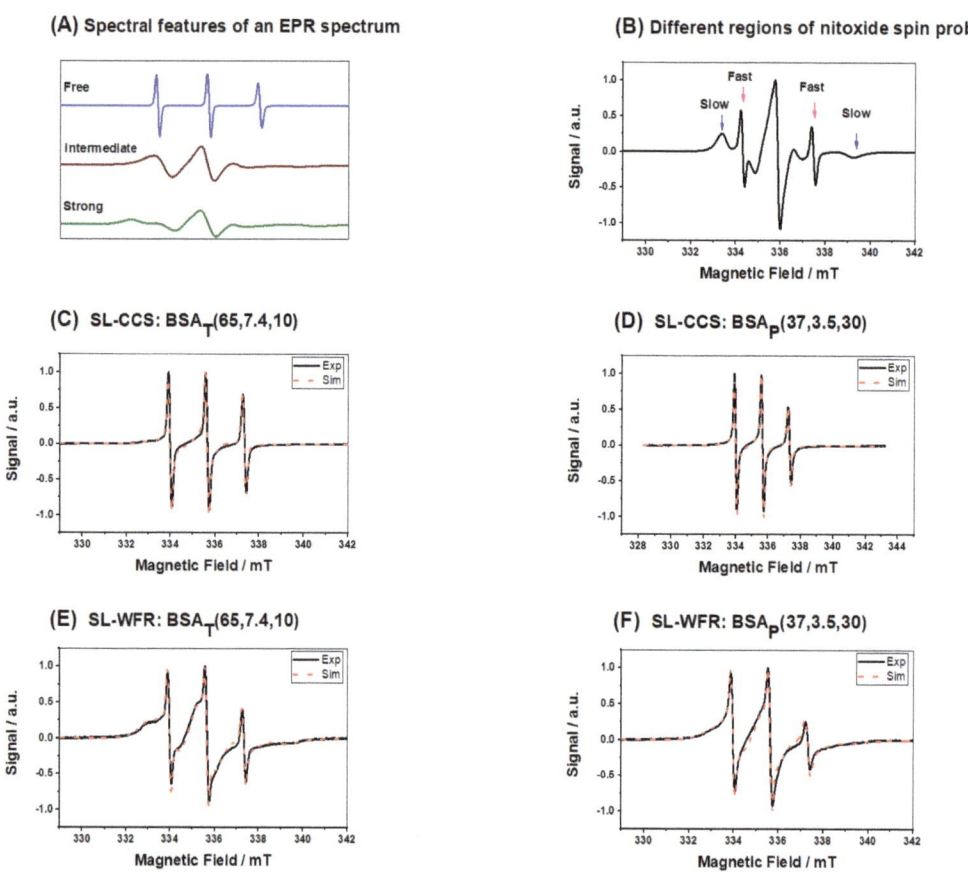

**Figure 3.** (**A**) Simulated components of EPR spectra; (**B**) different regions of nitroxide spin probe; (**C**) SL-CCS loaded $BSA_T(65, 7.4, 10)$ at a 2:1 SL-CCS:BSA molar ratio; (**D**) SL-CCS loaded $BSA_p(37, 3.5, 30)$ at a 2:1 SL-CCS:BSA molar ratio; (**E**) SL-WFR loaded $BSA_T(65, 7.4, 10)$ at a 2:1 SL-WFR:BSA molar ratio; and (**F**) SL-WFR loaded $BSA_p(37, 3.5, 30)$ at a 2:1 SL-WFR:BSA molar ratio.

In Figures 4 and 5, the release profiles of SL-CCS and SL-WFR from BSA hydrogels are given at different ratios and by the two preparation methods (other release curves for hydrogels with lower incubation times can be found in the Supplementary Materials). Double integration of the first derivative CW EPR spectra can be used to determine the signal intensity of the spectra [52]. Therefore, in all release curves, the double integral of EPR spectra is plotted versus the release time intervals.

Table 1. Parameters gained from the simulation in Figure 3.

| Figure | Type of Released Components | Percentage | Correlation Time $\tau_c$ (ns) | Hyperfine Coupling Constant $a_{iso}$ (MHz) |
|---|---|---|---|---|
| C | Bound | 29% | 14.6 | 44.53 |
|  | Intermediate | 44% | 5.4 | 47.53 |
|  | Free | 26% | 0.11 | 46.86 |
| D | Bound | 10% | 14.5 | 44.53 |
|  | Intermediate | 54% | 4.76 | 47.53 |
|  | Free | 35% | 0.16 | 46.86 |
| E | Bound | 47% | 31 | 42.53 |
|  | Intermediate | 48% | 3.2 | 46.86 |
|  | Free | 3% | 0.061 | 47.13 |
| F | Bound | 36% | 31 | 42.53 |
|  | Intermediate | 56% | 3.2 | 46.86 |
|  | Free | 6% | 0.85 | 47.20 |

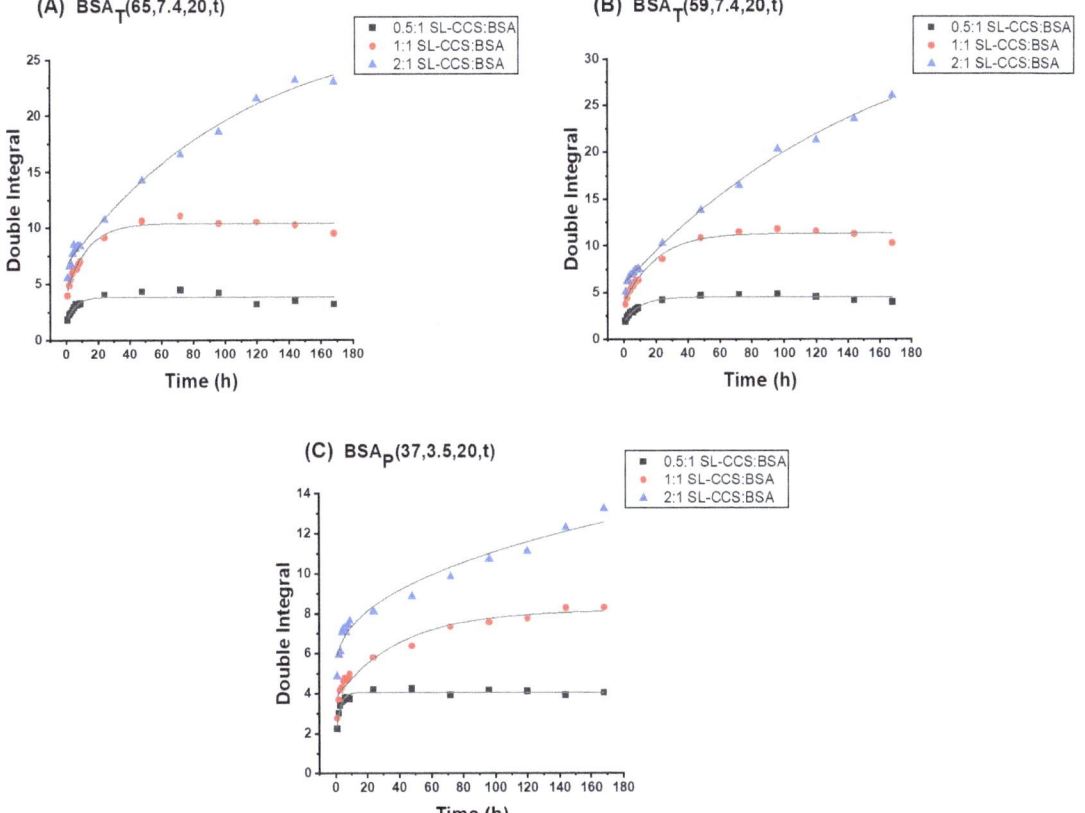

**Figure 4.** Release profiles of SL-CCS loaded BSA hydrogels at 0.5:1, 1:1 and 2:1 SL-CCS:BSA molar ratios: (**A**) $BSA_T$(65, 7.4, 20) hydrogel; (**B**) $BSA_T$(59, 7.4, 20) hydrogel; and (**C**) $BSA_P$(37, 3.5, 20) hydrogel. The curves are fitted.

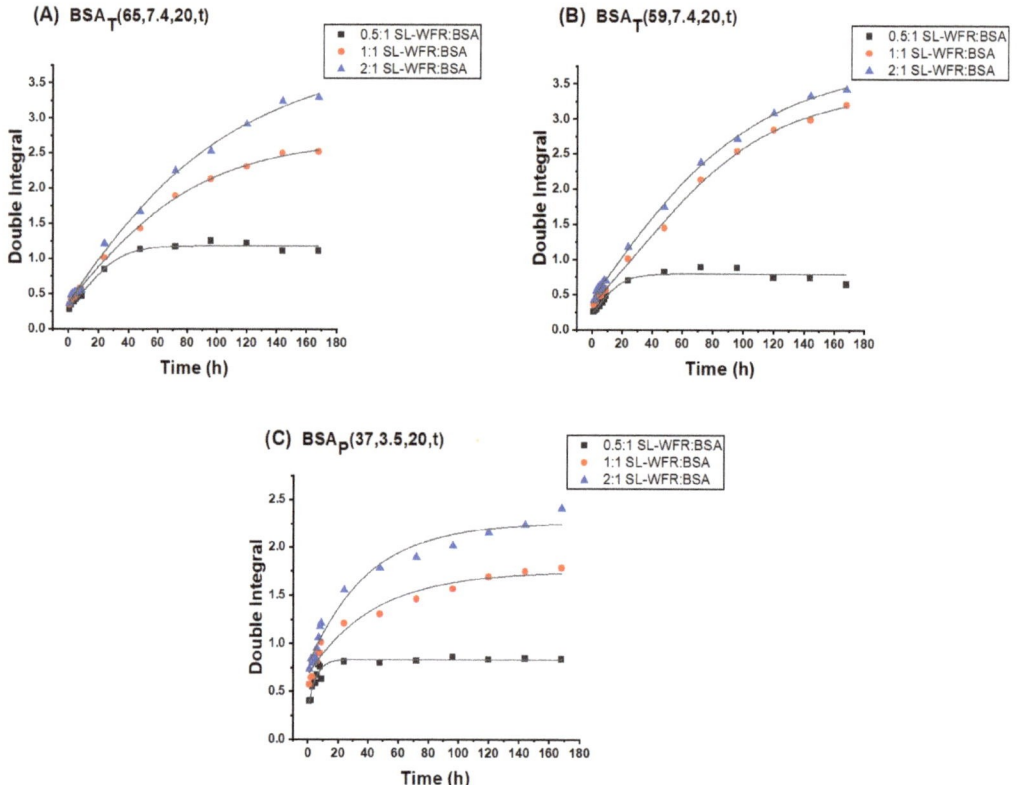

**Figure 5.** Release profiles of SL-WFR loaded BSA hydrogels with 0.5:1, 1:1 and 2:1 SL-CCS:BSA molar ratios: (**A**) $BSA_T$(65, 7.4, 20) hydrogel; (**B**) $BSA_T$(59, 7.4, 20) hydrogel; and (**C**) $BSA_P$(37, 3.5, 20) hydrogel. The curves are fitted.

It can be seen that all 0.5:1 and 1:1 ratios in the SL-CCS loaded BSA hydrogels prepared by different methods showed an initial fast release before reaching a plateau after 24 h. The initial release of large amounts of drug corresponds with the diffusion of release medium into the protein network, which dissolves the entrapped SL-CCS close to or at the surface of the hydrogel. However, the second and slower release is due to the depletion of drug in the inner part of gel matrix, which leads to the increase in the diffusion process length. In contrast, the kinetics of the SL-CCS:BSA 2:1 ratios almost corresponded to a zero-order release with an initial burst effect. It is possible that by increasing the ratio to 2:1, the binding sites from which the later release occurred are fully occupied and instead, the amount of drug between the hydrogel networks increases, which results in a drug release at a constant rate.

Figure 5 summarizes the SL-WFR release data. One can see an initial burst release for all samples, and a later sustained release only at the 0.5:1 SL-WFR:BSA molar ratio. The release from gels at 1:1 and 2:1 SL-WFR:BSA molar ratios first clearly followed the zero order kinetics and flattened after ~100h. Since BSA has only one high affinity binding site for SL-WFR, increasing the ratio to 1:1 and 2:1 resulted in the presence of a greater amount of freely moving SL-drug on the hydrogel surface and between the protein networks, which led to the linear release during the first five days; afterward, the release reached a certain level at which there was no more free SL-WFR available and the release of those from the binding site is initiated. We observed that all hydrogels with SL-CCS, regardless of molar ratios and preparation methods, had a higher release rate than SL-WFR loaded BSA gels, which may be attributed to the higher affinity of SL-WFR to albumin compared to SL-CCS.

Therefore, SL-WFR tends to attach to the binding pockets of BSA for longer periods of time and shows a lower release rate.

The effect of initial drug loading and preparation methods on the release profile is also discussed in Figures 4 and 5. In all experimental systems, we found that the increase in the ratio of SL-pharmaceuticals to albumin led to a higher release rate. In addition, thermally induced hydrogels prepared at 65 °C and 59 °C, respectively, had higher release rates than pH-induced hydrogels. As explained above for the rheological characterization, electrostatically triggered hydrogels are less rigid compared to hydrogels formed by heating, which may lead to the assumption that these gels release their pharmaceuticals faster. However, we observed the opposite effect. This is possibly because there are stronger transient interactions/attachments between the pharmaceuticals and the increased protein surface under acidic conditions. These transient complexes could protect the hydrogel from fast degradation, which may lead to a slower release rate over time. However, when comparing the release rate of hydrogels prepared at 65 °C with the respective rate for the gel prepared at 59 °C, the results showed that hydrogels that formed below the BSA denaturation temperature (at 59 °C) had a slightly higher rate of release as these gels were mechanically less robust than those prepared at 65 °C.

Figure 6 shows the effect of incubation time on the release behavior of BSA hydrogels incorporated with different ratios of SL-CCS (other ratios of SL-CCS and SL-WFR loaded hydrogels are available in the Supplementary Materials). It seems that increasing the incubation time from 3 min to 20 min slightly decreased the release rate. These results are in line with those of the rheological characterization, as a longer duration of gelation leads to more mechanically robust hydrogels. Consequently, the release rate can be tuned by changing the incubation time, which indicates the remarkable potential of BSA hydrogels for their implementation in controlled drug delivery applications.

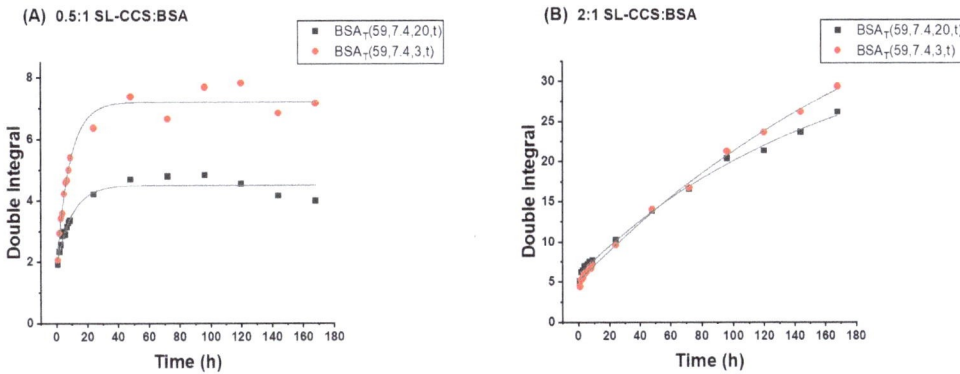

**Figure 6.** Release profiles of SL-CCS loaded BSA hydrogels prepared using heat induction at 59 °C with two different incubation times of 3 and 20 min at a (**A**) 0.5:1 SL-CCS:BSA molar ratio and (**B**) 2:1 SL-CCS:BSA molar ratio. The curves are fitted.

Figure 7 displays EPR spectra gained by analyzing the release medium. More molecular insights were obtained by spectral simulation, providing information on the fraction of SL-drugs strongly and intermediately bound to BSA and freely rotating SL-pharmaceuticals in the released solution (see Table 2). Results showed that 84% of SL-CCS rotated freely in PBS, 16% showed intermediate rotational motion, and there was no sign of tightly bound SL-CCS to BSA for the sample prepared by the heat-induced method at 65 °C by keeping the sample in a thermomixer for 20 min (the EPR spectra of the respective release experiment for samples prepared at 59 °C are available in the Supplementary Materials). The BSA hydrogel with SL-WFR prepared at the same temperature and incubation time showed an, in principal, similar release behavior. However, the percentage of freely tumbling SL-WFR decreased to 73% and that of the intermediate component increased to 26%. The percentage of strongly bound SL-drugs to BSA in the release medium increased when the hydrogels were prepared by the pH-induced method at 37 °C. For instance, 19% of SL-CCS and 46% of SL-WFR were released as they bind tightly to BSA. It must be mentioned that the percentage of released components in bound, intermediate, and free states was nearly constant during the different release time intervals for all samples, while in our previous work on fatty acid release, these percentages changed during the release experiment [20].

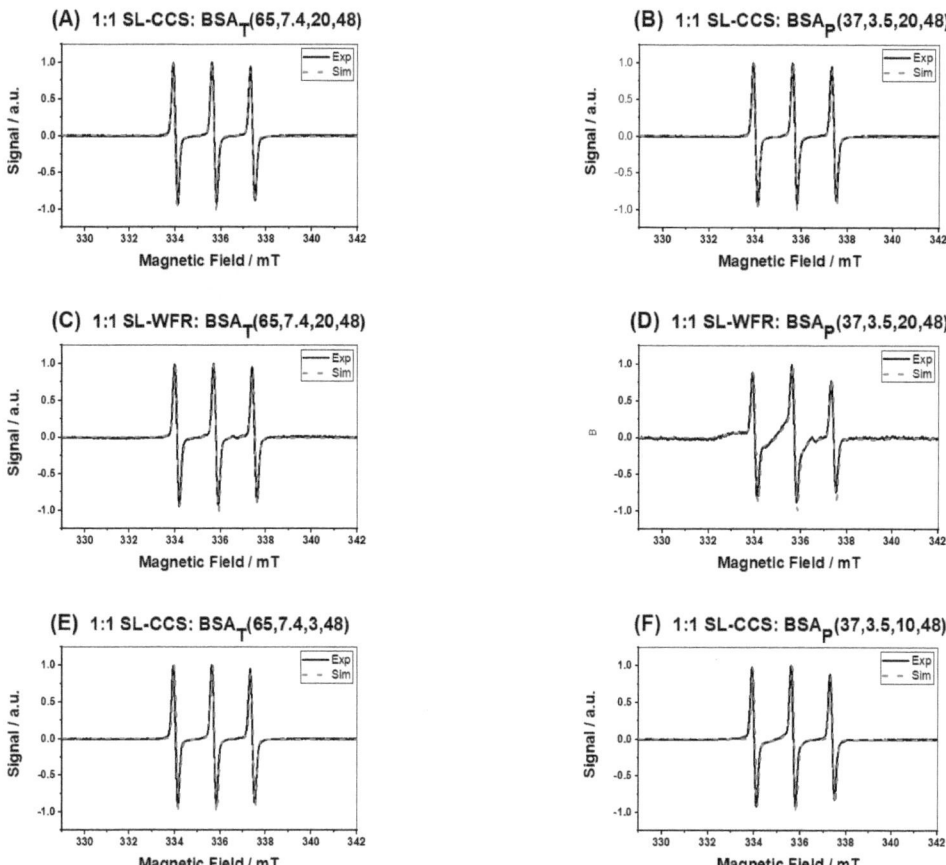

**Figure 7.** EPR spectra of release test after 48 h for SL-drugs loaded BSA hydrogels at a 1:1 molar ratio (**A**) SL-CCS:BSA$_T$(65, 7.4, 20, 48), (**B**) SL-CCS:BSA$_P$(37, 3.5, 20, 48), (**C**) SL-WFR:BSA$_T$(65, 7.4, 20, 48), (**D**) SL-WFR: BSA$_P$(37, 3.5, 20, 48), (**E**) SL-CCS:BSA$_T$(65, 7.4, 3, 48), and (**F**) SL-CCS:BSA$_P$(37, 3.5, 10, 48).

EPR spectra of the released components from BSA hydrogels with SL-CCS prepared with lower incubation times (3 min for the thermally induced hydrogel at 65 °C and 10 min for the pH-induced gel at 37 °C) are shown in Figure 7E,F. According to Table 2, we found that reducing the incubation time led to the release of a more intermediately immobilized SL-drug to BSA in the heat-induced gel and intermediately and strongly bound SL-CCS to BSA for the electrostatically triggered gel (see the Supplementary Materials the for release from hydrogels made at 59 °C and the whole data of SL-WFR incorporated BSA gels).

Table 2. Percentage of released components in different states gained from the spectral simulation in Figure 7.

| Figure | Type of Released Components | Percentage (Bound, Intermediate and Free) | Figure | Type of Released Components | Percentage (Bound, Intermediate and Free) |
|---|---|---|---|---|---|
| A | Bound | 0 | D | Bound | 46% |
|  | Intermediate | 16% |  | Intermediate | 31% |
|  | Free | 84% |  | Free | 22% |
| B | Bound | 19% | E | Bound | 0 |
|  | Intermediate | 16% |  | Intermediate | 20% |
|  | Free | 63% |  | Free | 80% |
| C | Bound | 0 | F | Bound | 24% |
|  | Intermediate | 26% |  | Intermediate | 19% |
|  | Free | 73% |  | Free | 55% |

*3.3. Monitoring of Release Behavior by Means of EPR Imaging*

We applied electron paramagnetic resonance imaging (EPRI) to study the spatial localization of a spin probe in a nondestructive way and followed the position of the probes inside the slowly dissolving gels not in the release medium. This technique combines spectral information with the spatial distribution of paramagnetic species, which permits monitoring of the changes in the property in different parts of the investigated sample [52,53].

Figure 8A shows a spectral-spatial two dimensional EPR image (absorption mode, not the standard CW EPR first-derivative mode) of a SL-CCS loaded BSA hydrogel. The intensity and spectral dimensions of a typical EPR spectrum are plotted along the z- and y-axes, respectively; the spatial dimension is shown along the x-axis. By applying spatial cuts, it is possible to obtain information on intensity distributions at certain positions. Figure 8B depicts the central spatial cut of dry SL-CCS loaded $BSA_T$(65, 7.4, 3) and release of SL-CCS from the BSA hydrogel during the first 4 h. It can be seen that the signal amplitude decreased over time, which illustrates the release of the SL-pharmaceutical from the hydrogel. Moreover, the EPR signal intensities slightly shifted to the right (bottom of the hydrogel) with release time, indicating that release occurs from the gel surface.

The amount of SL-pharmaceuticals inside the BSA hydrogel was calculated by double integration of the central spatial cuts. Figure 8C displays the amount of SL-CCS inside the BSA hydrogels prepared by the pH-induced method after exposure to the PBS buffer. For a better comparison, all of the samples were normalized by dividing each data point by the highest double integral value, the dry samples, for each of the ratios. We can see that the hydrogel at a 0.5:1 SL-CCS:BSA had the lowest amount of spin probe inside the gel due to the lowest initial drug content, while increasing the drug loading percentage led to a higher drug quantity in hydrogels over the whole release period. Figure 8D,E shows the effect of preparation methods on the release profile of SL-CCS and SL-WFR from BSA hydrogels. According to the double integral values, heat induced gels contained lower amount of drugs, while pH-induced hydrogels preserved a higher quantity of drug within their networks. These results are in agreement with the CW-EPR measurements, as hydrogels thermally induced at 65 °C and 59 °C showed higher release rates in comparison to the electrostatically triggered hydrogels. As explained in the CW-EPR section, acidic conditions may induce more interactions between pharmaceuticals and the protein surface, which results in a higher protein protection from fast degradation and lower release rate over time. Furthermore, all hydrogels with different ratios of SL-CCS or SL-WFR prepared with different methods showed that they released almost 80% of their drug contents during the first 24 h. The sustained release phase in all experimental samples is thought to involve the penetration of PBS into the protein networks, leading to the final dissolution of the drug in the inner part of the BSA chains. However, the results from CW-EPR showed zero-order kinetics for some ratios. It is possible that the difference in hydrogel quantities, sample holders used for CW-EPR and EPRI, or incubation times needed for gel formation leads to different release patterns.

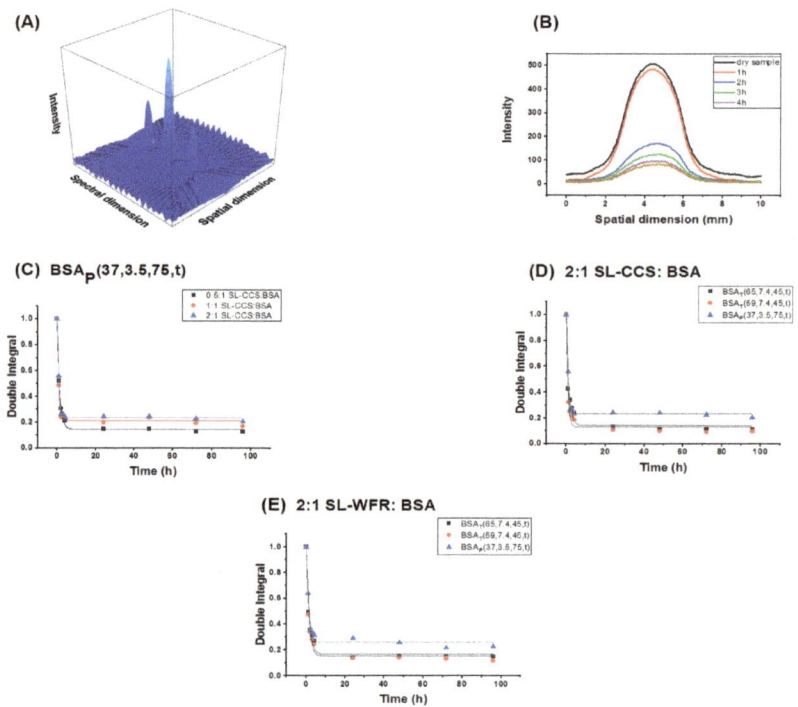

**Figure 8.** (**A**) 2-D spectral-spatial image of the BSA hydrogel with SL-CCS at a spin probe:BSA 1:1 molar ratio prepared by the heat induced method at 65 °C. (**B**) Central spatial cut (a) top and (b) bottom of the dry SL-CCS loaded $BSA_T(65, 7.4, 45)$ and release of SL-CCS from the BSA hydrogel during the first 4 h. Double integration of central spatial cuts of (**C**) SL-CCS:$BSA_P(37, 3.5, 75, t)$ at different molar ratios, (**D**) 2:1 SL-CCS:BSA molar ratio prepared with heat and pH induced methods, and (**E**) 2:1 SL-WFR:BSA molar ratio prepared with heat and pH induced methods. The curves are fitted.

### 3.4. Analyzing the Released Components with DLS

To better understand the components released over time, we determined the hydrodynamic radii and correlation functions using dynamic light scattering (DLS). Figure 9 displays the intensity–time correlation function of the released medium. We recorded pronounced autocorrelation functions and high scattering intensities, implying the presence of highly defined particles in PBS buffer. Figure 9A shows the autocorrelation functions from different release times from the heat induced SL-CCS incorporated BSA hydrogel prepared at 59 °C. We found that all autocorrelation functions decayed almost at the same time, indicating the release of at least one particle with the same size over release time periods. Figure 9B shows the effect of changing the incubation time on the size of the released components for hydrogels made with the same concentration, preparation method, and release time. It can clearly be seen that a sample with higher incubation time (20 min) decayed faster, which correlates with the release of smaller particles. These results are in good agreement with the rheological characterization and CW-EPR spectroscopy as hydrogels prepared with lower incubation times are mechanically less robust, which may result in the release of larger albumin derivatives formed during the gelation process. Furthermore, results from the simulation of the EPR spectra showed slightly higher percentages of SL-CCS and SL-WFR intermediately bound to BSA released from the hydrogels with lower incubation times (see Supplementary Materials). Further information about the release of SL-WFR from BSA hydrogels with different incubation times and behavior of the hydrodynamic radius can be found in the Supplementary Materials.

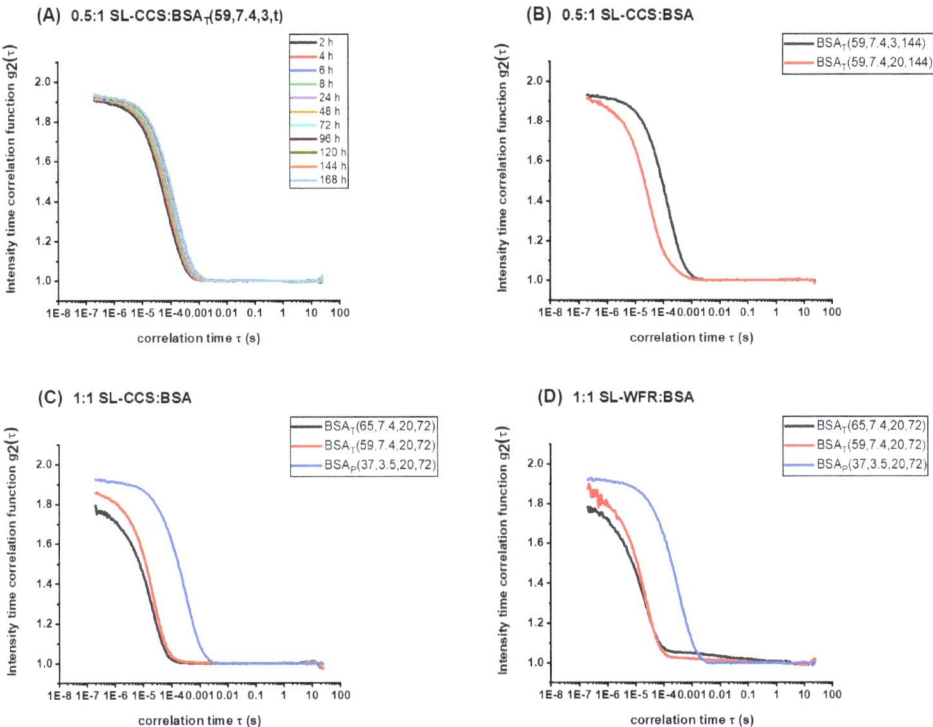

**Figure 9.** Intensity time correlation functions for (**A**) 0.5:1 SL-CCS:BSA$_T$(59, 7.4, 3) molar ratio during different release times, (**B**) SL-CCS:BSA$_T$(59, 7.4, 3, 144) and SL-CCS:BSA$_T$(59, 7.4, 20, 144) at a 0.5:1 molar ratio, (**C**) SL-CCS:BSA$_T$(65, 7.4, 20, 72), SL-CCS:BSA$_T$(59, 7.4, 20, 72) and SL-CCS:BSA$_P$(37, 3.5, 20, 72) at a 1:1 molar ratio, and (**D**) SL-WFR:BSA$_T$(65, 7.4, 20, 72), SL-WFR:BSA$_T$(59, 7.4, 20, 72), and SL-WFR: BSA$_P$(37, 3.5, 20, 72) at a 1:1 molar ratio.

Figure 9C,D shows the autocorrelation functions of SL-CCS and SL-WFR release from the BSA hydrogels after 72 h and the gels prepared with both thermally and pH induced methods by keeping the samples in the thermomixer for 20 min (results on the lower incubation time of SL-drug incorporated BSA hydrogels are given in the Supplementary Materials). As can be seen in both figures, the autocorrelation functions of the electrostatically triggered hydrogels displayed a slower decay those of the hydrogels prepared by the heat induced method at 65 °C and 59 °C. As discussed in the rheology section, the addition of acid to a precursor solution of BSA led to a mechanically weak hydrogel. Moreover, according to Table 2, the percentage of SL-pharmaceuticals strongly immobilized to BSA in the release medium increased when the hydrogels were prepared by the pH-induced method. We observed the same behavior in the DLS measurements. The existence of strongly bound SL-drugs, which are larger structures than intermediately and freely tumbling ones, results in the slower decay of the autocorrelation function. However, if—like in thermally-induced hydrogels—only freely rotating and intermediately BSA-bound SL-pharmaceuticals are released from thermally induced hydrogels, leading to the fast decay of the autocorrelation function for these samples. Therefore, these results complement all the earlier results by adding the perspective on the (larger) structures that are actually released into the release medium.

## 4. Conclusions

In the present work, BSA hydrogels with good mechanical properties were prepared as delivery hosts for pharmaceutical applications. The whole gelation procedures, namely thermally and pH induced methods, have previously been explained in detail [19]. SL-CCS and SL-WFR were loaded into BSA hydrogels at different molar ratios to evaluate the applicability of these structures as drug delivery systems. The results suggest that the drug release rate gained from double integration of EPR spectra is dependent on the type of drug, drug ratios, incubation time, and gelation method. We found that SL-CCS had a much higher release rate than SL-WFR. In general, higher drug concentrations, lower incubation times, and heat induced hydrogels prepared below BSA denaturation temperature resulted in a higher rate of release. Furthermore, the drug release pattern from these hydrogels showed that they can be used where the fast onset of release is required. The drug loading can affect the release behavior as lower ratios indicated the second sustained release phase, while higher ratios showed zero-order kinetics. Analyzing the hydrolytic degradation of hydrogels in the presence and absence of drugs as well as the SEM images of gels will be part of future work.

Additionally, EPR spectroscopy and DLS were applied to shed more light onto the interaction of SL-pharmaceuticals with BSA hydrogels as well as the nature and size of the released structures. We have shown that differences in chemical substitutions of SL-CCS and SL-WFR and binding capacities of BSA for SL-pharmaceuticals can deeply affect drug–protein interactions. Since a higher percentage of SL-WFR is attached strongly and intermediately to BSA hydrogels, more of these components are released compared to the SL-CCS incorporated BSA hydrogel, in which a higher percentage of freely tumbling SL-drug was found in the release medium. Moreover, a higher percentage of SL-CCS/SL-WFR intermediately (in case of thermally and pH induced hydrogels) and strongly (for electrostatically-triggered gels) bound to BSA was released from less rigid hydrogels due to faster penetration of water into the gel network. This led to the expedited release of albumin dimers or individual proteins when compared to the mechanically robust hydrogels. We hope that this study aids in paving the way to employing the full potential of BSA hydrogels as a suitable controlled release system and their implementation in biomedical applications.

**Supplementary Materials:** The following are available online at https://www.mdpi.com/article/10.3390/pharmaceutics13101661/s1, Figure S1: Storage (G′) and loss (G″) moduli as a function of time for different ratios of CCS:BSA at 59 °C, pH 7.4, Figure S2: Storage (G′) and loss (G″) moduli as a function of time for different ratios of WFR:BSA at (A) 65 °C, pH 7.4, (B) 59 °C, pH 7.4 and (C) 37 °C, pH 3.5, Figure S3: SL-CCS loaded (A) BSAT(65, 7.4, 10) at a 0.5:1 SL-CCS:BSA molar ratio, (B) BSAT(65, 7.4, 10) at a 1:1 SL-CCS:BSA molar ratio, (C) BSAT(59, 7.4, 10) at a 0.5:1 SL-CCS:BSA molar ratio, (D) BSAT(59, 7.4, 10) at a 1:1 SL-CCS:BSA molar ratio, (E) BSAT(59, 7.4, 10) at a 2:1 SL-CCS:BSA molar ratio, (F) BSAP(37, 3.5, 30) at a 0.5:1 SL-CCS:BSA molar ratio and (G) BSAP(37, 3.5, 30) at a 1:1 SL-CCS:BSA molar ratio, Figure S4: SL-WFR loaded (A) BSAT(65, 7.4, 10) at a 0.5:1 SL-WFR:BSA molar ratio, (B) BSAT(65, 7.4, 10) at a 1:1 SL-WFR:BSA molar ratio, (C) BSAT(59, 7.4, 10) at a 0.5:1 SL-WFR:BSA molar ratio, (D) BSAT(59, 7.4, 10) at a 1:1 SL-WFR:BSA molar ratio, (E) BSAT(59, 7.4, 10) at a 2:1 SL-WFR:BSA molar ratio, (F) BSAP(37, 3.5, 30) at a 0.5:1 SL-WFR:BSA molar ratio and (G) BSAP(37, 3.5, 30) at a 1:1 SL-WFR:BSA molar ratio, Figure S5: Release profiles of SL-CCS loaded BSA hydrogels with 0.5:1, 1:1 and 2:1 SL-CCS:BSA molar ratios (A) BSAT(65, 7.4, 3) hydrogel, (B) BSAT(59, 7.4, 3) hydrogel and (C) BSAP(37, 3.5, 10) hydrogel. The curves are fitted, Figure S6: Release profiles of SL-WFR loaded BSA hydrogels with 0.5:1, 1:1 and 2:1 SL-WFR:BSA molar ratios (A) BSAT(65, 7.4, 3) hydrogel, (B) BSAT(59, 7.4, 3) hydrogel and (C) BSAP(37, 3.5, 10) hydrogel. The curves are fitted, Figure S7: Release profiles of SL-CCS and SL-WFR loaded BSA hydrogels prepared with heat induced method at 59 °C with two different incubation times of 3 and 20 min at a (A) 0.5:1 SL-CCS:BSA molar ratio, (B) 0.5:1 SL-WFR:BSA molar ratio, (C) 1:1 SL-WFR:BSA molar ratio and (D) 2:1 SL-WFR:BSA molar ratio, Figure S8: EPR spectra of release test after 48 h for SL-drugs loaded BSA hydrogels at a 1:1 molar ratio (A) SL-CCS:BSAT(59, 7.4, 20, 48) and (B) SL-WFR:BSAT(59, 7.4, 20, 48), Figure S9: EPR spectra of release test after 48 h for SL-drugs loaded BSA hydrogels at a 1:1 molar ratio (A) SL-CCS:BSAT(59, 7.4, 3, 48), (B) SL-WFR:BSAT(65, 7.4, 3, 48), (C) SL-WFR:BSAT(59, 7.4, 3, 48) and (D) SL-WFR:BSAT(37, 3.5, 10, 48), Figure S10: Intensity time correlation functions for 0.5:1 SL-WFR:BSAT(59, 7.4, 3) molar ratio during different release times, Figure S11: Intensity time correlation functions for different concentrations of (A) SL-CCS diluted with 10× PBS and (B) SL-WFR diluted with 10× PBS, Figure S12: (A) Intensity time correlation functions for different concentrations of BSA solution diluted by 10× PBS and (B) hydrodynamic radius of different concentrations of BSA solution diluted by 10× PBS, Figure S13: Intensity time correlation functions of (A) SL-CCS:BSAT(59, 7.4, 3, 144) and SL-CCS:BSAT(59, 7.4, 20, 144) at a 1:1 molar ratio and (B) SL-CCS:BSAT(59, 7.4, 3, 144) and SL-CCS:BSAT(59, 7.4, 20, 144) at a 2:1 molar ratio, Figure S14: Intensity time correlation functions of (A) SL-WFR:BSAT(59, 7.4, 3, 144) and SL-WFR:BSAT(59, 7.4, 20, 144) at a 0.5:1 molar ratio, (B) SL-WFR:BSAT(59, 7.4, 3, 144) and SL-WFR:BSAT(59, 7.4, 20, 144) at a 1:1 molar ratio and (C) SL-WFR:BSAT(59, 7.4, 3, 144) and SL-WFR:BSAT(59, 7.4, 20, 144) at a 2:1 molar ratio, Figure S15: Intensity time correlation functions for (A) SL-CCS:BSAT(65, 7.4, 3, 72), SL-CCS:BSAT(59, 7.4, 3, 72) and SL-CCS:BSAP(37, 3.5, 10, 72) at a 1:1 molar ratio and (B) SL-WFR:BSAT(65, 7.4, 3, 72), SL-WFR:BSAT(59, 7.4, 3, 72) and SL-WFR:BSAP(37, 3.5, 10, 72) at a 1:1 molar ratio, Table S1: Parameters gained from simulation of Figure S3, Table S2: Parameters gained from simulation of Figure S4, Table S3: Percentage of released components in different states gained from spectral simulation of Figure S8, Table S4: Percentage of released components in different states gained from spectral simulation of Figure S9.

**Author Contributions:** Conceptualization, D.H.; Data curation, N.S., K.M. and D.H.; Formal analysis, N.S. and K.M.; Funding acquisition, K.M. and D.H.; Investigation, N.S.; Project administration, D.H.; Resources, K.M.; Validation, N.S. and D.H.; Writing – original draft, D.H. All authors have read and agreed to the published version of the manuscript.

**Funding:** This research was funded by the European Social Funds (ESF) and the State of Saxony—Anhalt through the graduate school AgriPoly. DH acknowledges support by the Deutsche Forschungsgemeinschaft (DFG, German Research foundation)—project-ID 436494874—RTG 2670.

**Institutional Review Board Statement:** Not applicable.

**Informed Consent Statement:** Not applicable.

**Data Availability Statement:** Data are available from the authors upon request.

**Conflicts of Interest:** The authors declare no conflict of interest.

# References

1. Bhowmik, D.; Gopinath, H.; Kumar, B.P.; Duraivel, S.; Kumar, K.S. Controlled release drug delivery systems. *Pharm. Innov.* **2012**, *1*, 24–32.
2. Siepmann, J.; Siegel, R.A.; Rathbone, M.J. *Fundamentals and Applications of Controlled Release Drug Delivery*; Springer: New York, NY, USA, 2012; Volume 3.
3. Lee, J.H.; Yeo, Y. Controlled drug release from pharmaceutical nanocarriers. *Chem. Eng. Sci.* **2015**, *125*, 75–84. [CrossRef] [PubMed]
4. de Souza, L.E.; Eckenstaler, R.; Syrowatka, F.; Beck-Broichsitter, M.; Benndorf, R.A.; Mäder, K. Has PEG-PLGA advantages for the delivery of hydrophobic drugs? Risperidone as an example. *J. Drug Deliv. Sci. Technol.* **2021**, *61*, 102239. [CrossRef]
5. Janich, C.; Friedmann, A.; Silva, J.M.D.S.E.; De Oliveira, C.S.; De Souza, L.E.; Rujescu, D.; Hildebrandt, C.; Beck-Broichsitter, M.; Schmelzer, C.E.H.; Mäder, K. Risperidone-Loaded PLGA–Lipid Particles with Improved Release Kinetics: Manufacturing and Detailed Characterization by Electron Microscopy and Nano-CT. *Pharmceutics* **2019**, *11*, 665. [CrossRef] [PubMed]
6. Cao, Z.; Ma, Y.; Sun, C.; Lu, Z.; Yao, Z.; Wang, J.; Li, D.; Yuan, Y.; Yang, X. ROS-sensitive polymeric nanocarriers with red light-activated size shrinkage for remotely con-trolled drug release. *Chem. Mater.* **2018**, *30*, 517–525. [CrossRef]
7. Thanh, V.M.; Nguyen, T.H.; Tran, T.V.; Ngoc, U.T.P.; Ho, M.N.; Nguyen, T.T.; Chau, Y.N.T.; Le, V.T.; Tran, N.Q.; Nguyen, C.K.; et al. Low systemic toxicity nanocarriers fabricated from heparin-mPEG and PAMAM dendrimers for controlled drug release. *Mater. Sci. Eng.* **2018**, *82*, 291–298. [CrossRef]
8. Wells, C.M.; Harris, M.; Choi, L.; Murali, V.P.; Guerra, F.D.; Jennings, J.A. Stimuli-responsive drug release from smart polymers. *J. Func. Biomater.* **2019**, *10*, 34. [CrossRef]
9. Xiong, D.; Zhang, X.; Peng, S.; Gu, H.; Zhang, L. Smart pH-sensitive micelles based on redox degradable polymers as DOX/GNPs carriers for controlled drug release and CT imaging. *Colloids Surf. B* **2018**, *163*, 29–40. [CrossRef]
10. Lai, W.; Chen, C.; Ren, X.; Lee, I.S.; Jiang, G.; Kong, X. Hydrothermal fabrication of porous hollow hydroxyapatite microspheres for a drug delivery system. *Mater. Sci. Eng. C* **2016**, *62*, 166–172. [CrossRef]
11. Caccavo, D.; Cascone, S.; Lamberti, G.; Barba, A.A. Controlled drug release from hydrogel-based matrices: Experiments and modeling. *Int. J. Pharm.* **2015**, *486*, 144–152. [CrossRef]
12. Wang, Y.; Wang, J.; Yuan, Z.; Han, H.; Li, T.; Li, L.; Guo, X. Chitosan cross-linked poly (acrylic acid) hydrogels: Drug release control and mechanism. *Colloids Surf. B* **2017**, *152*, 252–259. [CrossRef]
13. Sharma, P.K.; Taneja, S.; Singh, Y. Hydrazone-linkage-based self-healing and injectable xanthan–poly (ethylene glycol) hydrogels for controlled drug release and 3D cell culture. *ACS Appl. Mater. Interfaces* **2018**, *10*, 30936–30945. [CrossRef]

14. Bhattarai, N.; Gunn, J.; Zhang, M. Chitosan-based hydrogels for controlled, localized drug delivery. *Adv. Drug Deliv. Rev.* **2010**, *62*, 83–99. [CrossRef] [PubMed]
15. Langer, R.; Peppas, N.A. Advances in biomaterials, drug delivery, and bionanotechnology. *AIChE J.* **2003**, *49*, 2990–3006. [CrossRef]
16. Haeri, H.H.; Jerschabek, V.; Sadeghi, A.; Hinderberger, D. Copper–Calcium Poly (Acrylic Acid) Composite Hydrogels as Studied by Electron Paramagnetic Resonance (EPR) Spectroscopy. *Macromol. Chem. Phys.* **2020**, *221*, 2000262. [CrossRef]
17. Arabi, S.H.; Aghelnejad, B.; Volmer, J.; Hinderberger, D. Hydrogels from serum albumin in a molten globule-like state. *Protein Sci.* **2020**, *29*, 2459–2467. [CrossRef]
18. Tada, D.; Tanabe, T.; Tachibana, A.; Yamauchi, K. Drug release from hydrogel containing albumin as crosslinker. *J. Biosci. Bioeng.* **2005**, *100*, 551–555. [CrossRef]
19. Arabi, S.H.; Aghelnejad, B.; Schwieger, C.; Meister, A.; Kerth, A.; Hinderberger, D. Serum albumin hydrogels in broad pH and temperature ranges: Characterization of their self-assembled structures and nanoscopic and macroscopic properties. *Biomater. Sci.* **2018**, *6*, 478–492. [CrossRef]
20. Sanaeifar, N.; Mäder, K.; Hinderberger, D. Nanoscopic Characterization of Stearic Acid Release from Bovine Serum Albumin Hydrogels. *Macromol. Biosci.* **2020**, *20*, 2000126. [CrossRef]
21. Junk, M.J.; Li, W.; Schlüter, A.D.; Wegner, G.; Spiess, H.W.; Zhang, A.; Hinderberger, D. EPR spectroscopic characterization of local nanoscopic heterogeneities during the thermal collapse of thermoresponsive dendronized polymers. *Angew. Chem. Int. Ed.* **2010**, *49*, 5683–5687. [CrossRef]
22. Reichenwallner, J.; Hinderberger, D. Using bound fatty acids to disclose the functional structure of serum albumin. *Biochim. Biophys. Acta* **2013**, *1830*, 5382–5393. [CrossRef] [PubMed]
23. Akdogan, Y.; Reichenwallner, J.; Hinderberger, D. Evidence for water-tuned structural differences in proteins: An approach emphasizing variations in local hydrophilicity. *PLoS ONE* **2012**, *7*, e45681. [CrossRef] [PubMed]
24. Elsadek, B.; Kratz, F. Impact of albumin on drug delivery—New applications on the horizon. *J. Control. Release* **2012**, *157*, 4–28. [CrossRef] [PubMed]
25. Haeri, H.H.; Tomaszewski, J.; Phytides, B.; Schimm, H.; Möslein, G.; Niedergethmann, M.; Hinderberger, D.; Gelos, M. Identification of Patients with Pancreatic Cancer by Electron Paramagnetic Resonance Spectroscopy of Fatty Acid Binding to Human Serum Albumin. *ACS Pharmacol. Transl. Sci.* **2020**, *3*, 1188–1198. [CrossRef]
26. Larsen, M.T.; Kuhlmann, M.; Hvam, M.L.; Howard, K.A. Albumin-based drug delivery: Harnessing nature to cure disease. *Mol. Cell Ther.* **2016**, *4*, 3. [CrossRef]
27. Arabi, S.H.; Haselberger, D.; Hinderberger, D. The effect of ethanol on gelation, nanoscopic, and macroscopic properties of serum albumin hydrogels. *Molecules* **2020**, *25*, 1927. [CrossRef]
28. Boye, J.I.; Alli, I.; Ismail, A.A. Interactions involved in the gelation of bovine serum albumin. *J. Agric. Food Chem.* **1996**, *44*, 996–1004. [CrossRef]
29. Baler, K.; Michael, R.; Szleifer, I.; Ameer, G.A. Albumin hydrogels formed by electrostatically triggered self-assembly and their drug delivery capability. *Biomacromolecules* **2014**, *15*, 3625–3633. [CrossRef]
30. Pápay, Z.E.; Kósa, A.; Böddi, B.; Merchant, Z.; Saleem, I.Y.; Zariwala, M.G.; Klebovich, I.; Somavarapu, S.; Antal, I. Study on the pulmonary delivery system of apigenin-loaded albumin nanocarriers with antioxidant activity. *J. Aerosol Med. Pulm. Drug Deliv.* **2017**, *30*, 274–288. [CrossRef] [PubMed]
31. Gharbavi, M.; Danafar, H.; Sharafi, A. Microemulsion and bovine serum albumin nanoparticles as a novel hybrid nanocarrier system for efficient multifunctional drug delivery. *J. Biomed. Mater. Res. A* **2020**, *108*, 1688–1702. [CrossRef]
32. de Redín, I.L.; Boiero, C.; Martínez-Ohárriz, M.C.; Agüeros, M.; Ramos, R.; Peñuelas, I.; Allemandi, D.; Llabot, J.M.; Irache, J.M. Human serum albumin nanoparticles for ocular delivery of bevacizumab. *Int. J. Pharm.* **2018**, *541*, 214–223. [CrossRef]
33. Golubeva, E.; Chumakova, N.A.; Kuzin, S.V.; Grigoriev, I.A.; Kalai, T.; Korotkevich, A.A.; Bogorodsky, S.E.; Krotova, L.I.; Popov, V.K.; Lunin, V.V. Paramagnetic bioactives encapsulated in poly(D, L-lactide) microparticles: Spatial distribution and in vitro release kinetics. *J. Supercrit. Fluids* **2020**, *158*, 104748. [CrossRef]
34. Eisenächer, F.; Schädlich, A.; Mäder, K. Monitoring of internal pH gradients within multi-layer tablets by optical methods and EPR imaging. *Int. J. Pharm.* **2011**, *417*, 204–215. [CrossRef]
35. Kroll, C.; Hermann, W.; Stösser, R.; Borchert, H.H.; Mäder, K. Influence of drug treatment on the microacidity in rat and human skin—an in vitro electron spin resonance imaging study. *Pharm. Res.* **2001**, *18*, 525–530. [CrossRef] [PubMed]
36. Khalil, S.K.H.; El-Feky, G.S.; El-Banna, S.T.; Khalil, W.A. Preparation and evaluation of warfarin-β-cyclodextrin loaded chitosan nanoparticles for transdermal delivery. *Carbohydr. Polym.* **2012**, *90*, 1244–1253. [CrossRef] [PubMed]
37. Mekaj, Y.H.; Mekaj, A.Y.; Duci, S.B.; Miftari, E.I. New oral anticoagulants: Their advantages and disadvantages compared with vitamin K antagonists in the prevention and treatment of patients with thromboembolic events. *Ther. Clin. Risk Manag.* **2015**, *11*, 967. [CrossRef]
38. Verhoef, T.I.; Redekop, W.K.; Daly, A.K.; Van Schie, R.M.; De Boer, A.; Maitland-van der Zee, A.H. Pharmacogenetic-guided dosing of coumarin anticoagulants: Algorithms for warfarin, acenocoumarol and phenprocoumon. *Br. J. Clin. Pharmacol.* **2014**, *77*, 626–641. [CrossRef] [PubMed]
39. Hauenschild, T.; Reichenwallner, J.; Enkelmann, V.; Hinderberger, D. Characterizing Active Pharmaceutical Ingredient Binding to Human Serum Albumin by Spin-Labeling and EPR Spectroscopy. *Chem. Eur. J.* **2016**, *22*, 12825–12838. [CrossRef]

40. Widder, K.; MacEwan, S.R.; Garanger, E.; Núñez, V.; Lecommandoux, S.; Chilkoti, A.; Hinderberger, D. Characterisation of hydration and nanophase separation during the temperature response in hydrophobic/hydrophilic elastin-like polypeptide (ELP) diblock copolymers. *Soft Matter* **2017**, *13*, 1816–1822. [CrossRef] [PubMed]
41. Herrling, T.; Fuchs, J.; Groth, N. Kinetic measurements using EPR imaging with a modulated field gradient. *J. Magn. Reson.* **2002**, *154*, 6–14. [CrossRef] [PubMed]
42. Kaszuba, M.; McKnight, D.; Connah, M.T.; McNeil-Watson, F.K.; Nobbmann, U. Measuring sub nanometre sizes using dynamic light scattering. *J. Nanopart. Res.* **2008**, *10*, 823–829. [CrossRef]
43. Nobbmann, U.; Connah, M.; Fish, B.; Varley, P.; Gee, C.; Mulot, S.; Chen, J.; Zhou, L.; Lu, Y.; Sheng, F.; et al. Dynamic light scattering as a relative tool for assessing the molecular integrity and stability of monoclonal antibodies. *Biotechnol. Genet. Eng. Rev.* **2007**, *24*, 117–128. [CrossRef] [PubMed]
44. Peppas, N.A.; Bures, P.; Leobandung, W.S.; Ichikawa, H. Hydrogels in pharmaceutical formulations. *Eur. J. Pharm. Biopharm.* **2000**, *50*, 27–46. [CrossRef]
45. Yan, C.; Pochan, D.J. Rheological properties of peptide-based hydrogels for biomedical and other applications. *Chem. Soc. Rev.* **2010**, *39*, 3528–3540. [CrossRef]
46. Hao, J.; Weiss, R. Viscoelastic and mechanical behavior of hydrophobically modified hydrogels. *Macromolecules* **2011**, *44*, 9390–9398. [CrossRef]
47. Yamasaki, K.; Maruyama, T.; Kragh-Hansen, U.; Otagiri, M. Characterization of site I on human serum albumin: Concept about the structure of a drug binding site. *Biochim. Biophys. Acta -Protein Struct. Mol. Enzymol.* **1996**, *1295*, 147–157. [CrossRef]
48. Lee, P.; Wu, X. Modifications of human serum albumin and their binding effect. *Curr. Pharm. Design* **2015**, *21*, 1862–1865. [CrossRef]
49. Khodarahmi, R.; Karimi, S.A.; Kooshk, M.R.A.; Ghadami, S.A.; Ghobadi, S.; Amani, M. Comparative spectroscopic studies on drug binding characteristics and protein surface hydrophobicity of native and modified forms of bovine serum albumin: Possible relevance to change in protein structure/function upon non-enzymatic glycation. *Spectrochim. Acta A Mol. Biomol. Spectrosc.* **2012**, *89*, 177–186. [CrossRef]
50. Reichenwallner, J.; Oehmichen, M.T.; Schmelzer, C.E.; Hauenschild, T.; Kerth, A.; Hinderberger, D. Exploring the pH-induced functional phase space of human serum albumin by EPR spectroscopy. *Magnetochemistry* **2018**, *4*, 47. [CrossRef]
51. Akdogan, Y.; Wu, Y.; Eisele, K.; Schaz, M.; Weil, T.; Hinderberger, D. Host–guest interactions in polycationic human serum albumin bioconjugates. *Soft Matter* **2012**, *8*, 11106–11114. [CrossRef]
52. Kempe, S.; Metz, H.; Mäder, K. Application of electron paramagnetic resonance (EPR) spectroscopy and imaging in drug delivery research–chances and challenges. *Eur. J. Pharm. Biopharm.* **2010**, *74*, 55–66. [CrossRef]
53. Capancioni, S.; Schwach-Abdellaoui, K.; Kloeti, W.; Herrmann, W.; Brosig, H.; Borchert, H.H.; Heller, J.; Gurny, R. In vitro monitoring of poly (ortho ester) degradation by electron paramagnetic resonance imaging. *Macromolecules* **2003**, *36*, 6135–6141. [CrossRef]

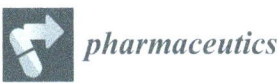

Article

# Albumin–Methotrexate Prodrug Analogues That Undergo Intracellular Reactivation Following Entrance into Cancerous Glioma Cells

Itzik Cooper [1,2,3,*], Michal Schnaider-Beeri [1,2,4], Mati Fridkin [5] and Yoram Shechter [6]

1. The Joseph Sagol Neuroscience Center, Sheba Medical Center, Tel Hashomer, Ramat Gan 52621, Israel; michal.beeri@sheba.health.gov.il
2. School of Psychology, Reichman University, Herzliya 4610101, Israel
3. The Nehemia Rubin Excellence in Biomedical Research—The TELEM Program, Sheba Medical Center, Tel Hashomer, Ramat Gan 52621, Israel
4. Department of Psychiatry, Mount Sinai School of Medicine, New York, NY 10029, USA
5. Department of Organic Chemistry, The Weizmann Institute of Science, Rehovot 76100, Israel; mati.fridkin@weizmann.ac.il
6. Department of Biomolecular Sciences, The Weizmann Institute of Science, Rehovot 76100, Israel; yoram.shechter@weizmann.ac.il
* Correspondence: itzik.cooper@sheba.health.gov.il

**Abstract:** A family of monomodified bovine serum albumin (BSA) linked to methotrexate (MTX) through a variety of spacers was prepared. All analogues were found to be prodrugs having low MTX-inhibitory potencies toward dihydrofolate reductase in a cell-free system. The optimal conjugates regenerated their antiproliferative efficacies following entrance into cancerous glioma cell lines and were significantly superior to MTX in an insensitive glioma cell line. A BSA–MTX conjugate linked through a simple ethylene chain spacer, containing a single peptide bond located 8.7 Å distal to the protein back bone, and apart from the covalently linked MTX by about 12 Å, was most effective. The inclusion of an additional disulfide bond in the spacer neither enhanced nor reduced the killing potency of this analogue. Disrupting the native structure of the carrier protein in the conjugates significantly reduced their antiproliferative activity. In conclusion, we have engineered BSA–MTX prodrug analogues which undergo intracellular reactivation and facilitate antiproliferative activities following their entrance into glioma cells.

**Citation:** Cooper, I.; Schnaider-Beeri, M.; Fridkin, M.; Shechter, Y. Albumin–Methotrexate Prodrug Analogues That Undergo Intracellular Reactivation Following Entrance into Cancerous Glioma Cells. *Pharmaceutics* **2022**, *14*, 71. https://doi.org/10.3390/pharmaceutics14010071

Academic Editor: Katona Gábor

Received: 30 November 2021
Accepted: 23 December 2021
Published: 28 December 2021

**Publisher's Note:** MDPI stays neutral with regard to jurisdictional claims in published maps and institutional affiliations.

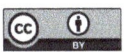

**Copyright:** © 2021 by the authors. Licensee MDPI, Basel, Switzerland. This article is an open access article distributed under the terms and conditions of the Creative Commons Attribution (CC BY) license (https://creativecommons.org/licenses/by/4.0/).

**Keywords:** cancer; albumin; disulfide; glioma; prodrug; conjugate

## 1. Introduction

Methotrexate (MTX) is an antiproliferative and immunosuppressive agent widely and effectively used against a broad spectrum of diseases, primarily cancerous tumors but also certain autoimmune diseases such as psoriasis and rheumatoid arthritis [1]. It facilitates its antiproliferative effects by inhibiting dihydrofolate-reductase (DHFR), a ubiquitous enzyme that catalyzes the reduction of folate to dihydrofolate (DHF) and then to tetrahydrofolate. The latter is a cofactor for de novo synthesis of thymidylate, purine, and glycine [2].

As with most antimetabolites, MTX is only partially selective for tumor cells and is toxic to all rapidly dividing normal cells, such as those of the intestinal epithelium and bone marrow [3]. Although relatively less toxic compared with other therapeutic agents, it is not devoid of side effects. In addition, a variety of tumor cells develop resistance to MTX upon treatment with agents, affecting several mechanistic pathways, including impaired transport of MTX into cells [4,5]. Solving these deficiencies and increasing MTX selectivity toward inflamed, diseased, or malignant tissues is therefore of primary clinical significance.

One of the approaches undertaken in recent years as an attempt to increase selectivity of chemotherapeutic agents was to link them covalently to macromolecules such as albumin.

Extravasation of albumin is upregulated about six-fold in inflamed, diseased, and malignant tissues [6,7]. If the covalently-linked MTX has low antiproliferative activity, this would create a rather profound clinical advantage, provided that the conjugate undergoes efficient intracellular reactivation following entrance into tumorigenic cells. The amide bond of MTX linked to the ε-amino group of lysine is chemically and enzymatically stable [8], and reactivation appears to be dependent on extensive intracellular proteolysis, as only MTX linked to short peptide fragments through its γ-carboxylate moiety regain significant antiproliferative efficacy (this study). Similarly, binding MTX to other macromolecules, such as anti-TNFα antibodies, might be clinically beneficial in autoimmune and inflammatory diseases such as arthritis, for example, where MTX is administrated at low dosages separately from anti-TNFα antibodies. Generating such an antibody–MTX conjugate may reduce side effects and improve efficacy as well as provide better treatment tolerance.

We thus initially searched for a chemical procedure to covalently link MTX to amino-containing molecules through the γ-carboxylate moiety of MTX. The linkage of such molecules to the α-carboxylate of MTX was documented to yield inactive analogues [9,10]. Secondly, we examined the possibility of introducing MTX to albumin through spacers containing disulfide bonds. Malignant tissues have elevated de novo synthesis of glutathione [11–13], and we wondered whether this would lead to increased selectivity and enhanced reduction-dependent release of active MTX in tumorigenic cells.

In this study, we describe our synthetic procedures for obtaining a variety of BSA–MTX conjugates, their cell-free DHFR-inhibitory potencies in the absence and in the presence of glutathione or cysteine, and their antiproliferative efficacies in several lines of cancerous cells relative to that of methotrexate. Two glioma cell lines are investigated here, for the first time, in the context of albumin conjugates to align with other research in our lab, in which new compounds and methods that enable blood–brain barrier (BBB) opening, and thus, the entrance of large therapeutic molecules such as albumin are being developed [14–18].

## 2. Experimental Procedures

### 2.1. Materials

Methotrexate, bovine serum albumin, cystamine dihydrochloride, hexamethyl diamine-dihydrochloride, dihydrofolate (DHF), N,N'dicyclohexylcarbodiimide (DCC), β-nicotinamide adenosine dinucleotide 2' phosphate (NADPH), reduced glutathione (GSH) oxidized glutathione (GSSG), and L-cysteine were purchased from Sigma (St. Louis, MO, USA). Methotrexate linked to a peptide (MTX–AYGRKKRRQRRR) was synthesized by the manual conventional solid-phase synthesis. An Fmoc (N-9-flurenylmethoxy carbonyl) strategy was employed through the peptide chain assembly. All other materials used in this study were of analytical grade.

### 2.2. Synthesis of MTX–Anhydride

Methotrexate (45.4 mg, 100 μM) dissolved in 0.7 mL dimethylformamide (DMF) and 95 μL from a solution of 1 M DCC in DMF (95 μM) was added. The reaction was carried out for 3 h at 25 °C. Dicyclohexylurea was filtered out. The MTX–anhydride formed was kept at 4 °C until used.

### 2.3. Synthesis of MTX–Dicystamine [MTX–CO$^γ$NH–(CH$_2$)$_2$–S–S–(CH$_2$)$_2$–NH$_2$]

Dicystamine di-HCl (100 μM) was dissolved in 0.7 mL DMF, neutralized with DIPEA, and combined with the solution of MTX–anhydride (150 μM in 0.7 mL DMF). The reaction mixture was stirred for 40 min, precipitated with ether, washed three times with ether, and desiccated. The solid material was suspended in H$_2$O and centrifuged. This procedure, which removes residual dicystamine and unreacted MTX, was repeated five times. The solid material was then lyophilized. MTX–CO$^γ$NH–(CH$_2$)$_3$–S–S–(CH$_2$)$_2$–NH$_2$ was obtained in 60% yield. It has a molar extinction coefficient similar to that of MTX ($\varepsilon_{305nm}$ = 22,700 and $\varepsilon_{372nm}$ = 7200). Calculated ESMS = 588 Da, found ESMS for M − H = 587.26 Da.

## 2.4. Synthesis of MTX–Hexamethyl-Amine and MTX–Glutathione

These derivatives were synthesized by the same procedure applied for MTX–dicystamine except that dicystamine was replaced with hexamethyldiamine-di-HCl or with GSSG. MTX–hexamethyl-amine [MTX–CO$^\gamma$NH(CH$_2$)$_6$–NH$_2$] and MTX–glutathione [MTX–CO$^\gamma$NH–GSSG] were obtained in 28 and 37% yields, respectively. Calculated ESMS for MTX–hexamethylamine is 552 Da, found for M + H = 553.41 Da, and M − H = 551.38 Da. Calculated ESMS for MTX–GSSG is 1048 Da, found M + H = 1049.4, and M − H = 1047.51.

## 2.5. Preparation of BSA–MTX Conjugates

MTX–dicystamine (4 μM) was dissolved in 50 μL DMF and combined with a solution of MAL–(CH$_2$)$_3$–COOSu (3 μM in 50 μL DMF). Following one hour of incubation, this reaction mixture was added in 9 aliquots (10 μL each) over a period of one hour to a stirred solution of BSA (3.0 mL, 70 mg/mL in 0.1 M HEPES buffer (pH 7.4). The reaction was carried out at 0 °C. The derivative thus obtained was dialyzed over a period of 3 days against H$_2$O, 0.03 M Na$_2$CO$_3$ (pH 10.3), and H$_2$O, and then lyophilized. BSA–S–S–MTX contains 0.7 ± 0.05 M MTX per mole BSA as determined by its absorbance at 372 nm using $\varepsilon_{372nm}$ = 7200. The protein concentration was determined by amino acid analysis following acid hydrolysis of a measured aliquot, calculated according to valine (36 residues) isoleucine (14 residues) and lysine (59 residues).

BSA–(CH$_2$)$_6$–MTX and BSA–GSSG–MTX were prepared essentially by the same procedure applied for BSA–S–S–MTX (previous section), except that MAL–(CH$_2$)$_3$–COOSu was linked to either MTX–hexamethylamine or to MTX–GSSG for obtaining either BSA–(CH$_2$)$_6$–MTX or BSA–GSSG–MTX, respectively. Analogues which contained covalently linked MTX in the range of 0.6 to 0.8 M MTX per mole of BSA were subjected to further studies.

## 2.6. Cleavage of BSA–(CH$_2$)$_6$–MTX with Cyanogen Bromide

BSA–(CH$_2$)$_6$–MTX (40 mg) was dissolved in 1.0 mL 70% formic acid. Solid cyanogen bromide (20 mg) was then added and incubated for 24 h at 25 °C. The reaction mixture was evaporated to dryness, dissolved in 1.0 mL H$_2$O, dialyzed for two days against H$_2$O, and lyophilized. Derivatives concentration and MTX content was obtained by quantitative amino-acid analysis and by the absorbance at 372 nm, as described in detail in the previous section.

## 2.7. Preparation of HSA(MTX)$_{40}$

HSA (67 mg, 1 μM) was dissolved in 10 mL of 0.1 M HEPES buffer pH 7.4, and MTX–anhydride (100 μM in 0.7 mL DMF) was added in 7 aliquots (100 μL each) over a period of 2 h at 0 °C to the stirred solution of the protein. The derivative thus obtained was dialyzed over a period of 3 days against H$_2$O, 0.03 M Na$_2$CO$_3$ (pH 10.3), and H$_2$O, and then lyophilized. HSA-(MTX)$_{40}$ contains 40 ± 3 M MTX per mole of HSA as determined by the absorbance at 372 nm ($\varepsilon_{372nm}$ = 7200). The protein content was determined by quantitative amino acid analysis following acid hydrolysis of a measured aliquot, calculated according to glycine (12 residues), alanine (62 residues), and valine (41 residues).

## 2.8. Partial Purification of DHFR from Chicken Liver

This was carried out by the procedure of Kaufman and Kemerer [19] with some modifications: Fresh chicken liver (20 g) was cut into pieces, homogenized in 0.1 M MnCl$_2$ and centrifuged. The supernatant was brought to pH 5–6 with HCl, and ZnSO$_4$ was added gradually to obtain a final concentration of 20 mM. The pH was elevated to pH 7.5–8 by the addition of solid NaHCO$_3$. The precipitate thus formed (about 87% of total protein) was removed by centrifugation. The proteins that remained in the supernatant were precipitated with 4.54 M ammonium sulfate. The precipitate was then dissolved in 50 mM Tris-HCl (pH 7.5) containing 0.1 M KCl and dialyzed for two days against the same buffer, and then frozen in aliquots at −80 °C until used. Partially purified DHFR prepared by this procedure has a specific activity of about 0.05 units/mg.

*2.9. Cell-Free Enzymatic Assay for DHFR*

The assay was based on DHFR-dependent reduction of dihydrofolate to tetrahydrofolate. In this process, NADPH is oxidized to NADP, and the extent of the oxidation is monitored by the decrease in absorbance at 340 nm [20]. Tubes containing 1.0 mL each of 0.05 M Tris-HCl buffer (pH 7.5) 0.5 M KCl, 0.137 mM NADPH, and 0.187 mM DHF were incubated for 1 h at 25 °C in the absence and the presence of partially purified DHFR (35 µg/mL) and increasing concentrations of MTX or its derivatives. The absorbance at 340 nm was then monitored. In a typical assay, absorbance at 340 nm amounted to $1.7 \pm 0.06$ and $0.65 \pm 0.06$ in the absence and the presence of DHFR. MTX inhibits DHFR with an $IC_{50}$ value of 55 nM. A methotrexate derivative yielding an $IC_{50}$ value of 0.55 µM was considered as having 10% of the inhibitory potency of the native folic acid antagonist.

*2.10. Maleimide–Thiol Exchange Assay*

BSA–S–MAL–$(CH_2)_3$–CONH–MTX (0.2 mM) was dissolved in 1.0 mL 0.1 M HEPES, pH 7.3, and transferred to a tube containing 7.5 mg GSH corresponding to 24 µM which are 100 molar excess over the conjugate. The solution was incubated for 7 h at 37 °C, followed by extensive dialysis and lyophilization. Absorbance was read at 372 nm.

*2.11. Cancer Cell Lines*

In this study, we used two glioma cell lines: (i) CNS-1; rat glioma; (ii) U251; human glioma. Cells were a generous gift from Dr. Yael Mardor from the Sheba Medical Center, Israel.

*2.12. Growth Inhibition Effects of BSA–MTX Analogues*

Cancer cell lines were grown in monoculture in 96-well plates in RPMI (CNS-1 cells) or DMEM containing 10% fetal bovine serum, 2 mM L-glutamine, penicillin (100 units/mL), and streptomycin (0.1 mg/mL) under humidified atmosphere containing 5% $CO_2$. Following 24 h or 48 h, MTX or BSA–MTX analogues were added to each plate to give a final MTX or HSA–MTX analogue concentration ranging from 1 nM to 10 µM. Cell viability was measured after 48 h using a standard MTT (3-(4,5-dimethylthiazol-2-yl)-2,5-diphenyltetrazolium bromide) assay, as described before [21].

*2.13. Statistical Analysis*

Statistical analysis was performed using the Prism (GraphPad) 6 software. Data are presented as the means ± standard error of the mean (SEM). Differences between two groups were assessed by an unpaired t-test and among three or more groups by a one-way analysis of variance followed by Tukey's multiple comparison test. A *p*-value of less than 0.05 was considered statistically significant.

## 3. Results

*3.1. Searching for a Chemical Procedure to Obtain Active MTX Derivatives Following the Covalent Introduction of Amino-Containing Nucleophiles*

Of the two carboxylates of MTX, the α carboxylate participating in binding to DHFR and its derivatization was documented to yield inactive analogues [9,10]. The γ carboxylate of MTX is more distal to the binding site of DHFR, and its derivatization can yield products with high or moderate affinity toward the enzyme [22,23]. In preliminary experiments, we found that the covalent linkage of MTX to the N-terminal position of a peptide (TAT, Table 1), synthesized by manual conventional peptide synthesis, yielded MTX–peptide having little MTX-inhibitory potency ($IC_{50} = 1.0 \pm 0.1$ µM, ~5.5% of MTX, summarized in Table 1), suggesting that a peptide-bond formation by the routine carbodiimide solid-phase synthesis takes place predominantly through the α-amino side chain of MTX.

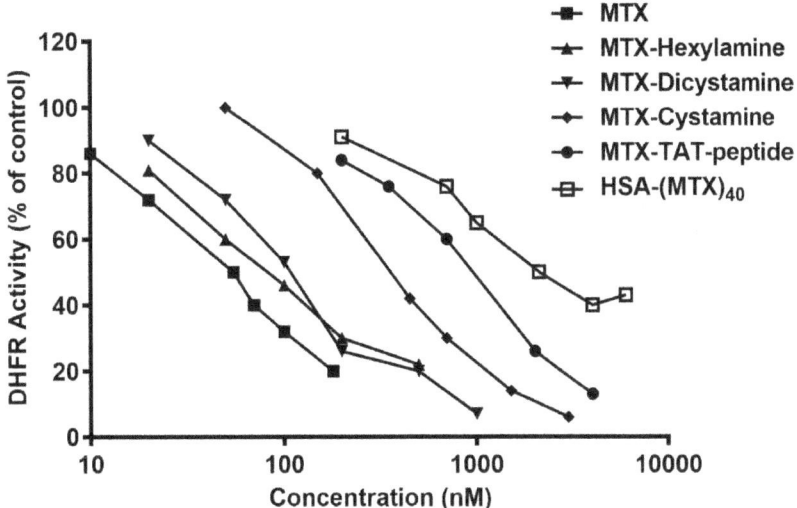

**Figure 1.** Inhibition of dihydrofolate reductase by MTX and MTX analogues. The indicated concentrations of MTX and its derivatives were analyzed for their potencies to inhibit the reduction of dihydrofolate to tetrahydrofolate by DHFR. In this process, NADPH is oxidized to NADP and the extent of this oxidation is monitored by the decrease in absorbance at 340 nm (experimental section). $OD_{340}$ amounted to $1.7 \pm 0.06$ in the absence of the enzyme (taken as 100% inhibition) and to $O.D_{340} = 0.65 \pm 0.06$ in its presence (taken as 100% activity).

**Table 1.** Dihydrofolate reductase inhibitory potencies of methotrexate-amino-containing derivatives.

| Derivative Designation | Abbreviated Structure | $IC_{50}$ nM | % Inhibition relative to MTX |
|---|---|---|---|
| Methotrexate | MTX | $55 \pm 4$ [a] | 100 |
| MTX–hexylamine | MTX–CONH–$(CH_2)_6$–$NH_2$ | $80 \pm 4$ | 69 |
| MTX–dicystamine | MTX–CONH–$(CH_2)_2$–S–S–$(CH_2)_2$–$NH_2$ | $110 \pm 12$ | 50 |
| MTX–cystamine | MTX–CONH–$(CH_2)_2$–SH | $340 \pm 11$ | 16.2 |
| MTX–TAT–peptide | MTX–AYGRKKRRQRRR | $1000 \pm 200$ | 5.5 |
| HSA–$(MTX)_{40}$ | HSA–$(NH–CO–MTX)_{40}$ | $2100 \pm 150$ | 2.6 |

[a] Determined under the experimental conditions specified in the legend to Figure 1.

Huang et al. investigated the reaction of aniline with α-amino-blocked L-glutamic acid anhydride. They found that this reaction yielded almost exclusively the γ-anilide isomer [24]. Based on that, we prepared MTX–anhydride by treating MTX with one equivalent of DCC in DMF. A stoichiometric amount of DCU was precipitated within a period of 0.5 h, indicating that MTX–anhydride was formed in a quantitative fashion under these experimental conditions (Scheme 1). The reaction of MTX–anhydride with low molecular-weight amino-containing nucleophiles (R–$CH_2$–$NH_2$) yielded analogues which preserved 16–69%, the DHFR inhibitory potency of MTX ($IC_{50}$ values in the range of 0.08–0.34 µM, Table 1). Out of the five MTX derivatives studied, MTX–CONH–$(CH_2)_6$–$NH_2$ was the most potent. It preserved 69% the potency of MTX ($IC_{50} = 0.08$ µM, Figure 1 and Table 1). Thus, linking amino-containing compounds up to a molecular weight of about 300 Da by this procedure yields fairly potent MTX derivatives. We next reacted human serum albumin (HSA) with MTX–anhydride obtaining HSA derivatives containing up to 40 M of MTX per mole of HSA linked to the amino side-chains of the protein (experimental procedure). HSA–$(MTX)_{40}$ had only 2.6% the inhibitory potency of MTX ($IC_{50} = 2.1 \pm 0.2$ µM, Figure 1 and Table 1), indicating that MTX linked to a macromolecule such as albumin through its γ-carboxylate moieties is, in principle, a prodrug, provided that such conjugates are capable of undergoing reactivation following entrance into tumorigenic cells.

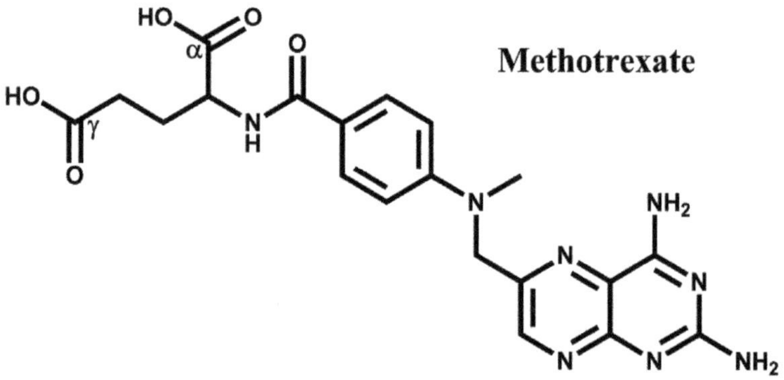

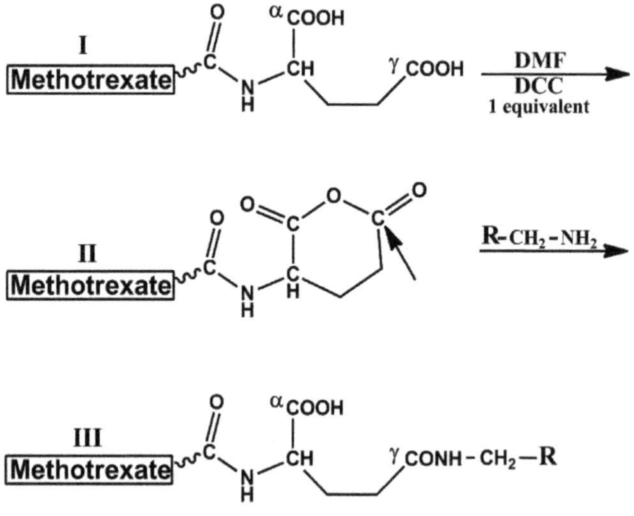

**Scheme 1.** The schematic synthetic procedure used to link amino-containing nucleophiles to the γ-carboxylate moiety of methotrexate. Methotrexate is initially treated with one equivalent of dicyclohexylcarbodiimide (DCC) to obtain the mixed anhydride (II). Amino-containing nucleophiles such as R–CH$_2$–NH$_2$ react preferentially with the γ-carbon (indicated by the arrow) to obtain γ-carboxylate-substituted derivatives (III) owing to the higher pKa (pKa~4.1) of the γ-carboxylate, as opposed to that of the α-carboxylate (pKa~2.1). A detailed description of this procedure can be found in Methods.

### 3.2. Preparing BSA–MTX Prodrug Analogues

Bovine serum albumin has a single cysteinyl moiety (cysteine 34), enabling introduction of MTX in a monomodified fashion, through a spacer maleimide (MAL) molecule linked to MTX through its γ-carboxylate moiety (experimental procedure). Three such analogues were prepared: BSA–S–S–MTX; [BSA–S–MAL–(CH$_2$)$_3$–CONH–(CH$_2$)$_2$–S–S–(CH$_2$)$_2$–NH$^γ$CO–MTX], BSA–GSSG–MTX; [BSA–S–MAL–(CH$_2$)$_3$–CO–NH–GSSG–NH$^γ$CO–MTX] and BSA–(CH$_2$)$_6$–NH$^\gamma$CO–MTX; [BSA–S–MAL–(CH$_2$)$_3$–CONH–(CH$_2$)$_6$–NH$^\gamma$CO–MTX] (Scheme 2). In the first two analogues, the spacer contains a disulfide bond. This was designed to evaluate whether the cells are equipped with cytosolic or endocytic disulfide bond-breaking machinery, and whether such activity would elevate the antiproliferative efficacy of those disulfide-containing analogues.

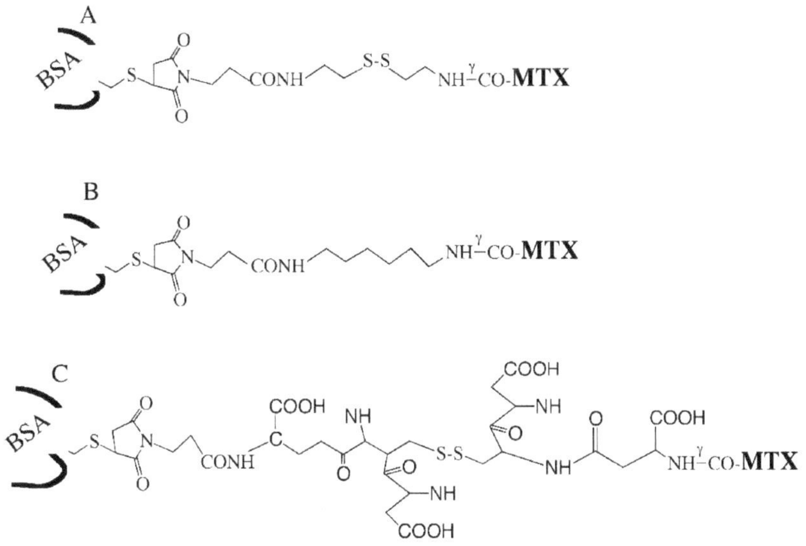

Scheme 2. Schematic presentation of the three monomodified analogues of BSA–MTX. (**A**) BSA–S–S–MTX, (**B**) BSA–(CH$_2$)$_6$–NH–$^\gamma$–CO–MTX, and (**C**) BSA–GSSG–NH–$^\gamma$–CO–MTX.

*3.3. BSA–MTX Analogues Are Prodrugs*

All three BSA–MTX analogues prepared had 2% to 7% the potency of MTX, to inhibit DHFR in a cell-free assay (summarized in Table 2). The disulfide-containing derivatives undergo 5- to 7-fold reactivation in the presence of 2mM dithioerythritol (Table 2). These analogues also undergo reactivation by reduced glutathione (GSH) and by L-cysteine (IC$_{50}$-value 0.8–1.2 mM for both, Figure 2). Glutathione and L-cysteine do not reactivate BSA–GSSG–MTX or BSA–S–S–MTX (not shown) at concentrations of 100 μM or lower (Figure 2). Thus, all three analogues expect to be systemically inactive, and therefore are nontoxic in body fluids, as those are devoid from significant amounts of disulfide-reducing agents such as GSH [12].

Table 2. Dihydrofolate reductase inhibitory potencies of BSA–MTX analogues. Reactivation by dithioerythritol (DTT).

| Derivative Designation | DHFR Inhibitory Potency (IC$_{50}$, nM) | % Activity Relative to MTX | Fold Reactivation by DTT |
|---|---|---|---|
| BSA–(CH$_2$)$_6$–MTX | 790 ± 30 | 7.0 | |
| BSA–S–S–MTX | 2750 ± 200 | 2.0 | |
| BSA–S–S–MTX + 2 mM DTT | 390 ± 30 | 14.1 | 7.05 |
| BSA–GSSG–MTX | 1750 ± 120 | 3.14 | |
| BSA–GSSG–MTX + 2 mM DTT | 340 ± 20 | 16.2 | 5.16 |

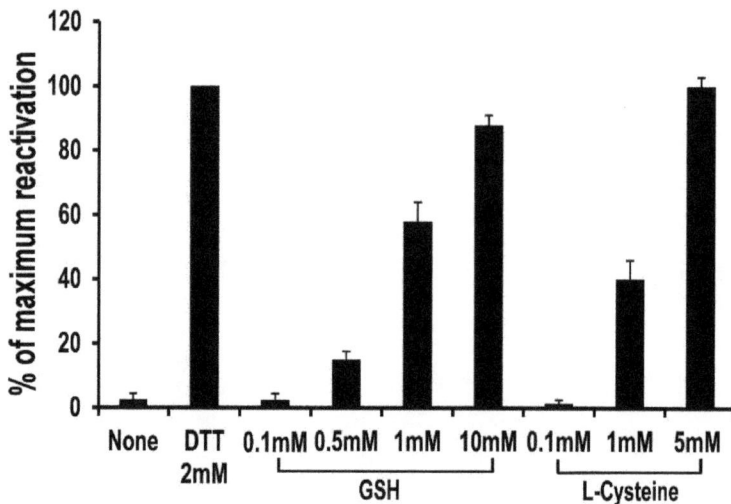

**Figure 2.** Reactivation of BSA–GSSG–MTX by reduced glutathione and L-cysteine. A solution of BSA–GSSG–MTX (50 μM in 0.1 M HEPES buffer, pH 7.4, 130 mM NaCl) was divided into plastic tubes (1.0 mL/tube) and incubated for 2 h at 25 °C in the absence and the presence of 2 mM DTT and the indicated concentrations of either GSH or L-cysteine. Samples were then analyzed for their DHFR inhibitory potencies and the $IC_{50}$ values were determined. Results are expressed as percent of maximal reactivation (obtained by preincubation with 2 mM DTT). Each point is the arithmetic mean of $n = 4$ tubes ± SEM.

### 3.4. Lack of Maleimide–Thiol Exchange of BSA–$(CH_2)_6$–MTX following Treatment with Reduced Glutathione (GSH)

Shen et al. [25] have demonstrated that SH-containing proteins, linked via maleimide to drugs, can undergo maleimide–thiol exchange if exposed to cysteine or to glutathione. To examine if such exchange takes place with BSA–S–MAL–$(CH_2)_3$–CONH–$(CH_2)_6$–NHCO–MTX, we incubated this derivative with 100 molar excess of GSH for a period of 7 h at pH 7.3, 37 °C. The conjugate was then dialyzed, lyophilized, and examined for its absorbance at 372 nm. As can be seen in Table 3, BSA–S–MAL–$(CH_2)_3$–CONH–MTX did not undergo significant maleimide–thiol exchange following prolonged incubation with 100-fold molar excess of GSH. This suggests that the maleimide linked to cysteine 34 of BSA is not exposed to the external medium.

**Table 3.** Lack of maleimide–thiol exchange of BSA–S–MAL–$(CH_2)_3$–CONH–MTX[a] following treatment with reduced glutathione (GSH).

| Treatment | Absorbance at 372 nm per mg Protein |
|---|---|
| Control | 0.479 ± 0.03 |
| GSH [a] | 0.487 ± 0.03 |

[a] BSA–S–MAL–$(CH_2)_3$–CONH–MTX (0.2 mM) dissolved in 1.0 mL 0.1 M HEPES, pH 7.3, and transferred to a tube containing 7.5 mg GSH corresponding to 24 μM which are 100 molar excess over the conjugate. The solution was incubated for 7 h at 37 °C, followed by extensive dialysis and lyophilization.

### 3.5. Selecting MTX-Sensitive and MTX-Insensitive Glioma Cell Lines for Studying the Antiproliferative Effects of BSA–MTX Analogues

The documented inhibitory effects of MTX in a variety of glioma cell lines has an average $EC_{50}$ of 2.4 μM with a large variation among different lines [26]. Following screening, we selected two glioma cell lines which differ significantly in their response to MTX. The first is an MTX-sensitive rat glioma cell line (CNS-1) with $EC_{50}$ (the effective concentration needed to obtain 50% of viable cells relative to untreated cells) of ~0.07 μM and 64% maximal effect (i.e., 36% viability in comparison to nontreated cells) within 48 h. The second cell line, the human glioma U251, is relatively insensitive to MTX. It has $EC_{50}$ of ~10 μM which is also the concentration needed to obtain a 49% maximum effect within 48 h of treatment (Figure 3).

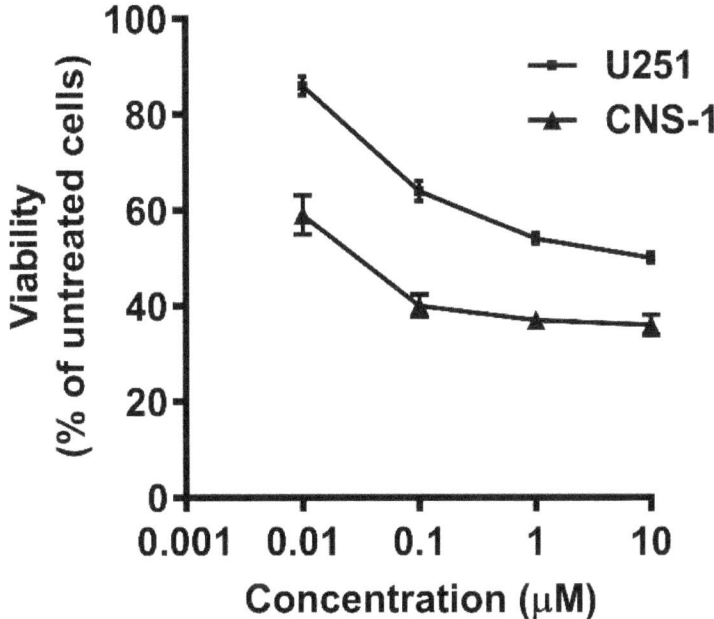

**Figure 3.** Viability of CNS-1 and U251 towards MTX. CNS-1 and U251 glioma cells were seeded in 96-well plates and MTX was applied a day later at the indicated concentrations. MTT assay was performed after 48 h. Viability is presented as mean ± SEM of each group in comparison to untreated cells. $n \geq 20$ from at least six different experiments. There is a significant difference of $p < 0.01$ between the two cell lines in all concentrations measured.

*3.6. Comparison of the Antiproliferative Potencies of the BSA–MTX Conjugates in the Insensitive and Sensitive Glioma Cell Lines*

Both BSA–MTX conjugates, BSA–S–S–MTX and BSA–$(CH_2)_6$–MTX, were found to be significantly more potent in the MTX-insensitive glioma cell line (Figure 4). As expected, those BSA–MTX analogues were less potent than MTX in the MTX-sensitive cell line. Nevertheless, at 10 μM (and to a lesser extent also at 1 μM), the BSA–MTX conjugates were significantly more inhibitory than MTX (Figure 4B).

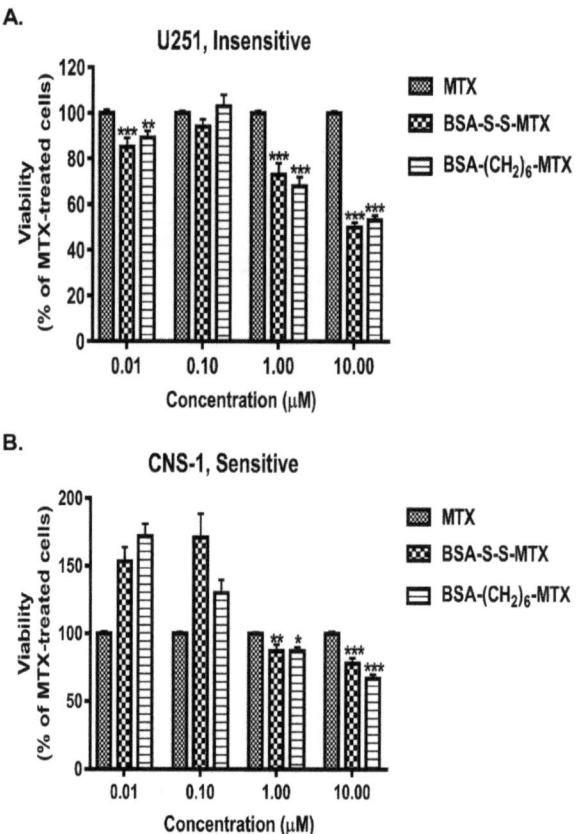

**Figure 4.** Viability of CNS-1 and U251 towards BSA–MTX derivatives. U251 (**A**) and CNS-1 (**B**) glioma cells were seeded in 96-well plates, and a day later, BSA–MTX derivatives were added at the concentrations shown. MTT assay was performed after 48 h to measure the viability of the cells. Viability of each conjugate was normalized to the viability of the cells treated with free MTX at each concentration. Data are presented as average mean ± SEM of each group in comparison to MTX-treated cells. $n \geq 20$ from at least three different experiments. * $p < 0.05$, ** $p < 0.01$, *** $p < 0.001$ vs. MTX-treated cells.

*3.7. Analyzing the Antiproliferative Potencies of Albumin–MTX Conjugates That Lost the Native Three-Dimensional Structure of the Protein*

We prepared two analogues of albumin–MTX in which the native structure of the carrier protein was disrupted, either by cleaving it at four sites with cyanogen bromide (CNBr-cleaved BSA–S–S–MTX) or derivatizing several of its amino side chains with MTX (HSA–MTX$_{40}$). Both analogues had negligible potency to inhibit DHFR in the cell-free system (Table 2). We next determined whether it is possible to regenerate activity in the glioma cell lines. Both analogues lost a significant amount of their antiproliferative potency and were significantly less effective in reducing the viability of the glioma cells in comparison to BSA–S–S–MTX (Figure 5). This was seen with both glioma cell lines in the concentration range of 1–10 µM at which BSA–S–S–MTX and BSA–(CH$_2$)$_6$–MTX are highly potent. Thus, it appears that preservation of the native structure of the carrier protein is required for either entry into those cell lines and/or obtaining the appropriate fragmentation requiring to turn those "silent" analogues into cytotoxic-active species.

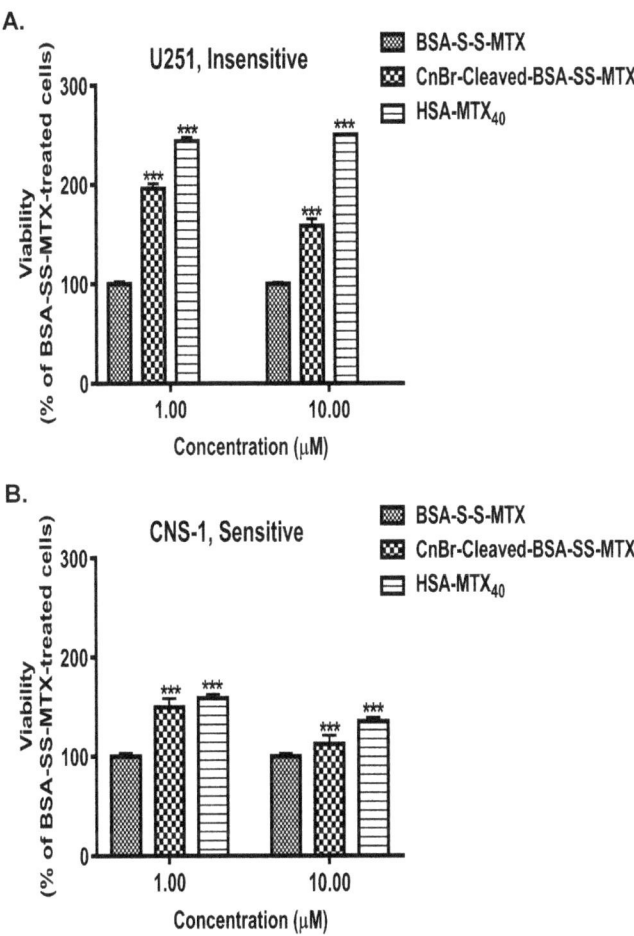

**Figure 5.** Viability of CNS-1 and U251 towards HSA–(MTX)$_{40}$ and CNBr-cleaved BSA–S–S–MTX. U251 (**A**) and CNS-1 (**B**) glioma cells were seeded in 96-well plates, and a day later, derivatives were added at the concentrations mentioned in the Figure. MTT assay was performed after 48 h to measure the viability of the cells. Viability of each conjugate was normalized to the viability of the cells treated with BSA–S–S–MTX at each concentration. Data are presented as average mean ± SEM of each group in comparison to BSA–S–S–MTX–treated cells. $n \geq 12$ from at least four different experiments. *** $p < 0.001$ vs. BSA–S–S–MTX–treated cells.

The inclusion of a disulfide bond in the spacer connecting MTX to BSA does not elevate the antiproliferative effect of the conjugate. As malignant tissues have elevated intracellular GSH, reaching concentrations as high as 10 mM [27,28] while the circulatory system possesses low reductive potency [29], it was logical to assume that BSA–MTX conjugates containing a disulfide bond will have increased selectivity and enhanced killing potency towards cancerous cell lines in general. We found that BSA–S–S–MTX is slightly less potent than BSA–(CH$_2$)$_6$–MTX, both in the sensitive and the insensitive glioma cell lines (Figure 4). This is in spite of the fact that GSH, at a concentration of 1 mM or higher, reactivated this conjugate, as shown by its efficacy to inhibit DHFR in the cell-free state (Figure 2). Thus, it suggests that the conjugate is not exposed at all to the cytosolic glutathione following internalization.

## 4. Discussion

In this study, we have engineered, synthesized, and studied conjugates of bovine-serum albumin linked to methotrexate (BSA–MTX conjugates). Those were found to be inactive antiproliferative prodrugs which efficiently regained their cytotoxic efficacy following entrance into cancerous cells. The antiproliferative efficacy of these conjugates was studied in cancerous cell lines of brain glioma origin, to complement another activity of our laboratory aiming to transfer chemotherapeutically active macromolecules from the blood to the brain via the blood–brain barrier (BBB) for treating major brain disorders such as glioblastoma multiforme [14–17].

The steps involved in preparing the appropriate BSA–MTX conjugates included the application of a chemical procedure enabling linkage of a variety of amino-containing nucleophiles (the spacers) to MTX with the preservation of a significant level of the DHFR-inhibitory potencies (Figure 1, Table 1, Scheme 1); the linkage of these MTX–spacer molecules to the single cysteinyl moiety of BSA, for obtaining monomodified analogues which preserve the native three-dimensional structure of the protein (Scheme 2); determining the DHFR inhibitory potency of these analogues in the cell-free state (Table 2); and studying their cytotoxic potencies in two types of glioma cell lines, one of which is insensitive to MTX (Figure 4A,B).

Of equal interest was to determine the efficacy of those glioma cell lines to regenerate the antiproliferative potencies of albumin–MTX analogues which lost their native three-dimensional configurations (Figure 5A,B).

The superiority of the BSA–MTX conjugates over that of MTX in the insensitive human glioma cell line (Figure 4A) is of profound interest to us. In theory, this superiority might be simply due to impaired MTX-transport into cells [30] which should not affect the albumin–MTX analogues, as they enter cells by the pathway of albumin-mediated endocytosis [31]. It should be noted, however, that this glioma cell line is only partially resistant to MTX (Figure 3); therefore, aberrations, downstream to MTX entry, such as the decrease in thymidylate synthase activity [32], a moderate elevation in the intracellular level of DHFR [33], or a decrease in the binding affinity of MTX to DHFR [23], might take place as well. Those three parameters were documented to be affected to the extent of 1.5- to 3-fold in a variety of other tumorigenic cells that were desensitized to MTX [34].

Although we assumed a priori that the inclusion of a disulfide bond in the spacer connecting MTX to the protein would be significantly beneficial, this assumption was found to be incorrect. Both BSA–S–S–MTX and BSA–$(CH_2)_6$–MTX showed essentially equipotent antiproliferative activity, both in the MTX-sensitive and the MTX-insensitive glioma cell lines (Figure 4), even though glutathione reactivated the conjugate in the cell-free state (Figure 2). It therefore appears that the internalized conjugate is not in contact at all with the cytosolic glutathione. We are currently investigating whether this finding is generally valid for endocytosed-disulfide-containing protein–toxin conjugates.

Scheme 3 combines our cell-free findings to those found in the cancerous cell lines. BSA–S–S–MTX is a prodrug conjugate having only 1.8% ($IC_{50}$ = 2.75 µM) the inhibitory potency of MTX toward DHFR (Table 2). In theory, the spacer arm connecting MTX to the protein can be endogenously cleaved at three sites (marked I, II, and III in the scheme). Site I, the peptide bond linking MTX via the γ-carboxylate moiety to the spacer, appeared quite uncleavable due to steric hindrance, as previously documented [8]. Site II (the disulfide bond) appears to be negligibly cleaved endogenously as well. BSA–$(CH_2)_6$–MTX, which lacks this disulfide bond, shows equipotent potency as BSA–S–S–MTX (Figure 4). Thus, the peptide bond at site III appeared to be the one which is predominantly cleaved endogenously in the tumorigenic cell lines yielding MTX–$CO^\gamma NH$–$(CH_2)_6$–$NH_2$, an MTX derivative which preserves 69% ($IC_{50}$ = 0.08 µM) of the DHFR-inhibitory potency of the native folate antagonist (Table 1). Thus, a simple spacer arm connecting MTX to albumin, made of ethylene-chain, and containing a single peptide bond-distal from the protein backbone by about 8.7 Å, and apart from the covalently linked MTX by about 12 Å, appears most appropriate to bridge cysteine 34 of albumin to MTX (Scheme 3B) for obtaining endogenously-reactivatable prodrug conjugate in the cancerous cell lines studied here. More complicated spacer arms, such as that obtained in our BSA–G–S–S–G–MTX analogue (Scheme 2) appears less promising. It showed low antiproliferative efficacy in the cancer cell lines (unpublished results). These findings also substantiate the poor endogenous efficacy of the tumorigenic cell lines to facilitate glutathione- or cysteine-dependent chemical reduction. Both GSH and cysteine are highly effective in reactivating the DHFR inhibitory potency of this analogue in the cell-free state (Figure 2).

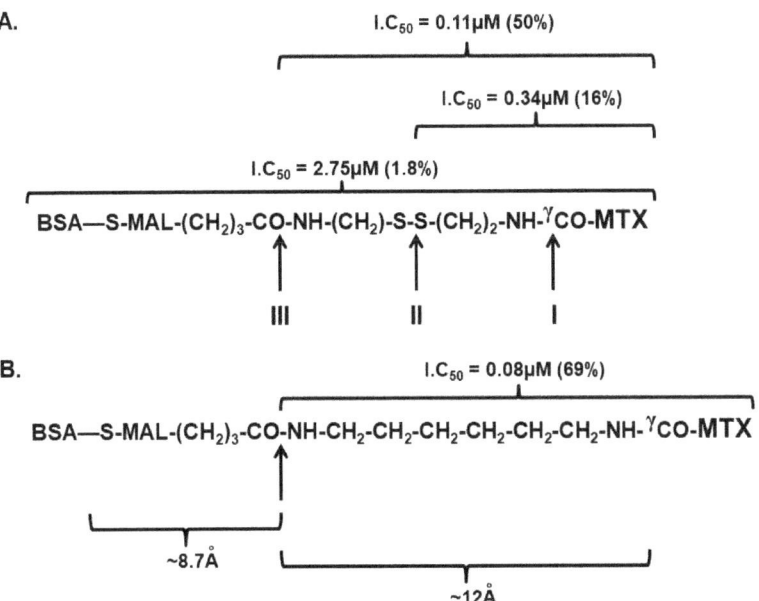

**Scheme 3.** Schematic presentation of the putative endogenously cleaved sites in the BSA–MTX conjugates studied. (**A**) BSA-S-S-MTX; Shown in parenthesis the inhibitory potencies of DHFR by the whole conjugate (I.C$_{50}$ = 2.75 µM) and the inhibitory potencies of the two potentially cleaved MTX containing fragments (I.C$_{50}$ = 0.34 µM and 0.11 µM respectively). (**B**) BSA-(CH$_2$)$_6$–MTX; Shown in upper parenthesis, the inhibitory potency of DHFR by the potentially cleaved MTX containing fragment (I.C$_{50}$ = 0.08 µM, 69 % the efficacy of non-modified MTX).

Interestingly, thiosuccinimide linkages are now known to be less robust than once thought, and may undergo maleimide–thiol exchange, for example, by cysteine or GSH present in the external medium [35,36]. This may constitute a drawback to protein–drug conjugates if they undergo such maleimide–thiol exchange. We studied whether such exchange takes place with BSA–S–MAL–(CH$_2$)$_3$–CONH–MTX, which was incubated for a prolonged period at pH 7.3, 37 °C with high concentrations of reduced glutathione (GSH). We found that such exchange does not occur with this conjugate (Table 3). Cysteine 34 of albumin is located in a deep hydrophobic crevice of 10–12 Å [37]. It therefore seems that the maleimide linked to this cysteine is buried within this crevice, and not exposed to this potential exchange.

Although not in the framework of this study, it appears to us that replacement of MTX therapy by albumin–MTX prodrug therapy is expected to minimize the acquired resistance to MTX which develops upon MTX treatment in cancerous cells. Such analogues that introduce MTX to the cell by an alternative pathway may therefore leave folate carrier free for folic acid entry. Endogenous albumin–MTX cannot be converted to MTX–glutamate or to MTX–polyglutamate by folylpolyglutamate synthetase—an event that prolongs the lifetime of MTX by entrapment [38]. With albumin–MTX, this prolongation is not required, and the induction of desensitization by decreasing the synthesis of MTX–polyglutamate for shortening lifetime of endogenous MTX becomes irrelevant. Dihydrofolate reductase (DHFR) is inhibited by nonmodified MTX at extremely low concentration [39], restricting the inhibitory effect of DHFR by albumin–MTX conjugate, solely to the folic acid-dependent cascade. Undesirable inhibition of RNA and protein synthesis by MTX might be avoided. Inhibition of DHFR per se can still lead to acquired resistance to MTX by increasing DHFR content and/or decrease thymidylate synthase activity. However, such albumin–MTX prodrug analogues preserve low level of active MTX in a continuous fashion, both externally and endogenously following permeation into the cells. This may prevent overdosing of MTX and the consequent side effects.

We have previously found that MTX–amino compounds, such as MTX–CONH–$(CH_2)_6$–$NH_2$, covalently linked to carboxylate moieties, such as PEG40–COOH, undergo unusual MTX-dependent acid-dependent peptide bond cleavage, catalyzed by the α-carboxylate moiety of MTX [40]. Unlike what we thought before, this peptide bond is not cleaved in BSA–$(CH_2)_6$–MTX at neutral pH value (Table 3). This is most likely due to the fact that this peptide bond is well located within the 10–12 Å hydrophobic crevice following the covalent linkage to cysteine 34 of BSA. This cleavage, however, expects to take place in an accelerated rate intracellularly due to either degradation of the conjugate and/or by the acidic pH of the lysosome, elevating the reactivation efficacy of those pro-drug conjugates in an intracellular fashion.

In conclusion, the following three conditions appear to be required to engineer the appropriate albumin–MTX prodrug analogues in the future: (i) MTX should be linked to the amino-containing spacer via its γ carboxylate moiety; (ii) the spacer should contain a readily cleavable bond in close proximity to the MTX; (iii) in agreement with previous studies [6,41], the conjugated albumins must preserve their native structure for undergoing extravasation by malignant tissues. As MTX is a drug used also in noncancerous application, such as arthritis, for example, the suggested binding technology might be used also for conjugating it to other macromolecules, such as anti-inflammatory monoclonal antibodies, to increase treatment efficacy and tolerance and to reduce side effects.

**Author Contributions:** I.C. planned and performed experiments and wrote the paper; M.S.-B. wrote the paper; M.F. planned the experiments; Y.S. planned and performed experiments and wrote the paper. All authors have read and agreed to the published version of the manuscript.

**Funding:** This work was supported by a joint Weizmann Institute of Science-Sheba Medical Center grant for Biomedical Research and from the Kimmelman Center of Biomolecular Structure and Assembly.

**Institutional Review Board Statement:** Not applicable.

**Informed Consent Statement:** Not applicable.

**Data Availability Statement:** The data that support the findings of this study are available from the corresponding authors, upon reasonable request.

**Acknowledgments:** We thank Michael Walker from the Weizmann Institute of Science for helpful discussions.

**Conflicts of Interest:** The authors declare no conflict of interest.

## Abbreviations

| | |
|---|---|
| BSA | bovine serum albumin |
| MTX | methotrexate |
| DHF | dihydrofolic acid |
| DHFR | dihydrofolate reductase |
| MAL–(CH$_2$)$_3$–COOSu | maleimidopropionic acid-$N$-hydroxysuccinimide ester |
| GSSG | oxidized glutathione |
| BSA–S–S–MTX | BSA–S–MAL–(CH$_2$)$_2$–CONH–(CH$_2$)$_2$–S–S–(CH$_2$)$_2$–NH$^\gamma$CO–MTX |
| BSA–GSSG–MTX | BSA–S–MAL–(CH$_2$)$_3$–CONH–GSSG–NH$^\gamma$CO–MTX |
| BSA–(CH$_2$)$_6$–MTX | BSA–S–MAL–(CH$_2$)$_3$–CONH–(CH$_2$)$_6$–NH$^\gamma$CO–MTX |
| MALDI-TOF | matrix-assisted laser desorption ionization time of flight |
| ESMS | electrospray single quadruple mass spectroscopy |
| DCC | $N,N'$ dicyclohexylcarbodiimide |
| GSH | reduced glutathione |
| DMF | dimethylformamide |
| DIPEA | $N,N'$ diisopropylethylamine |

## References

1. Abolmaali, S.S.; Tamaddon, A.M.; Dinarvand, R. A review of therapeutic challenges and achievements of methotrexate de-livery systems for treatment of cancer and rheumatoid arthritis. *Cancer Chemother. Pharmacol.* **2013**, *71*, 1115–1130. [CrossRef] [PubMed]
2. Genestier, L.; Paillot, R.; Quemeneur, L.; Izeradjene, K.; Revillard, J.-P. Mechanisms of action of methotrexate. *Immunopharmacology* **2000**, *47*, 247–257. [CrossRef]
3. Sirotnak, F.M.; Moccio, D.M. Pharmacokinetic basis for differences in methotrexate sensitivity of normal proliferative tissues in the mouse. *Cancer Res.* **1980**, *40*, 1230–1234. [PubMed]
4. Sirotnak, F.M.; Kurita, S.; Hutchison, D.J. On the nature of a transport alteration determining resistance to amethopterin in the L1210 leukemia. *Cancer Res.* **1968**, *28*, 75–80.
5. Hill, B.T.; Bailey, B.D.; White, J.C.; Goldman, I.D. Characteristics of transport of 4-amino antifolates and folate compounds by two lines of L5178Y lymphoblasts, one with impaired transport of methotrexate. *Cancer Res.* **1979**, *39*, 2440–2446. [PubMed]
6. Neumann, E.; Frei, E.; Funk, D.; Becker, M.D.; Schrenk, H.-H.; Müller-Ladner, U.; Fiehn, C. Native albumin for targeted drug delivery. *Expert Opin. Drug Deliv.* **2010**, *7*, 915–925. [CrossRef] [PubMed]
7. Levick, J.R. Permeability of rheumatoid and normal human synovium to specific plasma proteins. *Arthritis Rheum.* **1981**, *24*, 1550–1560. [CrossRef]
8. Fitzpatrick, J.J.; Garnett, M.C. Design, synthesis and in vitro testing of methotrexate carrier conjugates linked via oligopeptide spacers. *Anticancer Drug Des.* **1995**, *10*, 1–9.
9. Matthews, D.A.; Alden, R.A.; Bolin, J.T.; Filman, D.J.; Freer, S.T.; Hamlin, R.; Hol, W.G.; Kisliuk, R.L.; Pastore, E.J.; Plante, L.T.; et al. Dihydrofolate reductase from *Lactobacillus casei*. X-ray structure of the enzyme methotrexate.NADPH complex. *J. Biol. Chem.* **1978**, *253*, 6946–6954. [CrossRef]
10. Rosowsky, A.; Forsch, R.; Uren, J.; Wick, M. Methotrexate analogues. Synthesis of new gamma-substituted derivatives as dihydrofolate reductase inhibitors and potential anticancer agents. *J. Med. Chem.* **1981**, *24*, 1450–1455.
11. Ballatori, N.; Krance, S.M.; Notenboom, S.; Shi, S.; Tieu, K.; Hammond, C.L. Glutathione dysregulation and the etiology and progression of human diseases. *Biol. Chem.* **2009**, *390*, 191–214. [CrossRef]
12. Austin, C.D.; Wen, X.; Gazzard, L.; Nelson, C.; Scheller, R.H.; Scales, S.J. Oxidizing potential of endosomes and lysosomes limits intracellular cleavage of disulfide-based antibody-drug conjugates. *Proc. Natl. Acad. Sci. USA* **2005**, *102*, 17987–17992. [CrossRef]
13. Wang, J.; Li, S.; Luo, T.; Wang, C.; Zhao, J. Disulfide Linkage: A Potent Strategy in Tumor-Targeting Drug Discovery. *Curr. Med. Chem.* **2012**, *19*, 2976–2983. [CrossRef]
14. Cooper, I.; Sasson, K.; Teichberg, V.I.; Schnaider-Beeri, M.; Fridkin, M.; Shechter, Y. Peptide derived from HIV-1 TAT protein de-stabilizes a monolayer of endothelial cells in an in vitro model of the blood-brain barrier and allows permeation of high molecular weight proteins. *J. Biol. Chem.* **2012**, *287*, 44676–44683. [CrossRef]
15. Sharabi, S.; Guez, D.; Daniels, D.; Cooper, I.; Atrakchi, D.; Liraz-Zaltsman, S.; Last, D.; Mardor, Y. The application of point source electroporation and chemotherapy for the treatment of glioma: A randomized controlled rat study. *Sci. Rep.* **2020**, *10*, 2178. [CrossRef]
16. Sharabi, S.; Bresler, Y.; Ravid, O.; Shemesh, C.; Atrakchi, D.; Schnaider-Beeri, M.; Gosselet, F.; Dehouck, L.; Last, D.; Guez, D.; et al. Transient blood–brain barrier disruption is induced by low pulsed electrical fields in vitro: An analysis of permeability and trans-endothelial electric resistivity. *Drug Deliv.* **2019**, *26*, 459–469. [CrossRef]
17. Sharabi, S.; Last, D.; Daniels, D.; Fabian, I.D.; Atrakchi, D.; Bresler, Y.; Liraz-Zaltsman, S.; Cooper, I.; Mardor, Y. Non-Invasive Low Pulsed Electrical Fields for Inducing BBB Disruption in Mice-Feasibility Demonstration. *Pharmaceutics* **2021**, *13*, 169. [CrossRef]

18. Cooper, I.; Last, D.; Guez, D.; Sharabi, S.; Goldman, S.E.; Lubitz, I.; Daniels, D.; Salomon, S.; Tamar, G.; Tamir, T.; et al. Combined Local Blood–Brain Barrier Opening and Systemic Methotrexate for the Treatment of Brain Tumors. *Br. J. Pharmacol.* **2015**, *35*, 967–976. [CrossRef]
19. Kaufman, B.T.; Kemerer, V.F. Purification and characterization of beef liver dihydrofolate reductase. *Arch. Biochem. Biophys.* **1976**, *172*, 289–300. [CrossRef]
20. Kumar, A.A.; Kempton, R.J.; Anstead, G.M.; Freisheim, J.H. Fluorescent analogues of methotrexate: Characterization and interaction with dihydrofolate reductase. *Biochemistry* **1983**, *22*, 390–395. [CrossRef]
21. Cooper, I.; Malina, K.C.-K.; Cagnotto, A.; Bazzoni, G.; Salmona, M.; Teichberg, V.I. Interactions of the prion peptide (PrP 106-126) with brain capillary endothelial cells: Coordinated cell killing and remodeling of intercellular junctions. *J. Neurochem.* **2011**, *116*, 467–475. [CrossRef] [PubMed]
22. Piper, J.R.; Montgomery, J.A.; Sirotnak, F.M.; Chello, P.L. Syntheses of alpha- and gamma-substituted amides, peptides, and esters of methotrexate and their evaluation as inhibitors of folate metabolism. *J. Med. Chem.* **1982**, *25*, 182–187. [PubMed]
23. Miyachi, H.; Takemura, Y.; Kobayashi, H.; Ando, Y. Expression of variant dihydrofolate reductase with decreased binding affinity to antifolates in MOLT-3 human leukemia cell lines resistant to trimetrexate. *Cancer Lett.* **1995**, *88*, 93–99. [CrossRef]
24. Huang, X.; Day, N.; Luo, X.; Roupioz, Y.; Seid, M.; Keillor, J.W. Synthesis and characterization of a series of novel glutamic gamma-15N-anilide dipeptides. *J. Pept. Res.* **1999**, *53*, 126–133. [CrossRef]
25. Shen, B.-Q.; Xu, K.; Liu, L.; Raab, H.; Bhakta, S.; Kenrick, M.; Parsons-Reponte, K.L.; Tien, J.; Yu, S.-F.; Mai, E.; et al. Conjugation site modulates the in vivo stability and therapeutic activity of antibody-drug conjugates. *Nat. Biotechnol.* **2012**, *30*, 184–189. [CrossRef]
26. Wolff, J.E.A.; Trilling, T.; Mölenkamp, G.; Egeler, R.M.; Jürgens, H. Chemosensitivity of glioma cells in vitro: A meta analysis. *J. Cancer Res. Clin. Oncol.* **1999**, *125*, 481–486. [CrossRef] [PubMed]
27. Ortega, A.L.; Mena, S.; Estrela, J.M. Glutathione in Cancer Cell Death. *Cancers* **2011**, *3*, 1285–1310. [CrossRef] [PubMed]
28. Ames, B.N.; Gold, L.S.; Willett, W.C. The causes and prevention of cancer. *Proc. Natl. Acad. Sci. USA* **1995**, *92*, 5258–5265. [CrossRef]
29. Go, Y.-M.; Jones, D.P. Redox compartmentalization in eukaryotic cells. *Biochim. Biophys. Acta (BBA)–Gen. Subj.* **2008**, *1780*, 1273–1290. [CrossRef]
30. Spinella, M.J.; Brigle, K.E.; Sierra, E.E.; Goldman, I.D. Distinguishing between folate receptor-alpha-mediated transport and reduced folate carrier-mediated transport in L1210 leukemia cells. *J. Biol. Chem.* **1995**, *270*, 7842–7849. [CrossRef]
31. Wosikowski, K.; Biedermann, E.; Rattel, B.; Breiter, N.; Jank, P.; Löser, R.; Jansen, G.; Peters, G.J. In vitro and in vivo antitumor activity of methotrexate conjugated to human serum albumin in human cancer cells. *Clin. Cancer Res.* **2003**, *9*, 1917–1926. [PubMed]
32. Ayusawa, D.; Koyama, H.; Seno, T. Resistance to methotrexate in thymidylate synthetase-deficient mutants of cultured mouse mammary tumor FM3A cells. *Cancer Res.* **1981**, *41*, 1497–1501. [PubMed]
33. Banerjee, D.; Mayer-Kuckuk, P.; Capiaux, G.; Budak-Alpdogan, T.; Gorlick, R.; Bertino, J.R. Novel aspects of resistance to drugs targeted to dihydrofolate reductase and thymidylate synthase. *Biochim. Biophys. Acta (BBA)–Mol. Basis Dis.* **2002**, *1587*, 164–173. [CrossRef]
34. Cowan, K.H.; Jolivet, J. A methotrexate-resistant human breast cancer cell line with multiple defects, including diminished formation of methotrexate polyglutamates. *J. Biol. Chem.* **1984**, *259*, 10793–10800. [CrossRef]
35. Ravasco, J.M.J.M.; Faustino, H.; Trindade, A.; Gois, P.M.P. Bioconjugation with Maleimides: A Useful Tool for Chemical Biology. *Chem. A Eur. J.* **2019**, *25*, 43–59. [CrossRef] [PubMed]
36. Baldwin, A.D.; Kiick, K.L. Tunable Degradation of Maleimide–Thiol Adducts in Reducing Environments. *Bioconjugate Chem.* **2011**, *22*, 1946–1953. [CrossRef]
37. Carter, D.C.; Ho, J.X. Structure of Serum Albumin. In *Lipoproteins, Apolipoproteins, and Lipases*; Elsevier: Amsterdam, The Netherlands, 1994; pp. 153–203.
38. Assaraf, Y.G. Molecular basis of antifolate resistance. *Cancer Metastasis Rev.* **2007**, *26*, 153–181. [CrossRef] [PubMed]
39. Williams, M.N.; Poe, M.; Greenfield, N.J.; Hirshfield, J.M.; Hoogsteen, K. Methotrexate binding to dihydrofolate reductase from a methotrexate-resistant strain of *Escherichia coli*. *J. Biol. Chem.* **1973**, *248*, 6375–6379. [CrossRef]
40. Cooper, I.; Fridkin, M.; Shechter, Y. Conjugation of Methotrexate-Amino Derivatives to Macromolecules through Carboxylate Moieties Is Superior over Conventional Linkage to Amino Residues: Chemical, Cell-Free and In Vitro Characterizations. *PLoS ONE* **2016**, *11*, e0158352. [CrossRef]
41. Stehle, G.; Sinn, H.; Wunder, A.; Schrenk, H.H.; Schütt, S.; Maier-Borst, W.; Heene, D.L. The loading rate determines tumor targeting properties of methotrexate-albumin conjugates in rats. *Anti-Cancer Drugs* **1995**, *8*, 677–685. [CrossRef]

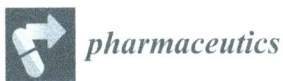

Article

# A Comparison of Evans Blue and 4-(*p*-Iodophenyl)butyryl Albumin Binding Moieties on an Integrin $\alpha_v\beta_6$ Binding Peptide

Ryan A. Davis [1], Sven H. Hausner [2], Rebecca Harris [2] and Julie L. Sutcliffe [1,2,3,*]

1. Department of Biomedical Engineering, University of California, Davis, CA 95616, USA; rydavis@ucdavis.edu
2. Department of Internal Medicine, Division of Hematology/Oncology, University of California, Davis, CA 95817, USA; shhausner@ucdavis.edu (S.H.H.); relharris@ucdavis.edu (R.H.)
3. Center for Molecular and Genomic Imaging, University of California, Davis, CA 95616, USA
* Correspondence: jlsutcliffe@ucdavis.edu; Tel.: +1-916-734-5536

**Abstract:** Serum albumin binding moieties (ABMs) such as the Evans blue (EB) dye fragment and the 4-(*p*-iodophenyl)butyryl (IP) have been used to improve the pharmacokinetic profile of many radiopharmaceuticals. The goal of this work was to directly compare these two ABMs when conjugated to an integrin $\alpha_v\beta_6$ binding peptide ($\alpha_v\beta_6$-BP); a peptide that is currently being used for positron emission tomography (PET) imaging in patients with metastatic cancer. The ABM-modified $\alpha_v\beta_6$-BP peptides were synthesized with a 1,4,7,10-tetraazacyclododecane-1,4,7,10-tetracetic acid (DOTA) chelator for radiolabeling with copper-64 to yield [$^{64}$Cu]Cu DOTA-EB-$\alpha_v\beta_6$-BP ([$^{64}$Cu]**1**) and [$^{64}$Cu]Cu DOTA-IP-$\alpha_v\beta_6$-BP ([$^{64}$Cu]**2**). Both peptides were evaluated in vitro for serum albumin binding, serum stability, and cell binding and internalization in the paired engineered melanoma cells DX3puro$\beta$6 ($\alpha_v\beta_6$ +) and DX3puro ($\alpha_v\beta_6$ −), and pancreatic BxPC-3 ($\alpha_v\beta_6$ +) cells and in vivo in a BxPC-3 xenograft mouse model. Serum albumin binding for [$^{64}$Cu]**1** and [$^{64}$Cu]**2** was 53–63% and 42–44%, respectively, with good human serum stability (24 h: [$^{64}$Cu]**1** 76%, [$^{64}$Cu]**2** 90%). Selective $\alpha_v\beta_6$ cell binding was observed for both [$^{64}$Cu]**1** and [$^{64}$Cu]**2** ($\alpha_v\beta_6$ (+) cells: 30.3–55.8% and 48.5–60.2%, respectively, vs. $\alpha_v\beta_6$ (−) cells <3.1% for both). In vivo BxPC-3 tumor uptake for both peptides at 4 h was 5.29 ± 0.59 and 7.60 ± 0.43% ID/g ([$^{64}$Cu]**1** and [$^{64}$Cu]**2**, respectively), and remained at 3.32 ± 0.46 and 4.91 ± 1.19% ID/g, respectively, at 72 h, representing a >3-fold improvement over the non-ABM parent peptide and thereby providing improved PET images. Comparing [$^{64}$Cu]**1** and [$^{64}$Cu]**2**, the IP-ABM-$\alpha_v\beta_6$-BP [$^{64}$Cu]**2** displayed higher serum stability, higher tumor accumulation, and lower kidney and liver accumulation, resulting in better tumor-to-organ ratios for high contrast visualization of the $\alpha_v\beta_6$ (+) tumor by PET imaging.

**Keywords:** albumin binding moieties; peptides; Evans blue; 4-(*p*-iodophenyl)butyric acid; integrin $\alpha_v\beta_6$; integrin $\alpha_v\beta_6$ binding peptide; improved pharmacokinetics; PET imaging

Citation: Davis, R.A.; Hausner, S.H.; Harris, R.; Sutcliffe, J.L. A Comparison of Evans Blue and 4-(*p*-Iodophenyl)butyryl Albumin Binding Moieties on an Integrin $\alpha_v\beta_6$ Binding Peptide. *Pharmaceutics* **2022**, *14*, 745. https://doi.org/10.3390/pharmaceutics14040745

Academic Editor: Katona Gábor

Received: 1 March 2022
Accepted: 25 March 2022
Published: 30 March 2022

**Publisher's Note:** MDPI stays neutral with regard to jurisdictional claims in published maps and institutional affiliations.

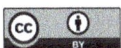

**Copyright:** © 2022 by the authors. Licensee MDPI, Basel, Switzerland. This article is an open access article distributed under the terms and conditions of the Creative Commons Attribution (CC BY) license (https://creativecommons.org/licenses/by/4.0/).

## 1. Introduction

The use of biologically active molecules such as peptides and antibodies continues to increase for both diagnosis and therapy [1–3]. Peptides are attractive platforms for diagnostics due to their ability to achieve high target binding affinity and in part due to their small size which results in short biological half-life and rapid clearance from non-target tissues, producing good target-to-non-target contrast, low toxicity, and generally low or absent immunogenicity [1]. Synthetic advantages of peptides include simple preparation and easy, flexible functionalization or chemical modification to further improve affinity, stability, selectivity, and overall pharmacokinetic properties [1,4]. However, some of the properties that are desirable for a diagnostic agent can hamper the translation to a therapeutic, which relies on a prolonged circulation for high and persistent uptake in the targeted tissue. Too rapid clearance can render the therapeutic ineffective, and poor clearance from non-target tissue can lead to off-target toxicity. Thus, peptides typically require fine-tuning for therapeutic applications to balance circulation time and provide high target accumulation with sufficient clearance from non-target tissues [5–7].

Chemical modifications of peptides offer a route to improving these pharmacokinetic properties; this includes incorporation of polyethylene glycol (PEG; PEGylation), glycosylation, or the formation of protein conjugates (e.g., with serum albumin) [4,8–11]. PEGylation is a convenient approach as PEGs are commercially available in a variety of molecular sizes, including mono-disperse PEGs with various functional groups for synthetic orthogonality [1,9]. PEGylation increases hydrophilicity (reducing kidney, lung, and liver accumulation) [12,13], provides increased stability (by protection from proteases), and reduces immunogenicity (by masking the peptide) [9,13]. The size and placement of the PEG on the peptides can significantly affect the pharmacokinetics and tumor accumulation [12–14]. Stability, circulation time, and tumor uptake of peptides can also be increased by chemical ligation ex vivo to serum albumin (taking advantage of albumin's size, long circulation time, and renal recycling) [8,15–17]. Alternatively, the same benefit can be achieved by direct attachment of a small albumin binding moiety (ABM) onto the peptide without substantially increasing the size. The ABM binds reversibly to albumin in the blood, thereby increasing circulation time and facilitating renal recycling, which, in turn, increases target tissue accumulation [8,15,16,18]. Several ABMs have been employed to modify pharmaceuticals currently used in the clinic, with some being used on their own, primarily for measuring plasma volume [16]; among the first ABMs used to modify pharmaceuticals were long-chain fatty acids, such as myristic and palmitic acid [5], and later other lipophilic molecules including benoxaprofen, phenytoin, ibuprofen, and naproxen [16].

More recently, two ABMs in particular, a fragment of Evans blue (EB) dye and the 4-(*p*-iodophenyl)butytryl (IP) group, have also been used to modify the pharmacokinetic profile of radiopharmaceuticals, in particular small molecules (folic acid and prostate specific membrane antigen (PSMA) agents) and peptides (octreotide, exendin-4, and cRGDfK) [10,11,16,18–20]. The EB-ABM was derived from Evans blue dye, a dye which has been used clinically for over 90 years to measure plasma volume and determine blood-brain barrier integrity [16,17,21]. The EB-ABM fragment was first used in 2004 as an MRI contrast agent for imaging blood vessels [22] and has since been used for a variety of applications, including determining blood volume, vascular permeability, and as a conjugate to enhance receptor targeting agents (small molecules and peptides) for both cancer imaging and therapy [9,17,23–26]. The IP-ABM has also been studied extensively to enhance radiopharmaceuticals (small molecules and peptides), where the group at the *para*-position of the aromatic ring of the IP-ABM can be tuned to adjust serum albumin affinity [15,27,28], and a neighboring aspartate residue (D) has been shown to provide a more sustained tumor retention [29]. Numerous preclinical studies have evaluated both ABMs and noted prolonged blood circulation, with an increase in tumor uptake that can also lead to a reduction of kidney accumulation [7,11,18].

The Sutcliffe laboratory has spent over a decade developing and optimizing an integrin $\alpha_v\beta_6$-binding peptide ($\alpha_v\beta_6$-BP) [30] to selectively target integrin $\alpha_v\beta_6$, an epithelium cell surface receptor that is absent or expressed in low levels in healthy adult epithelia, but is highly expressed in numerous challenging cancers, where it is associated with angiogenesis, proliferation, invasion, metastasis, and chemoresistance [31–41]. Thus, the integrin $\alpha_v\beta_6$ has been recognized as negative prognostic indicator with the expression levels correlating to poor prognosis and overall survival in many cancers [31–41]. During the optimization of the $\alpha_v\beta_6$-BP, the bi-terminal PEGylation with monodispersed PEG$_{28}$ of the 20 amino acid A20FMDV2-peptide (NAVPNLRGDLQVLAQKVART) derived from the integrin $\alpha_v\beta_6$-targeting foot and mouth disease virus, showed greatly improved integrin $\alpha_v\beta_6$ affinity and selectivity, and improved on the peptide's stability and tumor accumulation and retention [14]. Since then, further modifications have been tested in numerous preclinical models with an advancement of the peptide to >10-fold increase in tumor accumulation and the successful translation of the 4-[$^{18}$F]fluorobenzoyl labeled [$^{18}$F]$\alpha_v\beta_6$-BP into the clinic for PET imaging of a variety of cancers, including pancreatic adenocarcinoma [30]. Further optimization of $\alpha_v\beta_6$-BP continues towards an integrin $\alpha_v\beta_6$ targeted peptide receptor radionuclide therapy (PRRT).

Recently, Hausner et al. described the IP-ABM modified $\alpha_v\beta_6$-BP radiolabeled using 1,4,7-triazacyclo-nonane-N,N',N''-triacetic acid (NOTA) for aluminum [$^{18}$F]fluoride chelation, with the goals of improving the biodistributions and simplifying the fluorine-18 radiochemistry [42]. The [$^{18}$F]AlF NOTA-IP-ABM-$\alpha_v\beta_6$-BP had increased blood circulation and tumor accumulation that allowed for high-contrast PET imaging at 6 h post-injection (p.i.) [42], and >3.5-fold lower kidney retention than the very early generation [$^{18}$F]AlF NOTA-A20FMDV2-peptide [43]. Building on these data and to extend the imaging window beyond that of fluorine-18 ($t_{1/2}$ = 109.7 min), a copper-64 1,4,7,10-tetraazacyclododecane-1,4,7,10-tetracetic acid (DOTA) IP-ABM-$\alpha_v\beta_6$-BP ($t_{1/2}$ = 12.7 h) was prepared, which again resulted in an increased tumor accumulation that allowed PET imaging up to 72 h p.i. [44].

In the present study, we describe a head-to-head comparison of the $\alpha_v\beta_6$-BP modified with either EB-ABM or IP-ABM, with the goal to examine if fine tuning of the ABM could further increase tumor accumulation. Copper-64 radiolabeled [$^{64}$Cu]Cu DOTA-EB-$\alpha_v\beta_6$-BP ([$^{64}$Cu]1) and [$^{64}$Cu]Cu DOTA-IP-$\alpha_v\beta_6$-BP ([$^{64}$Cu]2), along with the non-$\alpha_v\beta_6$-targeting ABM controls [$^{64}$Cu]Cu DOTA-EB ([$^{64}$Cu]3) and [$^{64}$Cu]Cu DOTA-IP ([$^{64}$Cu]4; Figure 1) were synthesized. Peptides [$^{64}$Cu]1 and [$^{64}$Cu]2 were evaluated in vitro by competitive ELISA, serum stability, albumin binding assays, and cell binding and internalization assays with DX3puro$\beta$6 ($\alpha_v\beta_6$+), DX3puro ($\alpha_v\beta_6$−), and BxPC-3 ($\alpha_v\beta_6$+) cells (against controls [$^{64}$Cu]3 and [$^{64}$Cu]4), and in vivo by PET/CT imaging and biodistribution studies in mice bearing BxPC-3 xenograft tumors (4–72 h, p.i., against controls [$^{64}$Cu]3 and [$^{64}$Cu]4 at 4 h, p.i.).

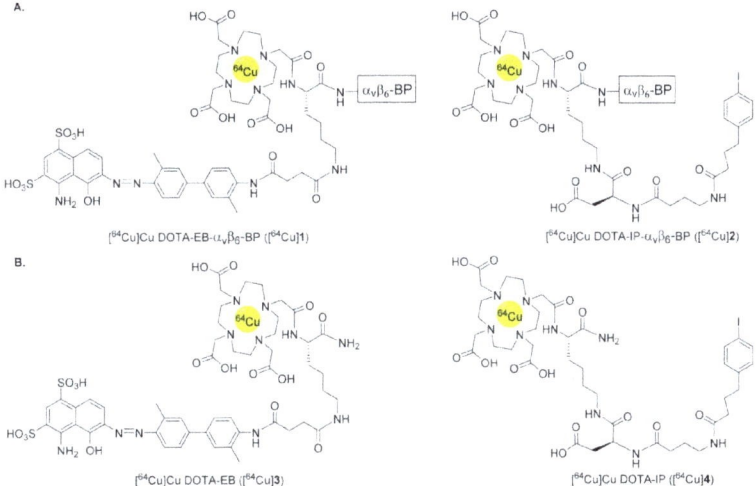

**Figure 1.** (**A**) Chemical structures of $^{64}$Cu-radiolabeled-ABM-$\alpha_v\beta_6$-BP: [$^{64}$Cu]Cu DOTA-EB-$\alpha_v\beta_6$-BP and [$^{64}$Cu]Cu DOTA-IP-$\alpha_v\beta_6$-BP ([$^{64}$Cu]1 and [$^{64}$Cu]2). (**B**) Chemical structures of $^{64}$Cu-radiolabeled non-targeting-ABM controls: [$^{64}$Cu]Cu DOTA-EB and [$^{64}$Cu]Cu DOTA-IP ([$^{64}$Cu]3 and [$^{64}$Cu]4). [$\alpha_v\beta_6$-BP = PEG$_{28}$-NAVPNLRGDLQVLAQRVART-PEG$_{28}$-CONH$_2$].

## 2. Materials and Methods

### 2.1. Materials and General Information

Amino acids N-terminally protected with a fluorenylmethyloxycarbonyl (Fmoc) protecting group and acid labile side chain protecting groups (trityl, Pbf, *tert*-butyl, or Boc) were purchased from Novabiochem (MA, USA) or GL Biochem (Shanghai, China). The orthogonally protected lysine with a 1-(4,4-dimethyl-2,6-dioxocyclohex-1-ylidene)-3-methylbutyl (ivDde) sidechain protecting group and an *N*-terminal Fmoc protecting group, Fmoc-Lys(ivDde)-OH was purchased from ChemPep (Wellington, FL, USA) and the reverse ivDde-Lys(Fmoc)-OH was purchased from EMD (MA, USA). The Fmoc-NH-PEG$_{28}$ carboxylic acid was purchased from Polypure (Oslo, Norway) and the chelator DOTA-tris(*tert*-butyl ester) was purchased from CheMatech (Dijon, France) and Macrocyclics (Plano, TX, USA). The coupling reagent 1-[bis(dimethylamino)methylene]-1*H*-1,2,3-triazolo[4,5-b]pyridinium 3-oxid hexafluorophosphate (HATU) was purchased from GL Biochem, and benzotriazol-1-yl-oxytripyrrolidinophosphoniumhexafluorophosphate (PyBOP) was purchased from Novabiochem. Ethylenediaminetetraacetic acid (EDTA), manganese chloride (MnCl$_2$), and Tris were purchased from Sigma-Aldrich (St. Louis, MO, USA). Tween 20 and sodium chloride (NaCl) were purchased from Fisher (Hampton, NH, USA). The non-fat dry milk powder was purchased from Raley's (West Sacramento, CA, USA). Anhydrous *N,N*-diisopropylethylamine (DIPEA) and hydrazine were purchased from Sigma-Aldrich and used without additional purification. Solvents *N,N*-dimethylformamide (DMF), dimethylsulfoxide (DMSO), acetonitrile (ACN), methanol (MeOH), dichloromethane (DCM), ethyl acetate (EtOAc), *n*-hexanes, and pyridine were purchased from EMD or Acros (NJ, USA). Water used was purified with a Millipore Integral 5 Milli-Q water system at 18.2 MΩ/cm resistivity through a 0.22 μm filter. All solid phase couplings were carried out by rotation in a fritted polypropylene reactor. Thin-layered chromatography (TLC) plates (silica gel 60 with 254 nm fluorescent indicator) from EMD were visualized by UV lamp at 254 nm and/or iodine staining (for the synthesis of **6**). Purification of compound **6** was carried out by normal phase flash column chromatography with silica gel (40–63 μm; Silicycle, QC, Canada). Characterization, purity, and stability were assessed by analytical C$_{12}$-reverse-phase (RP) high-pressure liquid chromatography (HPLC) column (Jupiter Proteo, 250 mm × 4.6 mm × 4 μm; Phenomenex, Torrance, CA, USA). A Semi-preparative C$_{18}$-RP-column (Proteo-Jupiter, 250 mm × 10 mm × 10 μm; Phenomenex) was used for purification as described in the Supporting Information (Table S3). All RP-HPLC were carried out on a Dionex Ultimate 3000 HPLC system or a Beckman Coulter Gold HPLC with the latter being used for all radio-RP-HPLC analysis. RP-HPLC were monitored by a UV detector at a wavelength of 220 nm; a serially connected gamma detector was used to monitor radioactivity. [$^{64}$Cu]CuCl$_2$ was from the University of Wisconsin Medical Physics Department (WIMR Cyclotron Labs, Madison, WI, USA). Tissue culture and cellular assays used Dulbecco's Modified Eagle Medium (DMEM), Roswell Park Memorial Institute (RPMI) 1640 medium, fetal bovine serum (FBS), bovine serum albumin (BSA), penicillin-streptomycin-glutamine (PSG), puromycin, and phosphate buffered saline (PBS; all: Gibco/Thermo Fisher). The DX3puroβ6 and DX3puro cells were a gift from Dr. John Marshall. The DX3puroβ6 and DX3puro cell lines were maintained in DMEM medium, supplemented with 10% FBS, 1% penicillin-streptomycin-glutamine, and 2 mg/mL-puromycin. The BxPC-3 cells were purchased from American Type Culture collection (ATCC, Manassas, VA, USA) and maintained in RPMI 1640 medium supplemented with 10% FBS and 1% penicillin-streptomycin-glutamine. Cells were kept in a humidified incubator at 37 °C under a 5%-carbon dioxide atmosphere. A Wizard 1470 or Wizard$^2$ 2470 automatic γ-counter (Perkin-Elmer, Waltham, MA, USA) was used to measure radioactivity samples. Mass spectrometry analysis was performed at the UC Davis Mass Spectrometry Facility using either a matrix assisted laser desorption ionization time of flight (MALDI-TOF) spectrometer (UltraFlextreme; Bruker, Billerica, MA, USA) in positive ionization mode with a sinapic acid matrix (Sigma-Aldrich), or with electrospray ionization (ESI) using a quadrupole ion-trap mass spectrometer (Orbitrap; ThermoFisher). Nuclear magnetic resonance (NMR) spectra were collected at the UC Davis NMR Facility on an 800 MHz Bruker instrument with the chemical shifts referenced to the residual solvent of deuterium oxide (D$_2$O, HOD 4.79 ppm).

## 2.2. Synthesis of EB-ABM 8

The synthesis of the Evans blue fragment (EB-ABM **8**) was based on previously described methods [7,17,45] (Scheme 1). In brief, *o*-tolidine **5** (531 mg, 2.5 mmol; TCI America, Inc., OR, USA) was dissolved in anhydrous pyridine (1 mL) followed by the addition of succinic anhydride (300 mg, 3.0 mmol) in DMF (1 mL) and allowed to react overnight at room temperature. The crude reaction mixture was concentrated under vacuum and purified by silica-gel column chromatography using a four solvent gradient system beginning with EtOAc/n-hexanes (1/1, $v/v$) to remove unreacted *o*-tolidine (**5**, yellow band). The solvent was then changed to 100% EtOAc before switching to MeOH/DCM (1/9, $v/v$) and gradually ramping to 3/7 ($v/v$) to obtain **6** (648 mg, rt = 0.13, 1:1 hexanes:EtOAc) as a white solid in 83% yield. Compound **6** was analyzed by analytical RP-HPLC and ESI mass spectrometry (Figure S17).

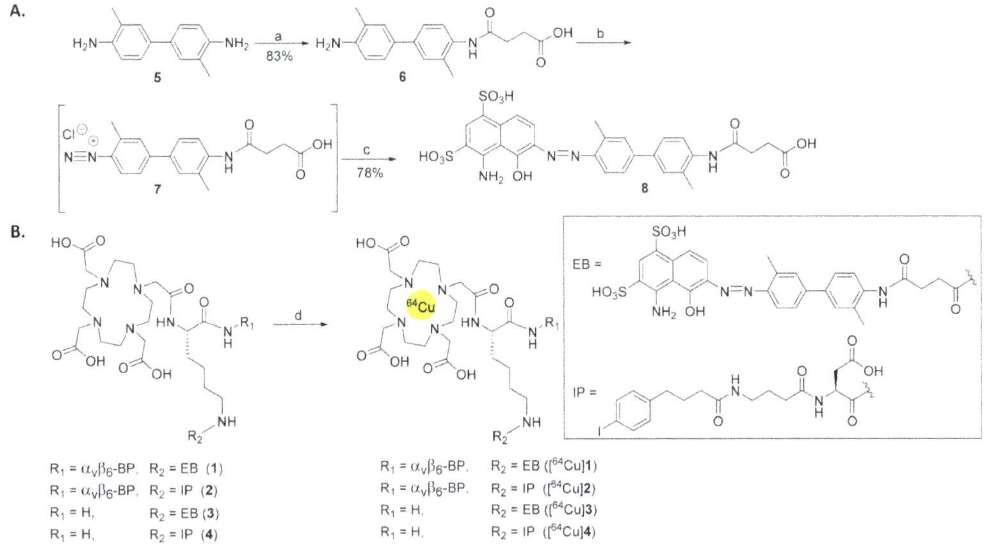

**Scheme 1.** (**A**) Synthetic route to modified EB-ABM **8**. (**B**) Radiochemical Synthesis of [$^{64}$Cu]**1**–**4**. a. Succinic anhydride, DMF, pyridine (1:1), b. NaNO$_2$, MeOH, HCl/H$_2$O, 0 °C, c. 1-amino-8-napthol-2,4-disulfonic acid, NaHCO$_3$, H$_2$O, 0 °C, d. [$^{64}$Cu]CuCl$_2$, NH$_4$OAc, 37 °C.

Compound **6** (300 mg, 0.96 mmol) was added to a 25 mL round bottom flask with stir bar containing MeOH (7 mL) and water (5 mL). The contents were cooled to 0 °C (ice/brine solution) and allowed to stir for 15 min prior to addition of concentrated hydrochloric acid 240 µL (HCl, 12.1 N; EMD). The diazonium formation of **7** was most successful when the addition of sodium nitrite was done in two portions; the first portion of sodium nitrite (NaNO$_2$, 70 mg, 1.01 mmol; Sigma-Aldrich) was allowed to react for 5 min before the addition of the second portion (NaNO$_2$, 70 mg, 1.01 mmol), after which the reaction was stirred an additional 30 min to generate **7** in situ, which was produced in better yields using the methanol co-solvent than water alone [46]. During in situ formation of **7**, sodium bicarbonate (350 mg, 4.17 mmol; EMD) was dissolved in water (4 mL) with 1-amino-8-napthol-2,4-disulfonic acid (377 mg, 1.18 mmol; TCI America, Inc.) in a separate 25 mL round bottom flask and the contents cooled in an ice/brine solution (~20 min). Next, the diazonium **7** reaction mixture (yellow) was cannulated into the 1-amino-8-napthol-2,4-disulfonic acid (brown-purple) solution by drop-wise addition over 20 min while maintaining both solutions at 0 °C. Upon complete addition of **7**, the reaction contents were allowed to stir for 3 h at 0 °C, and the crude reaction mixture was lyophilized and purified by semi-preparative RP-HPLC, and the collected material lyophilized. The EB-ABM **8** was afforded as a fluffy purple solid (480 mg, 78%) and was analyzed by analytical RP-HPLC, ESI mass spectrometry, and NMR (Figures S18 and S19).

### 2.3. Synthesis of DOTA-ABM-$\alpha_v\beta_6$-BPs 1 and 2

The $\alpha_v\beta_6$-BP (PEG$_{28}$-NAVPNLRGDLQVLAQRVART-PEG$_{28}$) was synthesized on NovaSyn TGR resin (NovaBiochem) and PEGylation was done using monodisperse Fmoc-amino-PEG-propionic acid (Fmoc-PEG$_{28}$-CO$_2$H; FW = 1544.8 g/mol) as previously described [30] using standard Fmoc-chemistry. After each coupling or deprotection the resin was rinsed with DMF (3×), MeOH (3×), and DMF (3×). The $\alpha_v\beta_6$-BP-resin was split in equal portions (100 mg, 0.0088 mmol) and further modified at the N-terminus for the synthesis of peptides 1 and 2. The DOTA-EB-$\alpha_v\beta_6$-BP 1 was generated by first removing the N-terminal Fmoc of the $\alpha_v\beta_6$-BP with 20% piperidine (Sigma-Aldrich) in DMF (2 × 10 min) followed by the addition of Fmoc-Lys(ivDde)-OH (50.6 mg, 0.088 mmol) using HATU (32.3 mg, 0.085 mmol) and DIPEA (30 μL, 0.172 mmol) in DMF (1 mL) for 2 h. The Fmoc was subsequently removed with 20% piperidine in DMF (2 × 10 min) and DOTA-tris(*tert*-butyl ester) (50.3 mg, 0.088 mmol) was coupled for 2 h to the N-terminus with HATU (32.3 mg, 0.085 mmol) and DIPEA (30 μL, 0.172 mmol) in DMF (1 mL). The removal of the ivDde lysine-sidechain protecting group was done with hydrazine (50 μL) in DMF (1 mL, 2 × 30 min) and the resin dried under vacuum. The EB-ABM 8 (60 mg, 0.093 mmol) was then coupled to the ε-amine of the sidechain of the DOTA-lysine on the $\alpha_v\beta_6$-BP-resin using PyBOP (125 mg, 0.24 mmol) and DIPEA (50 μL, 0.287 mmol) for 6 h to yield DOTA-EB-$\alpha_v\beta_6$-BP-resin 1 (Figure S4). The DOTA-EB-$\alpha_v\beta_6$-BP 1 was cleaved off the resin with concomitant removal of the protecting groups using trifluoroacetic acid (TFA, 2 mL; EMD), triisopropylsilane (TIPS, 50 μL; Alfa Aesar, Haverhill, MA, USA) and water (50 μL), concentrated, purified, and characterized by analytical RP-HPLC and MALDI-TOF (Figure S5). The IP-ABM containing-$\alpha_v\beta_6$-BP 2 was prepared as previously described [42,44] were upon removal the N-terminal Fmoc of the $\alpha_v\beta_6$-BP-resin, a ivDde-Lys(Fmoc)-OH was coupled. Completion of DOTA-IP-$\alpha_v\beta_6$-BP 2 was done by sequential coupling/deFmocing of (1) Fmoc-Asp(OtBu)-OH, (2) N-γ-Fmoc-γ-aminobutyric acid, and (3) 4-(*p*-iodophenyl)butyric acid using HATU and DIPEA for each coupling. Completion of DOTA-IP-$\alpha_v\beta_6$-BP 2 was achieved by removal of the N-terminal ivDde protecting group with 5%-hydrazine in DMF followed by attachment of DOTA-tris(*tert*-butyl ester) [44]. The completed DOTA-IP-$\alpha_v\beta_6$-BP 2 was cleaved, purified, and analyzed as described above for the DOTA-EB-$\alpha_v\beta_6$-BP 1 (Figure S8) [44].

### 2.4. Synthesis of Non-Targeting ABMs 3 and 4

Using Fmoc-chemistry with Rink AM resin (200 mg, 0.114 mmol; GL Biochem), DOTA-ABM non-targeting compounds 3 and 4 were synthesized by first coupling Fmoc-Lys(ivDde)-OH (196.6 mg, 0.342 mmol) using HATU (123.5 mg, 0.325 mmol) and DIPEA (100 μL, 0.574 mmol) in DMF (1 mL). The Fmoc was removed with 20% ($v/v$) piperidine in DMF (1 mL, 2 × 10 min) and DOTA-tris(*tert*-butyl ester) (80 mg, 0.140 mmol) was coupled for 2 h with HATU (50 mg, 0.132 mmol) and DIPEA (50 μL, 0.287 mmol). Following the ivDde protecting group removal with hydrazine (50 μL) in DMF (1 mL, 2 × 30 min), the resin was dried under vacuum and split into equal portions for synthesis of 3 and 4. For 3, the EB-ABM 8 (165 mg, 0.256 mmol) was coupled using PyBOP (166.5 mg, 0.32 mmol) and DIPEA (100 μL, 0.574 mmol) for 6 h. The EB-ABM 3 was cleaved off the resin, purified, and characterized by analytical RP-HPLC and MALDI-TOF (Figure S11). IP-ABM 4 was prepared by sequential coupling/deFmocing of (1) Fmoc-Asp(OtBu)-OH (90 mg, 0.219 mmol), (2) N-γ-Fmoc-γ-aminobutyric acid (70 mg, 0.215 mmol), and (3) 4-(*p*-iodophenyl)butyric acid (65 mg, 0.224 mmol) using HATU (78 mg, 0.205 mmol) and DIPEA (100 μL, 0.574 mmol) for each coupling. The IP-ABM 4 was then cleaved off the resin, purified, and characterized by analytical RP-HPLC and MALDI-TOF (Figure S14).

## 2.5. Radiochemical Synthesis of [$^{64}$Cu]1–4

DOTA-compounds **1–4** were dissolved in metal free water at 1 μg/μL, and the [$^{64}$Cu]CuCl$_2$ (1–10 μL of 0.5 M HCl, **1** and **2**: 174–255.3 MBq, **3** and **4**: 51–55 MBq) was diluted with 1.0 M ammonium acetate (NH$_4$OAc, Sigma-Aldrich) aqueous solution (pH = 8.0) to 0.27 μL/MBq. Peptides **1** and **2** were added to the NH$_4$OAc buffered [$^{64}$Cu]CuCl$_2$ such that the starting molar activity of the reaction was between 18.5 and 20 GBq/μmol. The starting molar activity for compounds **3** and **4** was between 15.9 and 17.1 GBq/μmol. The reaction mixtures were vortexed and warmed to 37 °C for 30 min. The radiochemical purity was assessed by quenching an aliquot of the reaction ($\leq$1 μL; 0.74–3.7 MBq) with 0.1 M EDTA (50 μL) and analyzed by analytical RP-HPLC. Product identity was confirmed by cold spike RP-HPLC, i.e., co-injection of the radiolabeled product with authenticated respective [$^{Nat}$Cu]Cu **1–4** reference standard of each compound (Figures S6, S9, S12 and S15). [$^{Nat}$Cu]Cu **1–4** reference standards were produced via reaction of DOTA-compounds **1–4** (0.1–0.5 mg) with excess CuCl$_2$ (Sigma-Aldrich, 1–6 mg) in water (50 μL) for 30 min at room temperature, and purified directly by RP-HPLC and confirmed by MALDI-TOF (Figures S7, S10, S13 and S16).

## 2.6. Integrin $\alpha_v\beta_6$ Affinity ELISA

Affinity for the integrin $\alpha_v\beta_6$ was determined by competitive binding ELISA of [$^{Nat}$Cu]**1** and [$^{Nat}$Cu]**2** against biotinylated-LAP (G&P Biosciences, Santa Clara, CA, USA) as previously described to determine the half-maximum inhibitory concentration (IC$_{50}$) [44]. Briefly, in a 96 well Nunc Immuno maxisorp plate, capturing anti-$\alpha_v$ antibody (P2W7, 5 μg/mL, Abcam, MA, USA) was plated (50 μL/well) at 37 °C for 1 h, washed with PBS (3×), and blocked overnight with blocking buffer (300 μL/well, 0.5% non-fat dry milk powder ($w/v$), 1% Tween 20, in PBS). It was then washed with wash buffer that consisted of 2 mmol/L of Tris buffer (pH = 7.6), 150 mmol/L sodium chloride, 1 mmol/L manganese chloride, and 0.1% Tween 20 ($v/v$) in deionized water (3×). Purified integrin $\alpha_v\beta_6$ (R&D Systems, Minneapolis, MN, USA) in conjugate buffer (50 μL/well, 20 mM Tris, 1 mM MnCl$_2$, 150 mM NaCl, 0.1% Tween, 0.1% milk powder in water) was then added to each well, incubated at 37 °C for 1 h, followed by washing using wash buffer 3×). Serial dilutions of each peptide stock of 2 mmol/L in 10% DMSO ($v/v$) into PBS and biotinylated natural ligand LAP were premixed in equal volumes and placed onto the plate in triplicate for each peptide concentration (50 μL/well) and allowed to incubate at 37 °C for 1 h then washed with wash buffer (3×). A 1:1000 dilution of ExtrAvidin Horseradish Peroxidase (HRP; Fisher, NH, USA) was added to each well (50 μL/well), incubated at 37 °C for 1 h, and then washed with wash buffer (3×). The ExtrAvidin HRP was detected with TMB One solution (50 μL/well; Promega Corp., Madison, WI, USA) for 10–15 min at room temperature. The reaction was stopped by adding 1N sulfuric acid (H$_2$SO$_4$, 50 μL/well; EMD, MA, USA) and the absorbance was measured in a Multiscan Ascent plate reader (Thermo Fisher, Waltham, MA, USA) at 450 nm. Half-maximal inhibitory concentration (IC$_{50}$) of peptides was determined by fitting to sigmoidal dose-response model in GraphPad Prism 8.0 (GraphPad, CA, USA). For the positive control no peptide was added and for the negative controls either no biotinylated-LAP or no integrin $\alpha_v\beta_6$ was added.

## 2.7. Cell Binding and Internalization Assay

Binding of [$^{64}$Cu]**1–4** and internalization to DX3puro, DX3puroβ6, and BxPC-3 cells were determined as previously described [44]. Prior to the experiment, the cells were analyzed by flow cytometry to confirm levels of integrin $\alpha_v\beta_6$ expression. Non-fat dry milk powder (0.5% $w/v$ in PBS) was used to pretreat the assay tubes to prevent non-specific binding. Aliquots of [$^{64}$Cu]**1–4** ($\leq$1 μL, 7.4–18.5 KBq) in 50 μL serum free medium (pH 7.2) were added to a cell suspension (3.75 × 10$^6$ cells in 50 μL serum free medium) and incubated for 1 h at room temperature in closed microfuge tubes ($n = 3$/cell line/compound) and gently agitated every 3 min to ensure mixing. The cells were pelleted by centrifugation at 200 (RCF) for 3 min and the supernatant collected. The cell pellet was washed with 0.5 mL serum free medium and the wash medium combined with the original supernatant. The cells were resuspended in 0.6 mL serum free medium for γ-counting. The fraction of bound radioactivity was determined with a γ-counter (by measuring cell pellet and combined supernatants). To determine the fraction of internalized radioactivity, the cells were re-pelleted, and re-suspended in acidic wash buffer (0.2 mol/L sodium acetate, 0.5 mol/L sodium chloride, pH 2.5, 300 μL, 4 °C, 5 min) to release surface-bound activity, followed by a wash with PBS (300 μL). The internalized fraction was determined with a γ-counter (cell pellet vs. radioactivity released into supernatant).

*2.8. Human and Mouse Serum Binding Assay and Stability Assay*

Serum protein binding of [$^{64}$Cu]1 and [$^{64}$Cu]2 was assessed following the previously reported method [42]. Peptides [$^{64}$Cu]1 and [$^{64}$Cu]2 were evaluated by ultrafiltration using Centrifree Ultrafiltration devices (EMD) according to the manufacturer's recommendations. Experiments were carried out in triplicate. The Centrifree Ultrafiltration devices were pretreated with PBS containing Tween 20 (5% $v/v$), followed by triplicate rinses with PBS. An aliquot of each peptide [$^{64}$Cu]1 or [$^{64}$Cu]2 in PBS ($\leq$25 μL, 20–60 KBq) was thoroughly mixed with 0.5 mL of serum at 37 °C in a microfuge tube. The mixture was incubated at 37 °C for 5 min, and an aliquot (50 μL) was transferred to a tube for γ-counting. The remaining sample was transferred to a Centrifree Ultrafiltration device and centrifuged for 40 min at 1500 (RCF) at ambient temperature (20–24 °C). An aliquot (50 μL) of the filtrate was transferred to a tube for γ-counting. For each radiolabeled peptide, a blank was run using 0.5 mL PBS/Tween 20 (5% $v/v$) instead of serum ($n$ = 3) to determine non-specific binding. Following γ-counting, the protein-bound radioactivity was calculated by subtracting the counts measured in the filtrate aliquot (i.e., not protein-bound) from the counts in the corresponding serum aliquot. The data are expressed as mean ± standard deviation of fraction of radioactivity bound to protein after subtraction of non-specific binding determined in the blank.

For serum stability, mouse serum or human serum (0.5 mL, both purchased from Sigma-Aldrich) was combined with an aliquot of each of the peptides [$^{64}$Cu]1 and [$^{64}$Cu]2 ($\leq$25 μL, 14.8–22.2 MBq) and incubated at 37 °C. At each time point (1, 4, and 24 h) an aliquot (50–200 μL) was taken, proteins precipitated with ethanol, and removed by pelleting at 1500 (RCF) for 4 min. The ethanol solution was diluted with water (1 mL) and analyzed by RP-HPLC as previously described [47].

*2.9. Biodistribution*

All animal procedures conformed to the Animal Welfare Act and were approved by the University of California, Davis Institutional Animal Care and Use Committee. Female athymic nu/nu-nude mice (6–8 weeks old) were purchased from Charles River Laboratories (Wilmington, MA, USA) and provided food and water on an ad libitum basis. BxPC-3 xenografts were implanted according to previous methods [42,44]. Briefly, BxPC-3 cells were evaluated by flow cytometry to confirm integrin $\alpha_v\beta_6$ expression levels, injected subcutaneously into the left flank [5 million in 100 μL of a 1:1 mixture of serum-free RPMI and GFR Matrigel (Corning, New York, NY, USA)], and allowed to grow for approximately 3 weeks until tumors reached a diameter of 0.5–1 cm.

For biodistribution studies the [$^{64}$Cu]1–4 (3.7–5.55 MBq) in PBS (100 μL, pH 7.2) was injected intravenously (i.v.) via catheter into the tail vein. Following a conscious uptake period, the mice were anesthetized (5% isoflurane), euthanized, and dissected ([$^{64}$Cu]1 and [$^{64}$Cu]2, $n$ = 3/radiolabeled peptide/time point; 4, 24, and 48 h p.i.; the 72 h time point was obtained from the imaging animals after the 72 h PET/CT scans; compounds [$^{64}$Cu]3 and [$^{64}$Cu]4, $n$ = 2/radiolabeled compound at 4 h p.i.). Tissues were rapidly collected, weighed, and radioactivity measured with a γ-counter. Decay-corrected radioactivity concentrations are expressed as the percentage of injected dose per gram of tissue (% ID/g). Data are reported as mean ± standard deviation (SD) (Figure S20, S21 and S25).

## 2.10. Blocking Biodistribution

For blocking studies, the metal free peptides **1** or **2** (~220 nmol, 1.3 mg in 100 µL PBS), respectively, were injected i.v. ($n$ = 1/peptide) as described above 10 min prior to the injection of matching radiolabeled [$^{64}$Cu]**1** or [$^{64}$Cu]**2** (3.7–5.55 MBq, 100 µL PBS). After a conscious 4 h uptake period, the animals were anesthetized, sacrificed, tissues rapidly collected, and analyzed as described above. Decay-corrected radioactivity concentrations are expressed as a percentage of injected dose per gram of tissue (% ID/g) (Figure S23).

## 2.11. PET-Imaging

For imaging studies, [$^{64}$Cu]**1** and [$^{64}$Cu]**2** (7.77–8.88 MBq) in PBS (100 µL, pH 7.2) were injected i.v. via a catheter into the tail vein of mice ($n$ = 3/radiolabeled peptide) anesthetized with 2–3% isoflurane in medical grade oxygen. Animals were imaged in a prone position two at a time side by side. PET/CT scans were acquired using Inveon scanners (Inveon DPET scanner and Inveon SPECT/CT scanner, Siemens Medical Solutions, Knoxville, TN, USA; PET scans: a static 15 min scan at 4 h p.i., static 30 min scans at 24 and 48 h p.i., and a static 1 h scan at 72 h p.i.) and analyzed as previously described using the Inveon Research Workplace software (Siemens) [42,44].

## 2.12. Statistical Analysis

Quantitative data are reported as mean ± standard deviation (SD). Statistical significance was determined by a paired two-tailed Student's $t$-test from the two independent sample means to give a significance value ($p$-value) at 95% confidence interval (CI). A $p$-value of <0.05 was considered statistically significant.

# 3. Results

## 3.1. Synthesis of EB-ABM 8

EB-ABM **8** was generated efficiently in three synthetic steps from o-tolidine **5** in an overall yield of 65% (Scheme 1A). EB-ABM **8** was characterized by analytical RP-HPLC with a retention time of 17.72 min; ESI-MS m/z [M + H]$^+$ for $C_{28}H_{27}N_4O_{10}S_2$ calc'ed 643.1163; found 643.1207, and by $^1$H NMR (Figures S18 and S19). $^1$H NMR (800 MHz, D$_2$O) δ 8.28 (s, 1H), 7.55 (d, $J$ = 9.4 Hz, 1H), 7.29–7.27 (m, 2H), 7.24–7.23 (m, 1H), 7.17–7.16 (m, 1H), 7.13–7.12 (m, 1H), 6.98–6.97 (m, 1H), 6.88 (d, 7.8 Hz, 1H), 2.64–2.61 (m, 4H), 2.12 (s, 3H), 1.96 (s, 3H).

## 3.2. Synthesis and Radiochemical Synthesis of [$^{64}$Cu]1–4

DOTA-compounds **1–4** were prepared in >97% isolated purity after RP-HPLC purification. DOTA-EB-$\alpha_v\beta_6$-BP **1** had an RP-HPLC retention time of 17.22 min with a MALDI-TOF m/z [M + Na]$^+$ for $C_{261}H_{460}N_{46}NaO_{102}S_2$ calc'ed 5958.1556; found 5958.1756 (Figure S5). DOTA-IP-$\alpha_v\beta_6$-BP **2** had an RP-HPLC retention time of 17.07 min with a MALDI-TOF m/z [M + H]$^+$ for $C_{251}H_{458}IN_{44}O_{98}$ calc'ed 5786.1314; found 5786.1209 (Figure S8). DOTA-EB-ABM **3** had an RP-HPLC retention time of 14.18 min with a MALDI-TOF m/z [M + H]$^+$ for $C_{50}H_{66}N_{11}O_{17}S_2$ calc'ed 1156.4074; found 1156.4079 (Figure S11). DOTA-IP-ABM **4** had an RP-HPLC retention time of 14.46 min with a MALDI-TOF m/z [M + H]$^+$ for $C_{40}H_{63}IN_9O_{13}$ calc'ed 1004.3585; found 1004.3590 (Figure S14).

The $^{64}$Cu-radiolabeled compounds ([$^{64}$Cu]**1–4**) were produced in near quantitative yields ($n$ = 2–4/compound/molar activity ranging between 16 and 20 GBq/µmol) by reaction of with [$^{64}$Cu]CuCl$_2$ in 1.0 M NH$_4$OAc-buffer (pH = 8) at 37 °C for 30 min (Scheme 1B). The radiochemical purities were ≥97% as determined analytical radio-RP-HPLC and compounds [$^{64}$Cu]**1–4** used without further purification. Analytical radio-RP-HPLC retention times were: [$^{64}$Cu]**1**—19.05 min (Figure S6); [$^{64}$Cu]**2**—18.68 min (Figure S9); [$^{64}$Cu]**3**—17.01 min (Figure S12); and [$^{64}$Cu]**4**—16.73 min (Figure S15).

## 3.3. Integrin $\alpha_v\beta_6$ Affinity ELISA

Competitive ELISA against biotinylated LAP, demonstrated that both ABM modifications of $\alpha_v\beta_6$-BP were well tolerated; [$^{Nat}$Cu]1 and [$^{Nat}$Cu]2 showed high integrin $\alpha_v\beta_6$-affinity as expressed by the half-maximum inhibitory concentrations (IC$_{50}$); [$^{Nat}$Cu]1 and [$^{Nat}$Cu]2: IC$_{50}$ = 14 ± 2 and 19 ± 5 nM, respectively) compared to DOTA-$\alpha_v\beta_6$-BP (IC$_{50}$ = 28 ± 3 nM) [44].

## 3.4. Cell Binding and Internalization Assay

Cell binding studies showed that [$^{64}$Cu]1 and [$^{64}$Cu]2 both bound to cells in an $\alpha_v\beta_6$-dependent manner at similar levels (DX3puroβ6 (+): [$^{64}$Cu]1 55.8 ± 3.0% of total radioactivity, [$^{64}$Cu]2 60.2 ± 3.9%; BxPC-3 (+): [$^{64}$Cu]1 30.3 ± 2.7%, [$^{64}$Cu]2 48.5 ± 3.5%; and the negative control DX3puro (−): [$^{64}$Cu]1 2.7 ± 0.5%, [$^{64}$Cu]2 3.1 ± 0.3%, Figure 2). This resulted in binding ratios for DX3puroβ6 (+) vs. DX3puro (−) of 20.7:1 for [$^{64}$Cu]1 and 19.4:1 for [$^{64}$Cu]2. Internalization into $\alpha_v\beta_6$-positive cells was also high ([$^{64}$Cu]1: 48.5–52.7% of the bound radioactivity, [$^{64}$Cu]2: 41.5–54.8%, Figure 2). The non-targeting control ABM conjugates [$^{64}$Cu]3 and [$^{64}$Cu]4 exhibited low, non-specific binding to all cell lines (≤4.3%; Figure S24).

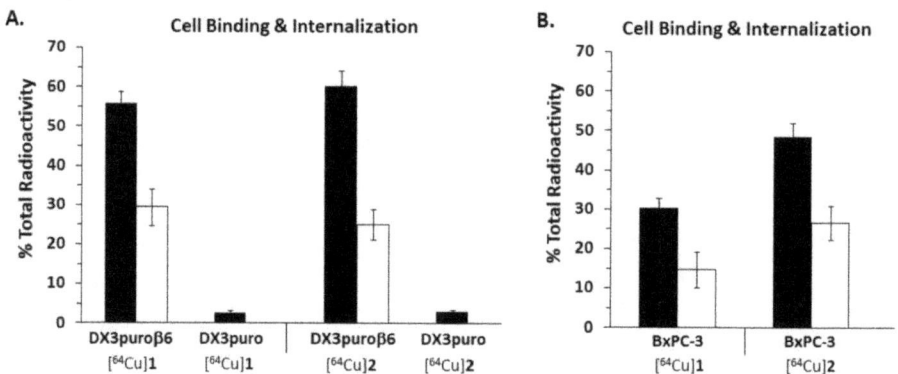

**Figure 2.** Cell binding (■) and internalization (□) for [$^{64}$Cu]Cu DOTA-EB-$\alpha_v\beta_6$-BP ([$^{64}$Cu]1) and [$^{64}$Cu]Cu DOTA-IP-$\alpha_v\beta_6$-BP ([$^{64}$Cu]2) for (**A**) DX3puroβ6 ($\alpha_v\beta_6$+) and DX3puro($\alpha_v\beta_6$−) cells and (**B**) BxPC-3 ($\alpha_v\beta_6$+) cells.

## 3.5. Human and Mouse Serum Binding Assay and Stability Assay

Serum albumin binding for [$^{64}$Cu]1 and [$^{64}$Cu]2 was similar, with higher binding to human serum protein (53.4 ± 0.9% and 63.3 ± 1.5%, respectively) than to mouse serum protein (41.9 ± 1.1% and 44.0 ± 0.1%, respectively; Figure 3A). The ABM modifications of [$^{64}$Cu]1 and [$^{64}$Cu]2 increased the serum albumin affinity as the [$^{64}$Cu]Cu DOTA-$\alpha_v\beta_6$-BP without an ABM modification showed <29% binding to either serum albumin [44]. Both peptides showed high stability in human serum at 37 °C ([$^{64}$Cu]1 1 h: 99% and 4 h: 89% intact; [$^{64}$Cu]2 1 h: 99% and 4 h: 93% intact) with some degradation apparent after 24 h ([$^{64}$Cu]1: 76% intact vs. [$^{64}$Cu]2: 90% intact, Figure 3B). In contrast, faster degradation was observed in mouse serum at 37 °C, and the stability was lower for [$^{64}$Cu]1 than for [$^{64}$Cu]2 at all-time points; [$^{64}$Cu]1 was 78% intact at 1 h, dropping to 58% at 4 h, and largely metabolized at 24 h (14% intact). By comparison, [$^{64}$Cu]2 was 92% and 83% intact at 1 h and 4 h, respectively, with 48% remaining intact at 24 h, a 3.4-fold higher stability than [$^{64}$Cu]1 (Figure 3C).

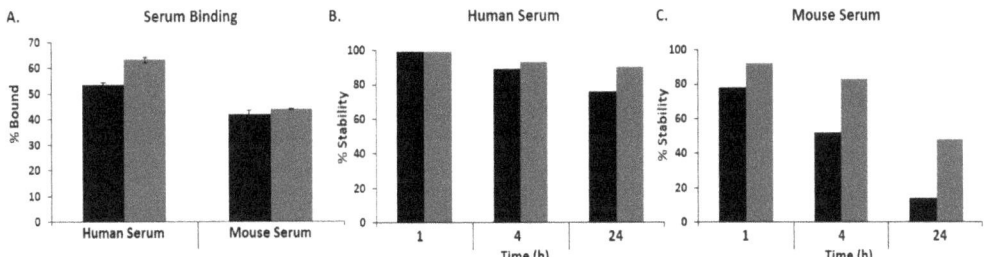

**Figure 3.** (**A**) Binding to human and mouse serum ($n$ = 3/compound/condition; bars: SD). (**B**) Stability in human serum at 37 °C. (**C**) Stability in mouse serum at 37 °C for [$^{64}$Cu]**1** (■) and [$^{64}$Cu]**2** (■).

*3.6. Biodistribution*

The biodistributions for [$^{64}$Cu]**1** and [$^{64}$Cu]**2** in the BxPC-3 tumor model showed good tumor uptake (4 h to 72 h: [$^{64}$Cu]**1** 5.29 ± 0.59 to 3.32 ± 0.46% ID/g, [$^{64}$Cu]**2** 7.60 ± 0.43 to 4.91 ± 1.19% ID/g, Figure 4). Overall, tumor uptake of [$^{64}$Cu]**2** appeared higher than of [$^{64}$Cu]**1**, particularly at the earliest time point, and relative tumor washout over the total observed time frame was similar for both peptides. The ABM modifications increased tumor accumulation by >3-to-4.5-fold compared to the [$^{64}$Cu]Cu DOTA-$\alpha_v\beta_6$-BP without an ABM, which had only 1.61 ± 0.70% ID/g at 4 h in the same BxPC-3 tumor model [44]. Clearance for [$^{64}$Cu]**1** and [$^{64}$Cu]**2** was primarily renal and the kidneys were the organ with the highest levels of radioactivity (Figure S20 and S21). Notably, [$^{64}$Cu]**1** showed more than double the kidney uptake of [$^{64}$Cu]**2** at 4 h, p.i. ([$^{64}$Cu]**1** 75.51 ± 7.26% ID/g; [$^{64}$Cu]**2** 33.56 ± 5.39% ID/g; $p = 0.0013$) and remained significantly higher for at least 48 h (>1.7-fold, $p < 0.05$), but both were cleared from the kidneys over time with accumulation dropping at 72 h ([$^{64}$Cu]**1** 19.97 ± 6.91% ID/g; [$^{64}$Cu]**2** 11.48 ± 1.02% ID/g; $p = 0.103$, Figure 4). Kidney accumulation for the ABM containing peptides [$^{64}$Cu]**1** and [$^{64}$Cu]**2** was initially higher than for the parent non-ABM containing [$^{64}$Cu]Cu DOTA-$\alpha_v\beta_6$-BP (20.37 ± 1.67% ID/g at 4 h to 6.81 ± 1.36% ID/g at 48 h) [44]. Some clearance for [$^{64}$Cu]**1** and [$^{64}$Cu]**2** was also observed through the gastrointestinal tract (GI), with the stomach having the highest uptake at 4 h, p.i. ([$^{64}$Cu]**1**: stomach 6.41 ± 0.64% ID/g, small intestines 4.72 ± 0.55% ID/g, large intestines 4.13 ± 0.10% ID/g, [$^{64}$Cu]**2**: stomach 18.07 ± 2.91% ID/g, small intestines 9.55 ± 1.21% ID/g, large intestines 9.83 ± 0.69% ID/g; Figure 4). Clearance from the GI tract was further confirmed by radioactivity measurements of fecal matter (4–72 h: [$^{64}$Cu]**1**: 3.03 ± 0.67 to 1.81 ± 0.74% ID/g; [$^{64}$Cu]**2**: 9.32 ± 1.08 to 2.29 ± 0.53% ID/g; Figure 4). The GI uptake for [$^{64}$Cu]**2** was more than double that of [$^{64}$Cu]**1** at the earliest time point, but both peptides dropped over time to below 3.2% ID/g at 72 h. The liver uptake was moderate (<3% ID/g) throughout for both peptides; but it increased to significantly higher levels for the EB-ABM containing peptide [$^{64}$Cu]**1**, beginning at 24 h, reaching >1.8-fold higher levels than [$^{64}$Cu]**2** at 72 h (2.36 ± 0.51% ID/g vs. 1.30 ± 0.13% ID/g, respectively; $p = 0.025$, Figure 4). Overall, the EB-ABM containing peptide [$^{64}$Cu]**1** had a less favorable pharmacokinetic profile with significantly higher uptake in the kidneys and liver, resulting in generally lower tumor-to-tissue ratios for [$^{64}$Cu]**1** compared to [$^{64}$Cu]**2**, most notably for the tumor-to-kidney ratio ([$^{64}$Cu]**1** 0.13 ± 0.06/1 to 0.19 ± 0.08/1 vs. [$^{64}$Cu]**2** 0.20 ± 0.06/1 to 0.44 ± 0.14/1), and the tumor-to-liver ratio ([$^{64}$Cu]**1** 2.39 ± 0.59/1 to 1.47 ± 0.47/1 vs. [$^{64}$Cu]**2** 2.72 ± 0.62/1 to 3.77 ± 0.72/1) (Figure S22).

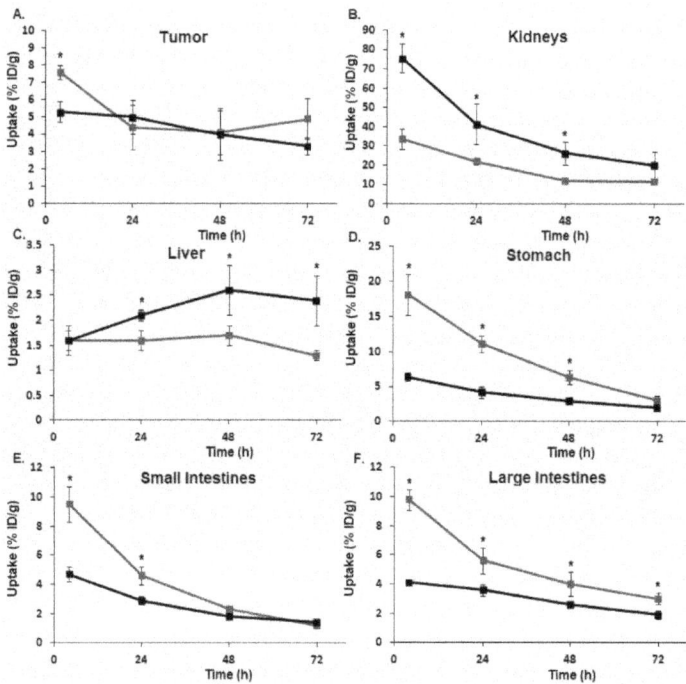

**Figure 4.** Biodistribution time activity plots for [$^{64}$Cu]1 (■) and [$^{64}$Cu]2 (■). (**A**) BxPC-3 tumors. (**B**) kidneys. (**C**) liver. (**D**) stomach. (**E**) small intestines. (**F**) large intestines (* $p \leq 0.05$).

The non-$\alpha_v\beta_6$-targeting ABM controls [$^{64}$Cu]3 and [$^{64}$Cu]4 were used to determine non-specific uptake and provide support that the enhanced tumor accumulation of ABM containing peptides [$^{64}$Cu]1 and [$^{64}$Cu]2 was due to integrin $\alpha_v\beta_6$ receptor mediated uptake. The biodistributions of the non-$\alpha_v\beta_6$-targeting ABM controls [$^{64}$Cu]3 and [$^{64}$Cu]4 at 4 h p.i. ($n$ = 2/compound) showed prolonged blood circulation with much higher blood accumulation (38.9 ± 10.4% ID/g and 9.5 ± 1.3% ID/g, respectively; Figure 5, Figure S25). This increased blood accumulation also led to higher systemic accumulation in other tissues, especially the highly perfused tissues such as the heart, muscle, liver, and lung (Figure 5, Figure S25), with the exception of the kidneys (18.6 ± 1.4% ID/g and 4.34 ± 0.61% ID/g, respectively). These distinctly different pharmacokinetic profiles of the non-integrin $\alpha_v\beta_6$-targeting [$^{64}$Cu]3 and [$^{64}$Cu]4 resulted in a low tumor-to-blood ratio of <0.9/1 compared to >4/1 for [$^{64}$Cu]1 and [$^{64}$Cu]2, a lower tumor-to-muscle ratio ranging from 5.6 to 6.3/1 for [$^{64}$Cu]3 and [$^{64}$Cu]4 compared to >8/1 for [$^{64}$Cu]1 and [$^{64}$Cu]2, and a lower tumor-to-liver ratio of 1.2–1.3/1 for [$^{64}$Cu]3 and [$^{64}$Cu]4 compared to 3.2–4.9/1 for [$^{64}$Cu]1 and [$^{64}$Cu]2 (Figure 5, Figure S26).

### 3.7. Blocking Biodistribution

Integrin $\alpha_v\beta_6$-dependence of the tumor uptake was further substantiated by blocking studies with pre-administration of the respective nonradioactive peptide, which reduced tumor uptake to 2.91% ID/g and 2.89% ID/g for [$^{64}$Cu]1 and [$^{64}$Cu]2, respectively (4 h; $\Delta$ = −45% and −62%, $p$ = 0.0124 and 0.0007, respectively; Figure S23).

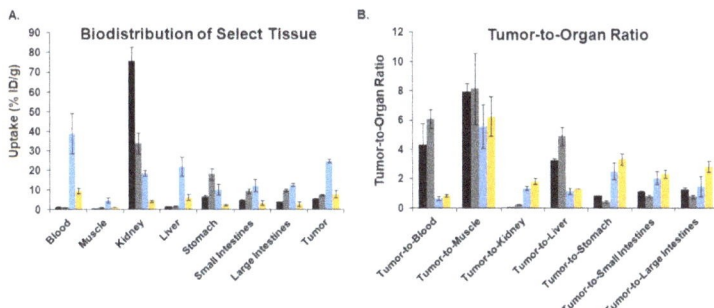

**Figure 5.** (**A**) Biodistribution of select tissues at 4 h p.i. for [$^{64}$Cu]1–4. (**B**) Tumor-to-organ ratios at 4 h p.i. for [$^{64}$Cu]1–4 [$^{64}$Cu]1 (■), [$^{64}$Cu]2 (▨), [$^{64}$Cu]3 (■), and [$^{64}$Cu]4 (■).

### 3.8. PET Imaging

Overall, the BxPC-3 tumors were clearly visualized by PET imaging with both peptides at all time points (Figure 6); the PET imaging also showed that [$^{64}$Cu]2 provided the clearest images based on its superior tumor-to-background ratios. Most notably, as previously discussed for the biodistribution data, the PET images for [$^{64}$Cu]1 had much higher kidney accumulation and higher levels of radiation in the liver, indicative of possible in vivo instability of [$^{64}$Cu]1, which had shown substantially higher degradation in mouse serum compared to [$^{64}$Cu]2.

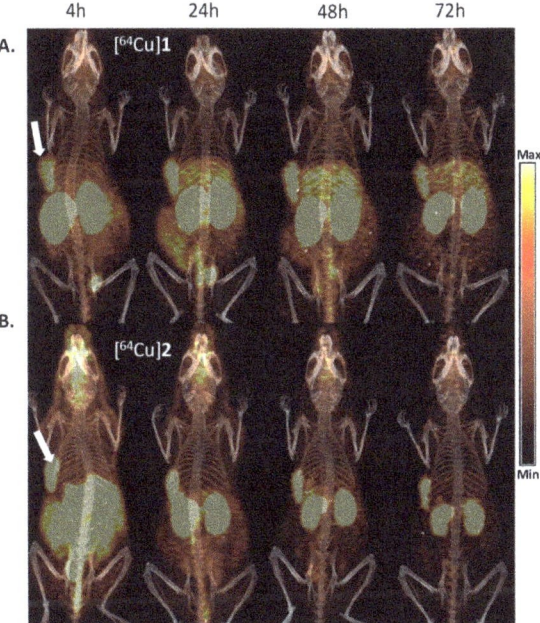

**Figure 6.** PET/CT imaging. Representative whole-body coronal maximum intensity projections (MIPs) of PET/CT images of mice bearing BxPC-3 xenograft tumors at 4 h, 24 h, 48 h, and 72 h p.i. of (**A**) [$^{64}$Cu]1 and (**B**) [$^{64}$Cu]2. Arrow: tumor. Decay corrected PET data are shown in color, CT data in gray.

## 4. Discussion

Cancer remains a leading cause of death globally [48,49]. Many cancers exhibit high expression of the cell surface receptor integrin $\alpha_v\beta_6$, and expression levels correlate with poor prognosis and reduced progression-free and overall survival [31,32,38]. Therefore, integrin $\alpha_v\beta_6$ has been identified as an important target both for imaging and treatment [50,51]. Receptor targeted delivery of radiopharmaceuticals is an important part of new approaches for improved cancer detection and therapy [48]. Peptides are attractive radiopharmaceuticals for both detection and treatment, because they are readily synthesized and can be chemically modified to optimize pharmacokinetics and metabolic stability. The addition of albumin binding moieties (ABMs) to numerous radiopharmaceuticals has demonstrated increased circulation time, reduced kidney uptake, and substantially increased tumor accumulation [18,52,53]. However, differences in the chemical structures of the ABM have been found at times to significantly affect the biodistribution, which ultimately determines target uptake, therapeutic efficacy, and off-target toxicity [52,54–56]. Thus, evaluation of different ABMs is important for optimal radiopharmaceutical performance towards the development of an $\alpha_v\beta_6$-targeted radiotherapeutic agent. Our laboratory continues to develop integrin $\alpha_v\beta_6$-targeting radiopharmaceuticals, including optimization of the core peptide structure [30] via PEGylation [14], and most recently the addition of an 4-(*p*-iodophenyl)butyryl (IP) ABM, which has demonstrated improved accumulation in tumors for both the [$^{18}$F]AlF NOTA and [$^{64}$Cu]Cu DOTA radiolabeled IP-ABM-$\alpha_v\beta_6$-BP compared to the parent non-ABM $\alpha_v\beta_6$-BP [42,44]. To further evaluate the choice of preferred ABM for $\alpha_v\beta_6$-BP, the comparison of the IP-ABM with another prominent ABM, the Evans blue fragment (EB-ABM), was explored. The synthesis of both $\alpha_v\beta_6$-BP peptides containing different ABMs, [$^{64}$Cu]**1** or [$^{64}$Cu]**2** (Scheme 1), was done efficiently using a solid-phase approach, which allowed installation of the respective ABM-peptide from the same batch of peptidyl-resin by first coupling an orthogonally protected lysine allowing for the attachment of the DOTA-chelator at the *N*-terminus and either the EB-ABM **8** or the IP-ABM at the sidechain. The IP-ABM included an aspartate (D) residue as it is reported to result in better tumor retention [28]. After removal from the resin and purification, both DOTA-ABM-$\alpha_v\beta_6$-BP peptides (**1** and **2**) were efficiently radiolabeled with copper-64 to yield [$^{64}$Cu]**1** and [$^{64}$Cu]**2** in high radiochemical purity >97%.

The ABM containing peptides [$^{64}$Cu]**1** and [$^{64}$Cu]**2** both demonstrated high tumor uptake at 4 h p.i., over 5% and 7.5% ID/g, respectively; representing a greater than 3- to-4.5-fold increase, respectively, from the non-ABM bearing [$^{64}$Cu]Cu DOTA-$\alpha_v\beta_6$-BP (1.61 ± 0.70% ID/g) [44]. The improvement in tumor accumulation was greater for the IP-ABM peptide [$^{64}$Cu]**2** than for the EB-ABM peptide [$^{64}$Cu]**1**, and was in concordance with the cell binding to both DX3puro$\beta$6 and BxPC-3 cells (Figure 2). Furthermore, the prolonged tumor uptake and retention (Figure 4A) were maintained for 72 h, and, in conjunction with rapid renal clearance, provided a high tumor-to-background ratio (Figure 5) and high contrast PET-images (Figure 6). Since the only difference between [$^{64}$Cu]**1** and [$^{64}$Cu]**2** is the ABM, and [$^{64}$Cu]**2** showed significantly higher stability in serum compared to [$^{64}$Cu]**1** (Figure 3), the observed differences in the tumor-to-background ratios could be attributed to the improved stability. This study adds to the growing number of literature reports describing improved tumor uptake following the incorporation of ABMs [4,7,11]. For example, the small molecule PSMA-617, a radiopharmaceutical targeting the prostate specific membrane antigen (PSMA), exhibited approximately a fivefold increase in tumor accumulation with the addition of an EB-ABM at 4 h and a twofold increase for the IP-ABM modified PSMA-617, compared to the unmodified (non-ABM bearing) PSMA-617; furthermore, the EB-ABM PSMA-617 maintained tumor accumulation over time (65.6–77.3% ID/g from 4 h to 48 h) [55]. In another study with PSMA-617, the addition of the IP-ABM also resulted in twofold higher accumulation in tumor tissue as compared to the non-ABM containing PSMA-617 agent (non-ABM PSMA-617: 38% ID/g vs. IP-ABM PSMA-617: 75.7% ID/g at 24 h) [28,57]. Other small molecule PSMA agents modified with ABMs have also shown improvements in tumor accumulation, with the EB-ABM MCG

PSMA agent having around a fourfold increase in tumor accumulation (MCG non-ABM: 10.9% ID/g vs. MCG-ABM: 40.4% ID/g at 24 h) [53] and an IP-ABM PSMA agent CTT1403 exhibiting >18-fold improvement in tumor accumulation (CTT1401 non-ABM: 2.2% ID/g vs. CTT1403-ABM: 40% ID/g at 24 h [54]. The addition of ABMs to other small molecule radiopharmaceuticals has also been shown to improve tumor accumulation with the small molecule radioligand folic acid modified with the IP-ABM having a threefold increase in tumor accumulation (ABM: 19.5% ID/g vs. non-ABM: 7% ID/g at 24 h, p.i.) with a considerably lower kidney accumulation (ABM: 28% ID/g vs. non-ABM: 70% ID/g at 4 h) [52,58].

Aside from small molecule radiopharmaceuticals, substantial benefits from the addition of ABMs to peptide radiopharmaceuticals have been shown; for example, the large peptide exendin-4 (39 amino acids), which targets the glucagon-like peptide 1 (GLP-1) receptor, when modified with the IP-ABM, demonstrated an improved stability and a twofold increase in tumor accumulation at 4 h, along with reduced kidney retention by more than half [7,59]. The small five amino acid integrin $\alpha_v\beta_3$ targeting cyclic peptide (cRGDfK) modified with EB-ABM and radiolabeled as [$^{64}$Cu]Cu NOTA-EB-cRGDfK displayed a >16-fold improvement (vs. [$^{64}$Cu]Cu NOTA-cRGDfK) in tumor accumulation in a U87MG glioblastoma tumor model (with ABM: 16.6% ID/g vs. non-ABM: <1.1% ID/g), but only had about a fivefold improvement in MDA-MB-435 melanoma and HT29 colorectal adenocarcinoma models [18]. The somatostatin receptor targeting peptide octreotide (TATE), which is eight amino acids in size, has seen some of the greatest improvements in tumor accumulation upon modification with an ABM. For example, the EB-ABM modified [$^{177}$Lu]Lu DOTA-EB-TATE provided a greater than eightfold increase in the tumor accumulation at 24 h (with ABM: 78.8% ID/g vs. non-ABM: 9.3% ID/g, respectively) [60] and the [$^{86}$Y]Y DOTA-EB-TATE showed a larger enhancement with a between 30- and 60-fold increase in tumor accumulation compared to [$^{86}$Y]Y DOTA-TATE, depending on the tumor model [6]. These studies paved the way for clinical trials where [$^{177}$Lu]Lu DOTA-EB-TATE showed an extended circulation which led to a 7.9-fold increase in tumor dose delivery [61]. Overall, these studies illustrate the potential benefits of including an ABM on targeted peptide receptor radionuclide therapy (PRRT).

The addition of either EB-ABM or the IP-ABM on the $\alpha_v\beta_6$-BP did significantly increase tumor accumulation (three-to-fivefold from the non-ABM-$\alpha_v\beta_6$-BP) and the overall clearance properties of the ABM-modified $\alpha_v\beta_6$-BP peptides [$^{64}$Cu]1 and [$^{64}$Cu]2 were similar with predominantly renal excretion. The organ with the highest accumulation was the kidneys, with the initial kidney uptake of the EB-ABM peptide [$^{64}$Cu]1 having more than double that of the IP-ABM peptide [$^{64}$Cu]2 (4 h: 75.5 ± 7.3% ID/g vs. 33.6 ± 5.4% ID/g, $p = 0.0013$), with both dropping to approximately one third of their initial value at 72 h p.i. (20.0 ± 6.9% ID/g and 11.4 ± 1.0% ID/g, respectively, $p = 0.10$, Figure 4). The introduction of the IP-ABM to the $\alpha_v\beta_6$-BP significantly reduced kidney accumulation, which we hypothesize is due to the higher stability of the IP-ABM [$^{64}$Cu]2 over the EB-ABM [$^{64}$Cu]1. These data are promising and indicate that renal toxicity would be less of a concern for PRRT of $\alpha_v\beta_6$-BP agents using the IP-ABM. The observed effects of the different ABMs on kidney uptake and retention are comparable to other radiopharmaceutical ABM-adducts, for example, the ABM modified peptide [$^{177}$Lu]Lu DOTA-TATE showed that the IP-ABM-analogue also provided lower kidney accumulation that was more rapidly cleared (dropping from ~20% ID/g at 4 h to ~5% ID/g at 72 h) compared to the EB-ABM-analogue (~30% ID/g at 4 h to ~15% ID/g at 72 h) [29,60]. This similar kidney accumulation and retention trend was also observed with the small molecule PSMA-617 agent, where the EB-PSMA-617 had considerably higher kidney accumulation and retention compared to the IP-PSMA-617, which had rapid kidney clearance (EB-PSMA-617: >20% ID/g at 4 h, which remained at 48 h vs. IP-ABM-PSMA-617: ~10% ID/g at 4 h dropping to <5% ID/g at 48 h) [55]. Both [$^{64}$Cu]1 and [$^{64}$Cu]2 also displayed some secondary clearance through the gastrointestinal (GI) tract and excretion of radioactivity in the feces (Figures S20 and S21). The IP-ABM modified peptide [$^{64}$Cu]2 had higher GI accumulation, with the highest uptake in the stomach of 18.1 ± 2.9% ID/g at 4 h, though, gratifyingly, both peptide's GI accumulation dropped down to less than one-fifth of their respective original value (≤3.2% ID/g at 72 h, Figure 4).

The non-$\alpha_v\beta_6$-targeting ABM controls [$^{64}$Cu]3 and [$^{64}$Cu]4 were used to evaluate non-specific uptake and demonstrate that the enhanced tumor accumulation of [$^{64}$Cu]1 or [$^{64}$Cu]2 resulted from integrin $\alpha_v\beta_6$ receptor mediated uptake, as opposed to the enhanced permeability and retention (EPR) effect. As expected, [$^{64}$Cu]3 and [$^{64}$Cu]4 largely remained in the blood, thus mostly acting as blood pool imaging agents with high blood accumulation of 39.0% ID/g and 9.5% ID/g, respectively, at 4 h (Figure S25) and mirrored other similar non-targeted ABMs, such as the EB-ABM compound [$^{64}$Cu]Cu NOTA-EB (NEB, ~15% ID/g at 4 h, dropping to ~10% ID/g at 1 d) [16,23]. Compared to the ABM peptides [$^{64}$Cu]1 and [$^{64}$Cu]2, accumulation of [$^{64}$Cu]3 and [$^{64}$Cu]4 generally increased in organs with high blood flow (viz. heart, liver, and lungs; Figure 5A) but was lower in the kidneys (though the EB compound was still higher than the IP compound with 18.6% ID/g and 4.3% ID/g, respectively, at 4 h; Figure 5A), highlighting the effect of both the properties of the ABM as well as the targeting peptide moiety on kidney uptake. Both non-targeted [$^{64}$Cu]3 and [$^{64}$Cu]4, due to their much higher blood accumulation (>9–39-fold higher than [$^{64}$Cu]1 and [$^{64}$Cu]2) and longer blood residence time, provided much higher tumor accumulation at 4 h than the two peptides [$^{64}$Cu]1 and [$^{64}$Cu]2 (Figure 5A). However, the non-targeted [$^{64}$Cu]3 and [$^{64}$Cu]4 showed minimal binding (<4.3%) in cell binding studies to both the $\alpha_v\beta_6$-expressing and $\alpha_v\beta_6$-null cells (Figure S24), thus their higher tumor accumulation compared to [$^{64}$Cu]1 and [$^{64}$Cu]2 was attributed to the EPR effect (which, together with the long circulation, resulted in the expectedly low tumor-to-blood ratios of <0.9/1 (Figure 5B, Figure S26). By comparison, [$^{64}$Cu]1 and [$^{64}$Cu]2 showed high and $\alpha_v\beta_6$-dependent cell binding (>30–60% binding; ~20:1 for DX3puroβ6 (+)/DX3puro (−) cells), and in vivo tumor uptake was efficiently blocked by the pre-administration of metal free **1** and **2**, respectively, supporting integrin $\alpha_v\beta_6$-dependent tumor accumulation (Figure S23). Taken together, the tumor uptake observed for the integrin $\alpha_v\beta_6$-binding peptides [$^{64}$Cu]1 and [$^{64}$Cu]2 was attributed to specific targeting of the integrin $\alpha_v\beta_6$ receptor. Both ABM modified $\alpha_v\beta_6$-BP peptides had improved pharmacokinetic profiles from the parent peptide and overall [$^{64}$Cu]2 demonstrated a more favorable biodistribution. Tumor retention of [$^{64}$Cu]1 and [$^{64}$Cu]2 was good over the three day study period, with each retaining about two-thirds of the original (4 h) uptake at 72 h p.i. The PET image quality improved, most notably for [$^{64}$Cu]2 over time after the initial uptake period (i.e., after 24 h p.i.) as a result of faster washout from non-target tissues (Figure 6). The high absolute tumor uptake of [$^{64}$Cu]2, its efficient binding and internalization to $\alpha_v\beta_6$-expressing cells (Figure 2), and its better serum stability (Figure 3) demonstrate the potential of using the [$^{64}$Cu]2 as an integrin $\alpha_v\beta_6$-targeted peptide receptor radionuclide therapy (PRRT) agent where the copper-64 is replaced by a therapeutic radioisotope such as lutetium-177.

## 5. Conclusions

The effect of Evans blue (EB) and 4-(p-iodophenyl)butyryl (IP)-based albumin binding moieties (ABMs) on the pharmacokinetics of $\alpha_v\beta_6$-BP, a peptide targeting the cancer-associated cell surface receptor integrin $\alpha_v\beta_6$ was investigated. The albumin binding moieties on $\alpha_v\beta_6$-BP did not interfere with integrin $\alpha_v\beta_6$ affinity or selectivity in vitro. In vivo in a BxPC-3 pancreatic tumor xenograft mouse model, the IP-ABM-modified $\alpha_v\beta_6$-BP [$^{64}$Cu]2 had a considerably more favorable pharmacokinetic profile compared to the EB-ABM-modified $\alpha_v\beta_6$-BP [$^{64}$Cu]1, with higher tumor uptake, reduced kidney and liver uptake, and improved tumor-to-background ratios that led to a clearer tumor visualization by PET imaging. Furthermore, the IP-ABM-modified $\alpha_v\beta_6$-BP [$^{64}$Cu]2 had superior serum stability, making it a lead candidate for future integrin $\alpha_v\beta_6$-targeted imaging and therapy studies.

**Supplementary Materials:** The following are available online at https://www.mdpi.com/article/10.3390/pharmaceutics14040745/s1, S1–S26. Table S1–S3: Table of Contents, Table S3: RP-HPLC methods, Figure S4: Schematic for solid phase reaction of EB-ABM **8** to peptidyl resin of DOTA-K(NH$_2$-$\alpha_v\beta_6$-BP to produce DOTA-EB-$\alpha_v\beta_6$-BP **1** after cleavage and pictorial of the reaction of **8** with peptidyl resin of DOTA-K(NH$_2$)-$\alpha_v\beta_6$-BP, Figure S5: RP-HPLC and MALDI-TOF of DOTA-EB-$\alpha_v\beta_6$-BP **1**, Figure S6: Radio-RP-HPLC of [$^{64}$Cu]**1** and co-injection radio-RP-HPLC of [$^{Nat}$Cu]**1** and [$^{64}$Cu]**1**, Figure S7: MALDI-TOF of [$^{Nat}$Cu]**1**, Figure S8: RP-HPLC and MALDI-TOF of DOTA-IP-$\alpha_v\beta_6$-BP **2**, Figure S9: Radio-RP-HPLC of [$^{64}$Cu]**2** and co-injection radio-RP-HPLC of [$^{Nat}$Cu]**2** and [$^{64}$Cu]**2**, Figure S10: MALDI-TOF of [$^{Nat}$Cu]**2**, Figure S11: RP-HPLC and MALDI-TOF of DOTA-EB-ABM **3**, Figure S12: Radio-RP-HPLC of [$^{64}$Cu]**3** and co-injection radio-RP-HPLC of [$^{Nat}$Cu]**3** and [$^{64}$Cu]**3**, Figure S13: MALDI-TOF of [$^{Nat}$Cu]**3**, Figure S14: RP-HPLC and MALDI-TOF of DOTA-IP-ABM **4**, Figure S15: Radio-RP-HPLC of [$^{64}$Cu]**4** and co-injection radio-RP-HPLC of [$^{Nat}$Cu]**4** and [$^{64}$Cu]**4**, Figure S16: MALDI-TOF of [$^{Nat}$Cu]**4**, Figure S17: RP-HPLC and ESI-FTMS of compound **6**, Figure S18: RP-HPLC and ESI-FTMS of EB-ABM **8**, Figure S19: $^1$H NMR and COSY of EB-ABM **8**, Figure S20: Biodistribution of [$^{64}$Cu]**1**, Figure S21: Biodistribution of [$^{64}$Cu]**2**, Figure S22: Tumor-to-organ ratios from 4 h to 72 h p.i. of [$^{64}$Cu]**1** and [$^{64}$Cu]**2**, Figure S23: Blocking biodistribution of [$^{64}$Cu]**1** and [$^{64}$Cu]**2**, Figure S24: Cell binding assay for [$^{64}$Cu]**3** and [$^{64}$Cu]**4**, Figure S25: Biodistribution of [$^{64}$Cu]**3** and [$^{64}$Cu]**4**, Figure S26: Summary of Tumor-to-organ ratios at 4 h for [$^{64}$Cu]**1–4**.

**Author Contributions:** Conceptualization, J.L.S. and R.A.D.; methodology, R.A.D. and S.H.H.; formal analysis, J.L.S., R.A.D. and S.H.H.; synthesis and radiolabeling with copper-64, R.A.D.; compound characterization and purification and formulation, R.A.D.; serum stability assay, R.A.D.; cell culture, R.H.; cell binding assay and serum binding assays, S.H.H. and R.A.D.; biodistribution, S.H.H., R.H. and R.A.D.; resources, J.L.S.; data curation, R.A.D.; writing—original draft preparation, R.A.D.; writing—review and editing, R.A.D., J.L.S. and S.H.H.; supervision, J.L.S.; funding acquisition, J.L.S. All authors have read and agreed to the published version of the manuscript.

**Funding:** This research was funded by National Institutes of Health's National Cancer Institute, grants number R01CA199725 and R50CA211556-01.

**Institutional Review Board Statement:** Radioactive work was conducted under radioactive use authorization 9098 managed by University of California, Davis Radiation Safety Services. All animal and biological research were conducted under biological use authorization R1580 and all animal work was conducted in accordance with procedures pre-approved by the Institutional of Animal Care and Use Committee (IACUC) at the University of California, Davis which is regulated by several independent resources. Accreditation and oversight has been approved since 1966 by AAALAC #000029 and by the Office of Laboratory Animal Welfare (OLAW) #D16-00272 (A3433-01).

**Informed Consent Statement:** Not applicable.

**Data Availability Statement:** Additional data supporting the reported results can be found in the Supplementary Materials (S1–S26).

**Acknowledgments:** We would like to thank the Center for Molecular and Genomic Imaging at UC Davis, Charles Smith and Sarah Tam for their technical support of injections during animal studies and running of the PET/CT scanners.

**Conflicts of Interest:** The authors declare the following competing financial interest(s): S. H. Hausner is a co-inventor of intellectual property related to $\alpha_v\beta_6$-BP. J. L. Sutcliffe is founder and CEO of and holds ownership interest (including patents) in Luminance Biosciences, Inc., and is a co-inventor of intellectual property related to $\alpha_v\beta_6$-BP. The funding agencies had no role in the design of the study; in the collection, analyses, or interpretation of data; in the writing of the manuscript, or in the decision to publish the results.

## References

1. Davis, R.A.; Hausner, S.H.; Sutcliffe, J.L. Peptides as radiopharmaceutical vectors. In *Radiopharmaceutical Chemistry*; Lewis, J.S., Windhorst, A.D., Zeglis, B.M., Eds.; Springer International Publishing: Cham, Switzerland, 2019; pp. 137–162.
2. Trier, N.; Hansen, P.; Houen, G. Peptides, antibodies, peptide antibodies and more. *Int. J. Mol. Sci.* **2019**, *20*, 6289. [CrossRef] [PubMed]
3. Kręcisz, P.; Czarnecka, K.; Królicki, L.; Mikiciuk-Olasik, E.; Szymański, P. Radiolabeled peptides and antibodies in medicine. *Bioconjugate Chem.* **2021**, *32*, 25–42. [CrossRef] [PubMed]

4. Zorzi, A.; Linciano, S.; Angelini, A. Non-covalent albumin-binding ligands for extending the circulating half-life of small biotherapeutics. *Med. Chem. Commun.* **2019**, *10*, 1068–1081. [CrossRef] [PubMed]
5. Zorzi, A.; Middendorp, S.J.; Wilbs, J.; Deyle, K.; Heinis, C. Acylated heptapeptide binds albumin with high affinity and application as tag furnishes long-acting peptides. *Nat. Commun.* **2017**, *8*, 16092. [CrossRef] [PubMed]
6. Tian, R.; Jacobson, O.; Niu, G.; Kiesewetter, D.O.; Wang, Z.; Zhu, G.; Ma, Y.; Liu, G.; Chen, X. Evans blue attachment enhances somatostatin receptor subtype-2 imaging and radiotherapy. *Theranostics* **2018**, *8*, 735–745. [CrossRef]
7. Chen, H.; Wang, G.; Lang, L.; Jacobson, O.; Kiesewetter, D.O.; Liu, Y.; Ma, Y.; Zhang, X.; Wu, H.; Zhu, L.; et al. Chemical conjugation of Evans blue derivative: A strategy to develop long-acting therapeutics through albumin binding. *Theranostics* **2016**, *6*, 243–253. [CrossRef]
8. Dennis, M.S.; Zhang, M.; Meng, G.Y.; Kadkhodayan, M.; Kirchhofer, D.; Combs, D.; Damico, L.A. Albumin binding as a general strategy for improving the pharmacokinetics of proteins. *J. Biol. Chem.* **2002**, *277*, 35035–35043. [CrossRef]
9. Jacobson, O.; Kiesewetter, D.O.; Chen, X. Albumin-binding Evans blue derivatives for diagnostic imaging and production of long-acting therapeutics. *Bioconjugate Chem.* **2016**, *27*, 2239–2247. [CrossRef]
10. Lau, J.; Jacobson, O.; Niu, G.; Lin, K.-S.; Bénard, F.; Chen, X. Bench to bedside: Albumin binders for improved cancer radioligand therapies. *Bioconjugate Chem.* **2019**, *30*, 487–502. [CrossRef]
11. Brandt, M.; Cardinale, J.; Giammei, C.; Guarrochena, X.; Happl, B.; Jouini, N.; Mindt, T.L. Mini-review: Targeted radiopharmaceuticals incorporating reversible, low molecular weight albumin binders. *Nucl. Med. Biol.* **2019**, *70*, 46–52. [CrossRef]
12. Gao, H.; Luo, C.; Yang, G.; Du, S.; Li, X.; Zhao, H.; Shi, J.; Wang, F. Improved in vivo targeting capability and pharmacokinetics of $^{99m}$Tc-Labeled isoDGR by dimerization and albumin-binding for glioma imaging. *Bioconjugate Chem.* **2019**, *30*, 2038–2048. [CrossRef] [PubMed]
13. Cheng, T.-L.; Chuang, K.-H.; Chen, B.-M.; Roffler, S.R. Analytical measurement of PEGylated molecules. *Bioconjugate Chem.* **2012**, *23*, 881–899. [CrossRef] [PubMed]
14. Hausner, S.H.; Bauer, N.; Hu, L.Y.; Knight, L.M.; Sutcliffe, J.L. The effect of bi-terminal PEGylation of an integrin $\alpha_v\beta_6$–targeted $^{18}$F peptide on pharmacokinetics and tumor uptake. *J. Nucl. Med.* **2015**, *56*, 784–790. [CrossRef] [PubMed]
15. Müller, C.; Farkas, R.; Borgna, F.; Schmid, R.M.; Benešová, M.; Schibli, R. Synthesis, radiolabeling, and characterization of plasma protein-binding ligands: Potential tools for modulation of the pharmacokinetic properties of (radio) pharmaceuticals. *Bioconjugate Chem.* **2017**, *28*, 2372–2383. [CrossRef] [PubMed]
16. Liu, Z.; Chen, X. Simple bioconjugate chemistry serves great clinical advances: Albumin as a versatile platform for diagnosis and precision therapy. *Chem. Soc. Rev.* **2016**, *45*, 1432–1456. [CrossRef]
17. Niu, G.; Lang, L.; Kiesewetter, D.O.; Ma, Y.; Sun, Z.; Guo, N.; Guo, J.; Wu, C.; Chen, X. In vivo labeling of serum albumin for PET. *J. Nucl. Med.* **2014**, *55*, 1150–1156. [CrossRef]
18. Chen, H.; Jacobson, O.; Niu, G.; Weiss, I.D.; Kiesewetter, D.O.; Liu, Y.; Ma, Y.; Wu, H.; Chen, X. Novel "add-on" molecule based on Evans blue confers superior pharmacokinetics and transforms drugs to theranostic agents. *J. Nucl. Med.* **2017**, *58*, 590–597. [CrossRef]
19. Ehlerding, E.B.; Lan, X.; Cai, W. Albumin hitchhiking" with an Evans blue analog for cancer theranostics. *Theranostics* **2018**, *8*, 812–814. [CrossRef]
20. Liu, Y.; Wang, G.; Zhang, H.; Ma, Y.; Lang, L.; Jacobson, O.; Kiesewetter, D.O.; Zhu, L.; Gao, S.; Ma, Q.; et al. Stable Evans blue derived exendin-4 peptide for type 2 diabetes treatment. *Bioconjugate Chem.* **2016**, *27*, 54–58. [CrossRef]
21. Saunders, N.R.; Dziegielewska, K.M.; Møllgård, K.; Habgood, M.D. Markers for blood-brain barrier integrity: How appropriate is Evans blue in the twenty-first century and what are the alternatives? *Front. Neurosci.* **2015**, *9*, 385. [CrossRef]
22. Yamamoto, T.; Ikuta, K.; Oi, K.; Abe, K.; Uwatoku, T.; Murata, M.; Shigetani, N.; Yoshimitsu, K.; Shimokawa, H.; Katayama, Y. First functionalized MRI contrast agent recognizing vascular lesions. *Anal. Sci.* **2004**, *20*, 5–7. [CrossRef] [PubMed]
23. Zhang, J.; Lang, L.; Zhu, Z.; Li, F.; Niu, G.; Chen, X. Clinical translation of an albumin-binding PET radiotracer $^{68}$Ga-NEB. *J. Nucl. Med.* **2015**, *56*, 1609–1614. [CrossRef] [PubMed]
24. Zhang, F.; Xue, J.; Shao, J.; Jin, L. Compilation of 222 drugs' plasma protein binding data and guidance for study designs. *Drug Discov. Today* **2012**, *17*, 475–485. [CrossRef] [PubMed]
25. Wang, Y.; Lang, L.; Huang, P.; Wang, Z.; Jacobson, O.; Kiesewetter, D.O.; Ali, I.U.; Teng, G.; Niu, G.; Chen, X. In vivo albumin labeling and lymphatic imaging. *Proc. Natl. Acad. Sci. USA* **2015**, *112*, 208–213. [CrossRef]
26. Yao, L.; Xue, X.; Yu, P.; Ni, Y.; Chen, F. Evans blue dye: A revisit of its applications in biomedicine. *Contrast Media Mol. Imaging.* **2018**, *2018*, 10. [CrossRef]
27. Dumelin, C.E.; Trüssel, S.; Buller, F.; Trachsel, E.; Bootz, F.; Zhang, Y.; Mannocci, L.; Beck, S.C.; Drumea-Mirancea, M.; Seeliger, M.W.; et al. A portable albumin binder from a DNA-encoded chemical library. *Angew. Chem. Int. Ed.* **2008**, *47*, 3196–3201. [CrossRef] [PubMed]
28. Umbricht, C.A.; Benešová, M.; Schibli, R.; Müller, C. Preclinical development of novel PSMA-targeting radioligands: Modulation of albumin-binding properties to improve prostate cancer therapy. *Mol. Pharm.* **2018**, *15*, 2297–2306. [CrossRef]
29. Rousseau, E.; Lau, J.; Zhang, Z.; Uribe, C.F.; Kuo, H.-T.; Zhang, C.; Zeisler, J.; Colpo, N.; Lin, K.-S.; Bénard, F. Effects of adding an albumin binder chain on [$^{177}$Lu]Lu-DOTATATE. *Nucl. Med. Biol.* **2018**, *66*, 10–17. [CrossRef]

30. Hausner, S.H.; Bold, R.J.; Cheuy, L.Y.; Chew, H.K.; Daly, M.E.; Davis, R.A.; Foster, C.C.; Kim, E.J.; Sutcliffe, J.L. Preclinical development and first-in human imaging of integrin $\alpha_v\beta_6$-binding peptide in metastatic carcinoma. *Clinic. Cancer Res.* **2019**, *25*, 1206–1215. [CrossRef]
31. Wang, B.; Wang, W.; Niu, W.; Liu, E.; Liu, X.; Wang, J.; Peng, C.; Liu, S.; Xu, L.; Wang, L.; et al. SDF-1/CXCR4 axis promotes directional migration of colorectal cancer cells through upregulation of integrin $\alpha_v\beta_6$. *Carcinogenesis* **2013**, *35*, 282–291. [CrossRef]
32. Li, Z.; Lin, P.; Gao, C.; Peng, C.; Liu, S.; Gao, H.; Wang, B.; Wang, J.; Niu, J.; Niu, W. Integrin $\beta_6$ acts as an unfavorable prognostic indicator and promotes cellular malignant behaviors via ERK-ETS1 pathway in pancreatic ductal adenocarcinoma (PDAC). *Tumor. Biol.* **2016**, *37*, 5117–5131. [CrossRef] [PubMed]
33. Izabela, Ł.; Jacek, M. Integrins as a new target for cancer treatment. *Anti-Cancer Agents Med. Chem.* **2019**, *19*, 580–586.
34. Bandyopadhyay, A.; Raghavan, S. Defining the role of integrin $a_v b_6$ in cancer. *Curr. Drug Targets.* **2009**, *10*, 645–652. [CrossRef]
35. Ahmed, N.; Pansino, F.; Clyde, R.; Murthi, P.; Quinn, M.A.; Rice, G.E.; Agrez, M.V.; Mok, S.; Baker, M.S. Overexpression of $\alpha v\beta 6$ integrin in serous epithelial ovarian cancer regulates extracellular matrix degradation via the plasminogen activation cascade. *Carcinogenesis* **2002**, *23*, 237–244. [CrossRef]
36. Elayadi, A.N.; Samli, K.N.; Prudkin, L.; Liu, Y.-H.; Bian, A.; Xie, X.-J.; Wistuba, I.I.; Roth, J.A.; McGuire, M.J.; Brown, K.C. A peptide selected by biopanning identifies the integrin $\alpha_v\beta_6$ as a prognostic biomarker for nonsmall cell lung cancer. *Cancer Res.* **2007**, *67*, 5889–5895. [CrossRef] [PubMed]
37. Moore, K.M.; Thomas, G.J.; Duffy, S.W.; Warwick, J.; Gabe, R.; Chou, P.; Ellis, I.O.; Green, A.R.; Haider, S.; Brouilette, K.; et al. Therapeutic targeting of integrin $\alpha_v\beta_6$ in breast cancer. *J. Natl. Cancer Inst.* **2014**, *106*, 1–14. [CrossRef]
38. Zhang, Z.Y.; Xu, K.S.; Wang, J.S.; Yang, G.Y.; Wang, W.; Wang, J.Y.; Niu, W.B.; Liu, E.Y.; Mi, Y.T.; Niu, J. Integrin $\alpha_v\beta_6$ acts as a prognostic indicator in gastric carcinoma. *Clin. Oncol.* **2008**, *20*, 61–66. [CrossRef]
39. Hsiao, J.-R.; Chang, Y.; Chen, Y.-L.; Hsieh, S.-H.; Hsu, K.-F.; Wang, C.-F.; Tsai, S.-T.; Jin, Y.-T. Cyclic $\alpha v\beta 6$-targeting peptide selected from biopanning with clinical potential for head and neck squamous cell carcinoma. *Head Neck.* **2010**, *32*, 160–172. [PubMed]
40. Bates, R.C. The $\alpha_v\beta_6$ integrin as a novel molecular target for colorectal cancer. *Future Oncol.* **2005**, *1*, 821–828. [CrossRef]
41. Berghoff, A.S.; Kovanda, A.K.; Melchardt, T.; Bartsch, R.; Hainfellner, J.A.; Sipos, B.; Schittenhelm, J.; Zielinski, C.C.; Widhalm, G.; Dieckmann, K.; et al. $\alpha_v\beta_3$, $\alpha_v\beta_5$ and $\alpha_v\beta_6$ integrins in brain metastases of lung cancer. *Clin. Exper. Met.* **2014**, *31*, 841–851. [CrossRef]
42. Hausner, S.H.; Bauer, N.; Davis, R.A.; Ganguly, T.; Tang, S.Y.C.; Sutcliffe, J.L. The effects of an albumin binding moiety on the targeting and pharmacokinetics of an integrin $\alpha_v\beta_6$-selective peptide labeled with aluminum [$^{18}$F]fluoride. *Mol. Imaging Biol.* **2020**, *22*, 1543–1552. [CrossRef] [PubMed]
43. Hausner, S.H.; Bauer, N.; Sutcliffe, J.L. In vitro and in vivo evaluation of the effects of aluminum [$^{18}$F]fluoride radiolabeling on an integrin $\alpha_v\beta_6$-specific peptide. *Nucl. Med. Biol.* **2014**, *41*, 43–50. [CrossRef] [PubMed]
44. Ganguly, T.; Bauer, N.; Davis, R.A.; Hausner, S.H.; Tang, S.Y.; Sutcliffe, J.L. Evaluation of copper-64-labeled $\alpha_v\beta_6$-targeting peptides: Addition of an albumin binding moiety to improve pharmacokinetics. *Mol. Pharm.* **2021**, *18*, 4437–4447. [CrossRef] [PubMed]
45. Zhang, F.; Zhu, G.; Jacobson, O.; Liu, Y.; Chen, K.; Yu, G.; Ni, Q.; Fan, J.; Yang, Z.; Xu, F.; et al. Transformative nanomedicine of an amphiphilic camptothecin prodrug for long circulation and high tumor uptake in cancer therapy. *ACS Nano.* **2017**, *11*, 8838–8848. [CrossRef]
46. Favre-Besse, F.-C.; Poirel, O.; Bersot, T.; Kim-Grellier, E.; Daumas, S.; El Mestikawy, S.; Acher, F.C.; Pietrancosta, N. Design, synthesis and biological evaluation of small-azo-dyes as potent vesicular glutamate transporters inhibitors. *Eur. J. Med. Chem.* **2014**, *78*, 236–247. [CrossRef] [PubMed]
47. Tang, Y.C.; Davis, R.A.; Ganguly, T.; Sutcliffe, J.L. Identification, characterization, and optimization of integrin $\alpha v\beta 6$-targeting peptides from a one-bead one-compound (OBOC) library: Towards the development of positron emission tomography (PET) imaging agents. *Molecules* **2019**, *24*, 309. [CrossRef]
48. Padma, V.V. An overview of targeted cancer therapy. *BioMedicine* **2015**, *5*, e46. [CrossRef]
49. Siegel, R.L.; Miller, K.D.; Jemal, A. Cancer statistics. *CA Cancer J. Clin.* **2019**, *69*, 7–34. [CrossRef]
50. Willemieke, T.S.; Farina-Sarasquota, A.; Boonstra, M.C.; Prevoo, H.A.; Sier, C.F.; Mieog, J.S.; Morreau, J.; van Eijck, C.H.; Kuppen, P.J.; van de Velde, C.J.; et al. Selection of optimal molecular targets for tumor-specific imaging in pancreatic ductal adenocarcinoma. *Oncotarget* **2017**, *8*, 56816–56828.
51. Färber, S.F.; Wurzer, A.; Reichart, F.; Beck, R.; Kessler, H.; Wester, H.-J.; Notni, J. Therapeutic radiopharmaceuticals targeting integrin $\alpha_v\beta_6$. *ACS Omega.* **2018**, *3*, 2428–2436. [CrossRef]
52. Müller, C.; Struthers, H.; Winiger, C.; Zhernosekov, K.; Schibli, R. DOTA conjugate with an albumin-binding entity enables the first folic acid–targeted $^{177}$Lu-radionuclide tumor therapy in mice. *J. Nucl. Med.* **2013**, *54*, 124–131. [CrossRef] [PubMed]
53. Wang, Z.; Jacobson, O.; Tian, R.; Mease, R.C.; Kiesewetter, D.O.; Niu, G.; Pomper, M.G.; Chen, X. Radioligand therapy of prostate cancer with a long-lasting prostate-specific membrane antigen targeting agent $^{90}$Y-DOTA-EB-MCG. *Bioconjugate Chem.* **2018**, *29*, 2309–2315. [CrossRef] [PubMed]
54. Choy, C.J.; Ling, X.; Geruntho, J.J.; Beyer, S.K.; Latoche, J.D.; Langton-Webster, B.; Anderson, C.J.; Berkman, C.E. $^{177}$Lu-labeled phosphoramidate-based PSMA inhibitors: The effect of an albumin binder on biodistribution and therapeutic efficacy in prostate tumor-bearing mice. *Theranostics* **2017**, *7*, 1928–1939. [CrossRef] [PubMed]

55. Wang, Z.; Tian, R.; Niu, G.; Ma, Y.; Lang, L.; Szajek, L.P.; Kiesewetter, D.O.; Jacobson, O.; Chen, X. Single low-dose injection of Evans blue modified PSMA-617 radioligand therapy eliminates prostate-specific membrane antigen positive tumors. *Bioconjugate Chem.* **2018**, *29*, 3213–3221. [CrossRef] [PubMed]
56. Kuo, H.-T.; Lin, K.-S.; Zhang, Z.; Uribe, C.F.; Merkens, H.; Zhang, C.; Bénard, F. $^{177}$Lu-labeled albumin-binder–conjugated PSMA-targeting agents with extremely high tumor uptake and enhanced tumor-to-kidney absorbed dose ratio. *J. Nucl. Med.* **2021**, *62*, 521–527. [CrossRef] [PubMed]
57. Benešová, M.; Umbricht, C.A.; Schibli, R.; Müller, C. Albumin-binding PSMA ligands: Optimization of the tissue distribution profile. *Mol. Pharm.* **2018**, *15*, 934–946. [CrossRef]
58. Siwowska, K.; Haller, S.; Bortoli, F.; Benešová, M.; Broehn, V.; Bernhardt, P.; Schibli, R.; Müller, C. Preclinical comparison of albumin-binding radiofolates: Impact of linker entities on the in vitro and in vivo properties. *Mol. Pharm.* **2017**, *14*, 523–532. [CrossRef]
59. Kaeppeli, S.A.M.; Jodal, A.; Gotthardt, M.; Schibli, R.; Béhé, M. Exendin-4 derivatives with an albumin-binding moiety show decreased renal retention and improved GLP-1 receptor targeting. *Mol. Pharm.* **2019**, *16*, 3760–3769. [CrossRef]

60. Bandara, N.; Jacobson, O.; Mpoy, C.; Chen, X.; Rogers, B.E. Novel structural modification based on Evans blue dye to improve pharmacokinetics of a somastostatin-receptor-based theranostic agent. *Bioconjugate Chem.* **2018**, *29*, 2448–2454. [CrossRef]
61. Zhang, J.; Wang, H.; Jacobson, O.; Cheng, Y.; Niu, G.; Li, F.; Bai, C.; Zhu, Z.; Chen, X. Safety, pharmacokinetics, and dosimetry of a long-acting radiolabeled somatostatin analog $^{177}$Lu-DOTA-EB-TATE in patients with advanced metastatic neuroendocrine tumors. *J. Nucl. Med.* **2018**, *59*, 1699–1705. [CrossRef]

MDPI  
St. Alban-Anlage 66  
4052 Basel  
Switzerland  
Tel. +41 61 683 77 34  
Fax +41 61 302 89 18  
www.mdpi.com

*Pharmaceutics* Editorial Office  
E-mail: pharmaceutics@mdpi.com  
www.mdpi.com/journal/pharmaceutics

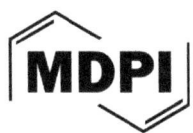

www.ingramcontent.com/pod-product-compliance
Lightning Source LLC
LaVergne TN
LVHW070624100526
838202LV00012B/715